Dietary Protein and Muscle in Aging People

Dietary Protein and Muscle in Aging People

Special Issue Editors

Matteo Cesari
Emanuele Marzetti

MDPI • Basel • Beijing • Wuhan • Barcelona • Belgrade

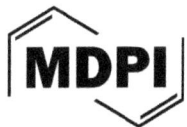

Special Issue Editors

Matteo Cesari
University of Milan
Italy

Emanuele Marzetti
Policlinico Universitario Agostino Gemelli
Italy

Editorial Office
MDPI
St. Alban-Anlage 66
4052 Basel, Switzerland

This is a reprint of articles from the Special Issue published online in the open access journal *Nutrients* (ISSN 2072-6643) in 2018 (available at: https://www.mdpi.com/journal/nutrients/special_issues/ Dietary_protein_and_muscle_in_aging_people).

For citation purposes, cite each article independently as indicated on the article page online and as indicated below:

LastName, A.A.; LastName, B.B.; LastName, C.C. Article Title. *Journal Name* **Year**, *Article Number*, Page Range.

ISBN 978-3-03897-457-4 (Pbk)
ISBN 978-3-03897-458-1 (PDF)

© 2018 by the authors. Articles in this book are Open Access and distributed under the Creative Commons Attribution (CC BY) license, which allows users to download, copy and build upon published articles, as long as the author and publisher are properly credited, which ensures maximum dissemination and a wider impact of our publications.

The book as a whole is distributed by MDPI under the terms and conditions of the Creative Commons license CC BY-NC-ND.

Contents

About the Special Issue Editors vii

Preface to "Dietary Protein and Muscle in Aging People" ix

Evasio Pasini, Giovanni Corsetti, Roberto Aquilani, Claudia Romano, Anna Picca, Riccardo Calvani and Francesco Saverio Dioguardi
Protein-Amino Acid Metabolism Disarrangements: The Hidden Enemy of Chronic Age-Related Conditions
Reprinted from: *Nutrients* **2018**, *10*, 391, doi:10.3390/nu10040391 1

Amanda V. Sardeli, Tiemy R. Komatsu, Marcelo A. Mori, Arthur F. Gáspari and Mara Patrícia T. Chacon-Mikahil
Resistance Training Prevents Muscle Loss Induced by Caloric Restriction in Obese Elderly Individuals: A Systematic Review and Meta-Analysis
Reprinted from: *Nutrients* **2018**, *10*, 423, doi:10.3390/nu10040423 12

Mary Ni Lochlainn, Ruth C. E. Bowyer and Claire J. Steves
Dietary Protein and Muscle in Aging People: The Potential Role of the Gut Microbiome
Reprinted from: *Nutrients* **2018**, *10*, 929, doi:10.3390/nu10070929 22

Bernhard Franzke, Oliver Neubauer, David Cameron-Smith and Karl-Heinz Wagner
Dietary Protein, Muscle and Physical Function in the Very Old
Reprinted from: *Nutrients* **2018**, *10*, 935, doi:10.3390/nu10070935 41

Xiao Song, Federico J. A. Perez-Cueto and Wender L. P. Bredie
Sensory-Driven Development of Protein-Enriched Rye Bread and Cream Cheese for the Nutritional Demands of Older Adults
Reprinted from: *Nutrients* **2018**, *10*, 1006, doi:10.3390/nu10081006 55

Deborah Agostini, Sabrina Donati Zeppa, Francesco Lucertini, Giosuè Annibalini, Marco Gervasi, Carlo Ferri Marini, Giovanni Piccoli, Vilberto Stocchi, Elena Barbieri and Piero Sestili
Muscle and Bone Health in Postmenopausal Women: Role of Protein and Vitamin D Supplementation Combined with Exercise Training
Reprinted from: *Nutrients* **2018**, *10*, 1103, doi:10.3390/nu10081103 76

Andreas Nilsson, Diego Montiel Rojas and Fawzi Kadi
Impact of Meeting Different Guidelines for Protein Intake on Muscle Mass and Physical Function in Physically Active Older Women
Reprinted from: *Nutrients* **2018**, *10*, 1156, doi:10.3390/nu10091156 97

Hélio José Coelho-Júnior, Luiz Milano-Teixeira, Bruno Rodrigues, Reury Bacurau, Emanuele Marzetti and Marco Uchida
Relative Protein Intake and Physical Function in Older Adults: A Systematic Review and Meta-Analysis of Observational Studies
Reprinted from: *Nutrients* **2018**, *10*, 1330, doi:10.3390/nu10091330 106

Hélio José Coelho-Júnior, Bruno Rodrigues, Marco Uchida and Emanuele Marzetti
Low Protein Intake Is Associated with Frailty in Older Adults: A Systematic Review and Meta-Analysis of Observational Studies
Reprinted from: *Nutrients* **2018**, *10*, 1334, doi:10.3390/nu10091334 122

Riccardo Calvani, Anna Picca, Federico Marini, Alessandra Biancolillo, Jacopo Gervasoni, Silvia Persichilli, Aniello Primiano, Hélio José Coelho-Junior, Maurizio Bossola, Andrea Urbani, Francesco Landi, Roberto Bernabei and Emanuele Marzetti
A Distinct Pattern of Circulating Amino Acids Characterizes Older Persons with Physical Frailty and Sarcopenia: Results from the BIOSPHERE Study
Reprinted from: *Nutrients* **2018**, *10*, 1691, doi:10.3390/nu10111691 . . . . **136**

About the Special Issue Editors

Matteo Cesari Cesari is Associate Professor of Geriatrics at the Università di Milano and Director of the Geriatric Unit at the Fondazione IRCCS Ca' Granda Ospedale Maggiore Policlinico (Milan, Italy). His research activities are focused on healthy aging and the management of frailty in "biologically old" individuals. He is listed by Clarivate Analytics among the worldwide Highly Cited Researchers (http://highlycited.com). Dr. Cesari is Editor-in-Chief of *The Journal of Frailty & Aging*, and Associate Editor of the *Journal of the American Medical Directors Association (JAMDA)*. He is the coordinator of the European Geriatric Medicine Society (EuGMS) Special Interest Group on "Frailty in older persons". Dr. Cesari has also been regularly collaborating with the World Health Organization on the themes of aging and integrated care in older people.

Emanuele Marzetti is a board-certified Geriatrician, Clinical Assistant Professor in Geriatrics, and leader of the orthogeriatric consultation team at the Department of Geriatrics, Neurosciences and Orthopaedics (Fondazione Policlinico Universitario "Agostino Gemelli", Università Cattolica del Sacro Cuore, Rome, Italy). He received his M.D. and Ph.D. degrees at the Università Cattolica del Sacro Cuore and a postdoctoral training in biochemistry of aging at the University of Florida (Gainesville, FL, USA). Dr. Marzetti serves as an Associate Editor for *Experimental Gerontology, The Journal of Frailty & Aging, JCSM Clinical Reports, and Frontiers in Medicine*. His research focuses on the mechanisms responsible for skeletal muscle and cardiovascular aging, with a special interest in mitochondrial pathophysiology, biomarker discovery, and the factors involved in the pathogenesis of frailty and disability in old age.

Preface to "Dietary Protein and Muscle in Aging People"

Over recent years, evidence has accumulated that protein intake above the current recommended dietary allowance (RDA, 0.8 g kg^{-1} d^{-1}) may help preserve muscle mass and function in old age. Opinion articles and consensus statements have argued that older people should be advised to ingest 1.0–1.5 g of protein kg^{-1} d^{-1}. This recommendation is mainly based on findings from observational studies showing that protein consumption above the RDA is associated with reduced risk of frailty, loss of lean body mass, slow walking speed, dynapenia, and poor balance. Notwithstanding, only a handful of clinical trials have tested the impact of specific protein ingestion regimens on body composition, physical performance, and frailty status of older people, with mixed results.

The purpose of this book was to convene experts and opinion leaders in nutrition, sarcopenia, frailty, and exercise science in the attempt to bring order in the field of protein requirements for muscle health in late life. The book showcases original articles, reviews, and meta-analyses addressing the relationship between dietary protein intake and muscle aging through clinical and translational approaches. Selected contributions also cover procedures aimed at increasing the palatability of protein supplements, the use of circulating amino acids as biomarkers for sarcopenia and frailty, and the impact of protein dysmetabolism in chronic conditions. The variety of the topics and the interdisciplinary content make the book appealing to a large readership, from clinicians interested in implementing nutritional interventions in their daily practice to researchers who may take cues for future studies on the subject.

Lastly, we would like to take to opportunity to thank the contributors, the reviewers, and the MDPI editorial staff, whose scientific excellence, time, and dedication made this book a reality.

Matteo Cesari, Emanuele Marzetti
Special Issue Editors

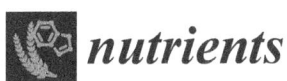

Review

Protein-Amino Acid Metabolism Disarrangements: The Hidden Enemy of Chronic Age-Related Conditions

Evasio Pasini [1,†], Giovanni Corsetti [2,*,†], Roberto Aquilani [3], Claudia Romano [2], Anna Picca [4], Riccardo Calvani [4] and Francesco Saverio Dioguardi [5]

1. Scientific Clinical Institutes Maugeri, IRCCS Lumezzane, Cardiac Rehabilitation Division, 25065 Lumezzane (Brescia), Italy; evpasini@gmail.com
2. Division of Human Anatomy and Physiopathology, Department of Clinical and Experimental Sciences, University of Brescia, Viale Europa, 11-25124 Brescia, Italy; cla300482@gmail.com
3. Department of Biology and Biotechnology, University of Pavia, 27100 Pavia, Italy; dottore.aquilani@gmail.com
4. Department of Geriatrics, Neurosciences and Orthopaedics, Catholic University of the Sacred Heart, 00198 Rome, Italy; anna.picca1@gmail.com (A.P.); riccardo.calvani@gmail.com (R.C.)
5. Department of Clinical Sciences and Community Health, University of Milan, 20122 Milan, Italy; fsdioguardi@gmail.com
* Correspondence: giovanni.corsetti@unibs.it; Tel.: +39-030-3717484; Fax: +39-030-3717486
† These authors contribute equally to this work.

Received: 15 February 2018; Accepted: 21 March 2018; Published: 22 March 2018

Abstract: Proteins are macro-molecules crucial for cell life, which are made up of amino acids (AAs). In healthy people, protein synthesis and degradation are well balanced. However, in the presence of hypercatabolic stimulation (i.e., inflammation), protein breakdown increases as the resulting AAs are consumed for metabolic proposes. Indeed, AAs are biochemical totipotent molecules which, when deaminated, can be transformed into energy, lipids, carbohydrates, and/or biochemical intermediates of fundamental cycles, such as the Krebs' cycle. The biochemical consequence of hyper-catabolism is protein disarrangement, clinically evident with signs such as sarcopenia, hypalbuminemia, anaemia, infection, and altered fluid compartmentation, etc. Hypercatabolic protein disarrangement (HPD) is often underestimated by clinicians, despite correlating with increased mortality, hospitalization, and morbidity quite independent of the primary disease. Simple, cheap, repeatable measurements can be used to identify HPD. Therefore, identification and treatment of proteins' metabolic impairment with appropriate measurements and therapy is a clinical strategy that could improve the prognosis of patients with acute/chronic hypercatabolic inflammatory disease. Here, we describe the metabolism of protein and AAs in hypercatabolic syndrome, illustrating the clinical impact of protein disarrangement. We also illustrate simple, cheap, repeatable, and worldwide available measurements to identify these conditions. Finally, we provide scientific evidence for HPD nutritional treatment.

Keywords: protein metabolism; sarcopenia; muscle wasting; amino acids; catabolism; inflammation

1. Metabolism of Proteins and Amino Acids: Essential Cellular Blocks

Proteins are macronutrients crucial for various cellular activities, as well as body metabolism. Protein synthesis is primarily controlled by amino acid (AA) availability in stoichiometric quantities proportional to the number of proteins needed for synthesis and energy requirements needed to sustain the synthetic process.

AAs serve many functions within the body. Being the only source of nitrogen for mammals, AA-derived nitrogen is pivotal for synthetizing precursors (purine and/or pyrimidine) of major energy molecules (i.e., ATP, ADP, IMP) and/or nucleic acids (i.e., DNA/RNA), and/or to produce compounds that can regulate major biochemical signaling pathways, such as nitric oxide (NO). Moreover, deamination of AAs released from skeletal muscle and/or circulating visceral proteins generate a carbon skeleton rich in oxygen and hydrogen suitable for subsequent biochemical transformation. This carbon skeleton can be used by the liver to produce glucose through gluconeogenesis and other macromolecules, such as lipids. The AA-derived carbon skeleton is also relevant in producing intermediaries fueling the Kreb's cycle that are thereafter transformed into energy and/or other metabolic intermediaries (Figure 1). Therefore, AAs can be considered "biochemical totipotent molecules" able to be converted into energy, carbohydrates, lipids, and biochemical intermediates, dependent on body metabolic demands [1,2] (Figure 2).

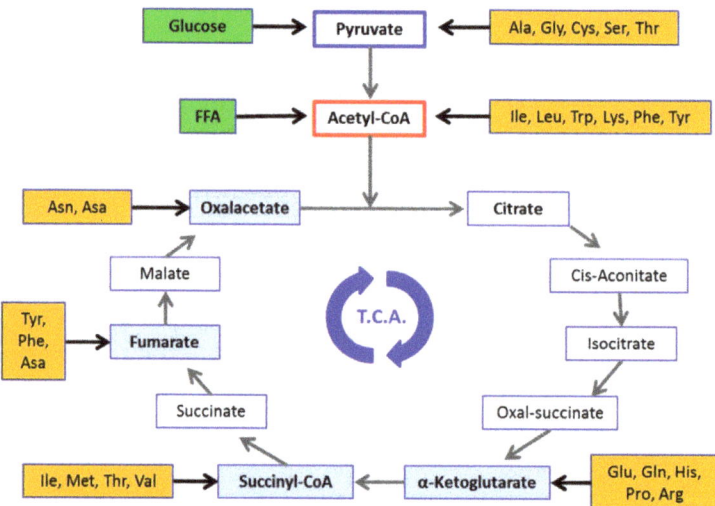

Figure 1. Amino acid-derived intermediates fueling the tri-carboxilic acid cycle (TCA) (Kreb's cycle). FFA = free fatty acids. Ala = alanine, Arg = arginine, Asa = aspartic acid, Asn = asparagine, Cys = cysteine, Gln = glutamine, Glu = glutamic acid, Gly = glycine, His = histidine, Ile = isoleucine, Leu = Leucine, Lys = lysine, Met = methionine, Phe = phenylalanine, Pro = proline, Ser = serine, Thr = threonine, Trp = tryptophan, Tyr = tyrosine, Val = valine.

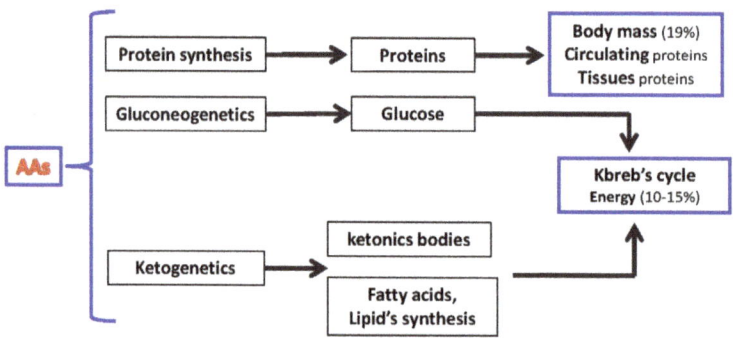

Figure 2. Amino acids (AAs) as biochemical totipotent molecules.

From a nutritional point of view, AAs are categorized as either "non-essential" (NEAAs) or "essential" (EAAs). NEAAs are synthetized within the body from carbohydrates and lipids deriving nitrogen from other AAs. EAAs, however, cannot be synthesized and need to be adequately introduced with the diet, and they are also the most relevant nutritional input for protein synthesis [3]. For instance, leucine is considered the primary nutritional regulator of muscle protein anabolism [4] due to its ability to trigger the mammalian target of the rapamycin (mTOR) pathway and inhibit the proteasome system [4].

Interestingly, under conditions such as injury, surgery, or chronic diseases, there is increased demand for AAs as a consequence of higher resting energy expenditure [5]. The consumption of EAAs into the Kreb's cycle and its competition with the oxidation of glucose or of fatty acids via β oxidation has been suggested as a strategy to maintain efficient energy production in pathological conditions. This is due to fat oxidation being less energy efficient than glycolysis and to the entry of AA-derived pyruvate into the mitochondrial Kreb's cycle [6].

Indeed, β oxidation, which is mostly cytoplasmic, reduces the ratio of ATP/available O_2, and obliges large amounts of EAAs to be used as intermediates of the Kreb's cycle. Interestingly, EAAs are used as substitutes for pyruvate-derived oxaloacetate shortened by the large amounts of NADH produced out of mitochondria due to β-oxidation [7].

Such a metabolic shift is one of the main alterations leading to an imbalance between nitrogen request and nitrogen intake observed in patients with chronic altered metabolic conditions and measured as the nitrogen balance. This ultimately triggers muscle and circulating protein disarrangement that become clinically evident in several muscle-wasting conditions (e.g., sarcopenia and cachexia) and/or hypoalbuminemia with or without anemia [8].

2. The Pathogenesis of Protein Disarrangement: The Hypermetabolic Syndrome

The pathophysiology of syndromes characterized by protein disarrangement is multi-factorial and dishomogeneous. Indeed, both the elderly and patients with chronic diseases (such as infections and sepsis) show a pattern of circulating mediators with altered ratios between catabolic molecules (e.g., TNF-α, cortisol, catecholamines, glucagons, cytokines) inducing protein degradation and anabolic factors (e.g., insulin, insulin-like growth factors, and growth hormone) that stimulate protein synthesis. Increased catabolic stimuli and the consequent impaired anabolic/catabolic stimulation is a condition that can be referred to as the "hypercatabolic syndrome" (HS). This severely impacts whole-body metabolism and causes an imbalance between nutritional input and synthetic/energy needs [9,10].

Muscle contractile proteins and circulating visceral proteins are the major reservoir of AAs within the body. Indeed, these proteins can be degraded by catabolic stimuli and/or physical exercises [11] and other AAs can be re-used by cells for de novo protein synthesis. However, a large amount of AAs are deaminated to produce energy and other metabolic intermediates via the Kreb's cycle and/or are released into the blood stream to maintain a ready-to-use pool of AAs [10] (Figure 3). In this context, the role of skeletal muscle and circulating visceral proteins goes well beyond that of ensuring posture maintenance and locomotion and transporting molecules or atoms.

The proteins of skeletal muscle and the circulatory system are in continuous turnover. Several studies indicate that about 250–350 g of proteins per day are metabolized in healthy individuals. However, this amount increases dramatically under conditions with higher metabolic demand. For instance, aged muscles have reduced anabolic response to low doses (e.g., less than 10 g) of EAAs [12]; yet, higher doses (e.g., 10–15 g, with at least 3 g of leucine) are sufficient to induce a protein anabolic response comparable to that observed in younger adults [12]. Therefore, it is recommended that older people consume food rich in high-quality proteins with higher proportions of EAAs, such as lean meat and other leucine-rich foods (e.g., soybeans, peanuts, chickpeas, and lentils) [13].

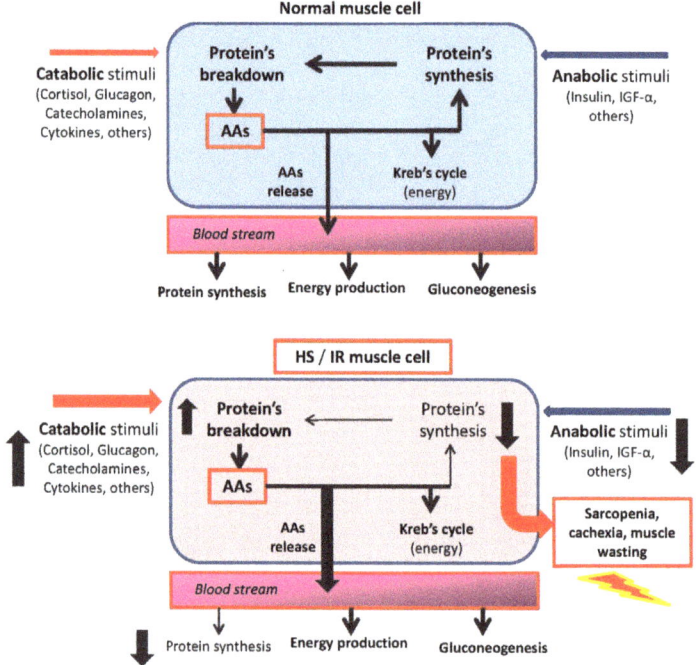

Figure 3. The fate of amino acids (AAs) in muscle cell: physiologic (**top**) and hypercatabolic syndrome (HS) and/or insulin resistance (IS) (**bottom**). The increase in catabolic stimuli enhances protein breakdown and AA release in the blood stream. These AAs are used almost exclusively for energy production and gluconeogenesis, but not for de novo protein synthesis. This favors the onset and aggravation of muscle wasting.

Recently, protein intake above the current recommended dietary allowance (RDA; 0.8 g/kg/day) has been proposed to preserve muscle health in later life [14–17]. It, therefore, appears appropriate to promote protein intake of 1.0–1.2 g/kg/day, while 1.2–1.5 g/kg/day of protein may be required in older adults with acute or chronic conditions [16–18]. Finally, older people with severe illnesses or overt malnutrition may need as much as 2.0 g/kg/day of protein [17].

It is also important to consider that HS induces "insulin resistance" (IR), a condition which reduces cytoplasmic and mitochondrial cell protein synthesis and impaired cell metabolism. This reinforces the protein-amino acid disarrangement [10,19].

3. Clinical Impact of Protein Disarrangements

Alterations in protein balance have been associated with muscle wasting in patients aged 65+, hospitalized for a variety of chronic disease conditions [20]. Furthermore, approximately 30% of patients with chronic heart failure exhibit reduced serum albumin (<3.5 g/dL) [21]. Notably, these conditions are related to increased morbidity, hospitalization, and mortality, independent of primary diseases, and so increases health-related costs and worse prognosis [11,22].

The central role of muscle proteins for the maintenance of whole-body metabolism, especially in response to stress (e.g., HS following chronic disease conditions) has recently gained support [23]. Indeed, the maintenance of muscle mass and protein metabolism has been suggested as being a relevant parameter to include in future studies because of its clinical relevance [23].

Therefore, the concept of dietary protein intake being calculated as a fixed and limited ratio (<20%) of total calories has also been questioned. Two major points should be considered: (1) nitrogen needs may significantly increase independent of caloric demand. This is often overlooked in large populations (i.e., the elderly with or without chronic diseases); and (2) nitrogen should not be calculated by using total protein nitrogen content, but by considering individual AAs. This is because dietary proteins are enriched in NEAAs, which are not fundamental to support global metabolism but do increase urea synthesis, and EAAs, which are crucial for refuelling proteins and global metabolism. Thus, insufficient intake of EAAs despite increased need may be a mechanism in obese patients with chronic disease (i.e., heart failure), further worsening protein metabolism [24].

Dietary intake providing adequate protein amount and, consequently, AAs to match organ demand, preserves the integrity of organs essential for life, as witnessed by peripheral muscle homeostasis and, ultimately, patient survival. Conversely, insufficient EAA intake induces muscle and circulating visceral protein degradation to release AAs to cope for this deficit. Thus, sarcopenia/muscle wasting and hypoalbuminemia become clinically evident.

HS also reduces the appetite, as well as nausea and digestive disorders in patients with chronic conditions leading to inadequate nutrition and consequent reduced availability of nutrients, including AAs [25]. Anamnesis would suggest that eating-related disorders can be found in chronic patients and specific therapeutic strategies can be implemented. Up to 50% of patients with severe chronic disease show altered protein metabolism, which is often underestimated by clinicians despite influencing cell life and having relevant clinical implications [25].

The consequences of protein disarrangement in various body organs and/or systems are illustrated in Figure 4. Altered protein metabolism in patients with chronic diseases, especially older ones, may increase the risk of developing life-threatening complications (e.g., infection due to reduced or circulating T cells and secretion of protein Ig or imbalance of the Na^+/K^+ ratio) with consequent water retention, respiratory failure, and pulmonary edema. Furthermore, cardiac dysfunction, ventricular arrhythmias, and renal insufficiency may also occur [25].

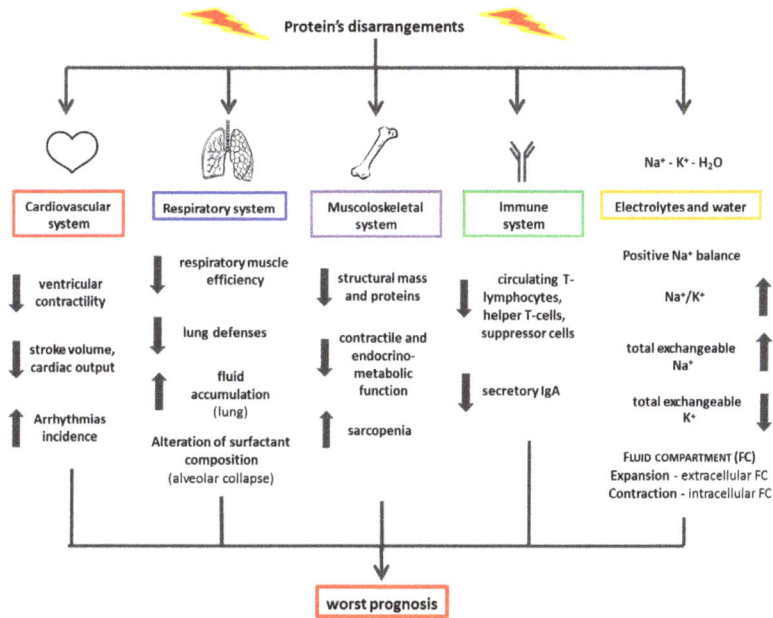

Figure 4. Effects of protein disarrangements on various systems and electrolyte balance.

4. Clinical Steps to Evaluate Protein Disarrangement

We have recently proposed a panel of practical and inexpensive tools for the clinical evaluation of protein disarrangement [26]. A set of indirect measurements evaluating body composition (anthropometric parameters), visceral protein composition (serum albumin, pre-albumin, transferrin, retinol binding protein, nitrogen balance), muscle protein degradation (serum or urinary excretion of 3-metil histidine), and immuno-competence (total lymphocyte count) has been proposed. However, a rapid, inexpensive, and easy assessment of protein disarrangements at the bedside is still lacking. As such, the evaluation of anthropometric parameters should be considered [26].

A simple way to evaluate body composition is to measure tricipital skin-fold thickness (TST, an index of fat mass) and arm muscle area (AMA, an index of lean mass) as described elsewhere [27,28]. Notably, TST and AMA are not modified by extracellular fluids, so they are useful tools even in patients with fluid retention. Interestingly, the presence of reduced AMA less than 5th percentile by age and sex, together with hypoalbuminemia, in the absence of liver and/or renal insufficiency, confirms the presence of muscle sarcopenia and altered protein metabolism. [29]

Whenever protein disarrangement associated with muscle wasting and hypoalbuminemia is suspected, the following additional evaluations can be considered.

4.1. Circulating Visceral Proteins

The concentration of serum proteins such as albumin, pre-albumin, transferrin, and retinol binding proteins are influenced by extra-cellular fluid composition.

Albumin concentration can be included in routine clinical blood measurements as it is easy to measure, non-invasive, and a repeatable marker. Its concentration correlates with worsening morbidity and mortality independent of the disease index [30]. Albumin half-life in circulation is about 20 days and the fractional replacement rate is 10% per day. In the absence of chronic stress, increased serum albumin levels appear within 14 days and a serum concentration <3.5 g/dL indicates impaired protein metabolism associated with muscle wasting [30]. Concentrations lower than 3.2 g/dL suggest more pronounced protein metabolism disarrangement. Notably, severe nephrosis, protein-losing enteropathy, or severe liver insufficiency reduce serum albumin concentrations. Consequently, these conditions should be excluded when albumin is used as an index of protein status.

Pre-albumin responds quickly to short-term (24–36 h) energy restriction and re-feeding. Repeated measurements of pre-albumin levels over a week could be a useful measure of both protein depletion and repletion. This is particularly useful to monitor treatment [30].

Transferrin correlates with mortality and is also influenced by iron metabolism. It has a half-life of about eight days and can, therefore, be used to monitor the effects of specific intervention.

Retinol-binding protein has a turnover of 12 h. Consequently, it is a measure of rapid protein metabolism modification.

4.2. Nitrogen Balance

Nitrogen balance (NB) is an indirect measure of dynamic processes of endogenous protein synthesis (anabolism) and demolition (catabolism). NB is expressed as: NB g/day = $N_I - N_V$ + 2 g. This formula includes nitrogen intake/supply in g/day (N_I) and urinary nitrogen excretion (N_V) in g/day + 20% N_V for non-urea N excretion. Two grams correspond to the nitrogen lost in feces and sweat.

NB is in equilibrium if its balance equals ± 1 g/day. NB > 1 g/day indicates prevalent protein synthesis. NB < 1 g/day suggests ongoing protein degradation with AAs used for general metabolic purpose instead of protein synthesis. Therefore, NB < 1 g/day represents an index of proteins disarrangement [8,26]. Notably, NB depends on urea excretion that is influenced by the daily amount of NEAAs that are routed to urea excretion. To obtain reliable information, this parameter should be monitored frequently.

4.3. 3-Methylistidine

Methylation of histidine is a marker of protein degradation derived from contractile actin and myosin. A simple and rapid method to estimate the fractional catabolic rate of myofibrillar protein is the evaluation of 3-methylhistidine: creatinine excretion in the urine. The presence of 3-MeH shows the presence of proteolysis over the immediate period-hours [8,31,32].

4.4. Blood Lymphocyte Count

The loss of circulating cell-mediated immune competence is present in patients with advanced heart failure with sarcopenia and metabolism disarrangements. Indeed, the lymphocyte count could be considered an indirect index of cell proliferation, protein synthesis, and energy availability and can be used to confirm protein and global metabolic impairment [33].

5. Possible Therapeutic Interventions

Protein intake and AA availability are key to maintaining protein synthesis in living organisms. Healthy individuals absorb AAs from the diet after protein digestion by pancreatic enzymes. However, the pancreas uses large amounts of AAs and energy to produce digestive enzymes [10]. The efficiency of pancreatic and mesenteric circulation may be progressively reduced in HS and/or in chronic diseases with water retention [34]. In addition, gut microbiota alterations and impaired intestinal function, including altered nutrient digestion and absorption, have been reported in patients with chronic disease [34]. These conditions lead to impaired AA digestion and absorption and, consequently, to reduced AA plasma levels that may become insufficient to maintaining protein synthesis and energy demand in HS patients [10]. In contrast, individual AAs derived from nutritional supplements are immediately available after absorption and transit into the bloodstream to be delivered to cells [35].

EAAs stimulate protein synthesis in both young and the elderly [36]. However, it has recently been shown that specific diets containing blends of individual EAAs in stoichiometric ratios are crucial for providing AAs for various metabolic needs, such as protein synthesis, mitochondrial biogenesis, and other important metabolic pathways crucial for cell life [6,37,38]. Indeed, specific EAA mixtures control protein synthesis in myocytes by activating AMP-activated protein kinase (AMPK) and mTOR, which regulate energy production/use, protein synthesis, cell proliferation, mitochondrial biogenesis, and anti-apoptotic process [39].

Clinical and experimental data suggest that oral supplements with specific individual EAA mixtures ensuring metabolic energy supply, administered traditionally, counteract protein disarrangement and cellular energy impairment without influencing renal function [40–43]. The clinical consequences of this is that the percentage of nitrogen and calories provided by diet should be calculated separately according to metabolic needs. Moreover, the amount of EAAs should be provided as a function of their intrinsic capacities to maintain proteins and body metabolism. In addition, individual AAs should be provided so they are not rapidly absorbed, thus increasing their blood viability [44].

Taken together, these observations could explain why previous studies were unable to show any effects of simple total protein dietary supplementation on protein and energy metabolism in patients with chronic diseases [45]. Such findings support the indication that the elderly need increased EAA to stimulate muscle protein synthesis. This also introduces the concept of evaluating protein AA composition (protein quality) [46]. A modification of the Dietary Guidelines of Americans (DG of A), which provides nutrient advice to avoid/reduce age-related nutritional problems, has been proposed as follows: (1) protein (and more importantly specific AAs) should be a part of the adult/aged people diet; (2) protein (and more importantly specific AAs) needs for adult/aged people should be proportional to body weight and/or clinical condition and not as a percentage of total energy intake; (3) most adult/aged people benefit from protein intake above the minimum recommended daily allowance. Indeed, to maintain healthy muscles and bones, at least 30 g of high-quality protein (and more importantly specific EAAs) should be ingested at more than one meal.

The effect of dietary administration of different EAAs blends has been actively investigated in the recent years [42–44]. Existing findings on the molecular pathways elicited by proteins and AA metabolism in chronic disease conditions could allow the development of therapeutic strategies to contrast metabolic impairment, especially in the elderly.

6. Conclusions

The evaluation of protein disarrangement deserves greater attention to manage chronic diseases, especially in old age (see Box 1). Readily available and inexpensive anthropometric and blood parameters, such as TST, AMA, and albuminemia, can be obtained routinely at the bedside. Additional research could unveil the causes of these conditions and monitor the outcome of specific therapeutic interventions.

Clinicians should consider protein homeostasis as essential to maintaining metabolic competence in patients with chronic diseases. This is fundamental for any further therapeutic approaches. The identification and treatment of protein metabolic impairment with appropriate therapies may be at least as important as any other evaluation and therapeutic strategy implemented in improving the prognosis of chronically ill patients.

Box 1. Main Messages from the text.

- Proteins are building blocks for living organisms consisting of amino acids (AAs).
- AAs are totipotent biochemical molecules essential for cellular activity.
- Pathological conditions increase protein/AA demand.
- Hypercatabolic syndromes, due to increased inflammation and catabolic hormones, cause significant changes in body metabolism and lead to an imbalance between nutritional input and synthetic/energy needs.
- Both circulating (i.e., albumin) and muscle proteins are a reservoir of AAs (above all, essential AAs) within the body.
- Altered protein metabolism in patients (especially those with chronic diseases and/or older), can increase the risk of developing life-threatening complications (e.g., infection, cardiac and/or renal dysfunction).
- The pathophysiology of conditions characterized by protein disarrangements (i.e., muscle wasting and/or hypoalbuminemia) need to be fully clarified to develop adequate therapeutic (nutritional) strategies.
- Clinicians need to consider protein metabolism as a critical aspect for the management of patients with chronic diseases.

Author Contributions: E.P., G.C. and F.S.D. designed research; E.P., G.C. and C.R. conducted research; R.A., A.P. and R.C. contributed to data interpretation and the drafting of the manuscript; E.P., G.C., C.R. and F.S.D. wrote the paper; G.C. and C.R. prepared figures; E.P. and F.S.D. had primary responsibility for the final content.

Conflicts of Interest: F.S.D. is the inventor and owner of US patent no. US6218420 B1: Compositions based on amino-acids for preventing and treating alimentary overload under conditions of high body nitrogen requirements, without causing calcium loss; no. US7973077 B2: Amino acid-based compositions for the treatment of pathological conditions distinguished by insufficient mitochondrial function and other patents pending on different amino acid based formulations. R.C. and E.M. are partners of the SPRINTT consortium, which is partly funded by the European Federation of Pharmaceutical Industries and Associations (EFPIA). E.M. served as a consultant for Huron Consulting Group, Genactis, and Novartis. R.C. served as a consultant from Novartis and Nutricia. All other authors have no competing financial interests to declare.

References

1. Lehninger, A.L. *Principles of Biochemistry*; Worth Publishers Inc.: New York, NY, USA, 1982.
2. Bischoffa, R.; Hartmut, S. Amino acids: Chemistry, functionality and selected non-post-translational modifications. *J. Proteom.* **2012**, *75*, 2275–2296. [CrossRef] [PubMed]

3. Mitchell, H.H.; Block, R.J. Some relationships between the amino acid contents of proteins and their nutritive values for the rat. *J. Biol. Chem.* **1946**, *163*, 599–620. [CrossRef] [PubMed]
4. Anthony, J.C.; Anthony, T.G.; Kimball, S.R.; Jefferson, L.S. Signalling pathways involved in translational control of protein synthesis in skeletal muscle by leucine. *J. Nutr.* **2001**, *131*, 856S–860S. [CrossRef] [PubMed]
5. Woolfson, A.M.J. Amino acids-their role as an energy source. *Proc. Nutr. Soc.* **1983**, *42*, 489–495. [CrossRef] [PubMed]
6. Dioguardi, F.S. Wasting and the substrate to energy controller pathway: A role for insulin resistance and amino acids. *Am. J. Cardiol.* **2004**, *93*, 6A–12A. [CrossRef] [PubMed]
7. Taegtmayer, H. Energy metabolism of the heart: From basic concepts to clinical applications. *Curr. Prob. Cardiol.* **1994**, *19*, 59–113. [CrossRef]
8. Aquilani, R.; Opasich, C.; Verri, M.; Boschi, F.; Febo, O.; Pasini, E.; Pastoris, O. Is nutritional intake adequate in chronic heart failure patients? *J. Am. Coll. Cardiol.* **2003**, *42*, 1218–1223. [CrossRef]
9. Anker, S.D.; Chaua, T.P.; Ponikowski, P.; Harrington, D.; Swan, J.W.; Kox, W.J.; Poole-Wilson, P.A.; Coats, A.J. Hormonal changes and catabolic/anabolic imbalance in chronic heart failure and their importance for cardiac cachexia. *Circulation* **1997**, *96*, 526–534. [CrossRef] [PubMed]
10. Pasini, E.; Aquilani, R.; Dioguardi, F.S.; D'Antona, G.; Gheorghiade, M.; Taegtmeyer, H. Hypercatbolic syndrome: Molecular basis and effects of nutritional supplementation with amino acids. *Am. J. Cardiol.* **2008**, *101*, 11E–15E. [CrossRef] [PubMed]
11. Aquilani, R.; Opasic, C.; Dossena, M.; Iadarola, P.; Gualco, A.; Arcidiaco, P.; Viglio, S.; Boschi, F.; Verri, M.; Pasini, E. Increased skeletal muscle amino acid release with light exercise in deconditioned patients with heart failure. *J. Am. Coll. Cardiol.* **2005**, *45*, 154–164. [CrossRef] [PubMed]
12. Katsanos, C.S.; Kobayashi, H.; Sheffield-Moore, M.; Aarsland, A.; Wolfe, R.R. Aging is associated with diminished accretion of muscle proteins after the ingestion of a small bolus of essential amino acids. *Am. J. Clin. Nutr.* **2005**, *82*, 1065–1073. [CrossRef] [PubMed]
13. Martone, A.M.; Marzetti, E.; Calvani, R.; Picca, A.; Tosato, M.; Santoro, L.; Di Giorgio, A.; Nesci, A.; Sisto, A.; Santoliquido, A.; Landi, F. Exercise and Protein Intake: A Synergistic Approach against Sarcopenia. *Biomed. Res. Int.* **2017**, 2672435. [CrossRef] [PubMed]
14. Fielding, R.A.; Vellas, B.; Evans, W.J.; Bhasin, S.; Morley, J.E.; Newman, A.B.; Abellan van Kan, G.; Andrieu, S.; Bauer, J.; Breuille, D.; et al. Sarcopenia: An undiagnosed condition in older adults. Current consensus definition: Prevalence, etiology, and consequences. International working group on Sarcopenia. *J. Am. Med. Dir. Assoc.* **2011**, *12*, 249–256. [CrossRef] [PubMed]
15. Volpi, E.; Campbell, W.W.; Dwyer, J.T.; Johnson, M.A.; Jensen, G.L.; Morley, J.E.; Wolfe, R.R. Is the optimal level of protein intake for older adults greater than the recommended dietary allowance? *J. Gerontol. A Biol. Sci. Med. Sci.* **2013**, *68*, 677–681. [CrossRef] [PubMed]
16. Morley, J.E.; Argiles, J.M.; Evans, W.J.; Bhasin, S.; Cella, D.; Deutz, N.E.P.; Doehner, W.; Fearon, K.C.H.; Ferrucci, L.; Hellerstein, M.K.; et al. Society for Sarcopenia, Cachexia, and Wasting Disease. Nutritional recommendations for the management of Sarcopenia. *J. Am. Med. Dir. Assoc.* **2010**, *11*, 391–396. [CrossRef] [PubMed]
17. Bauer, J.; Biolo, G.; Cederholm, T.; Cesari, M.; Cruz-Jentoft, A.J.; Morley, J.E.; Phillips, S.; Sieber, C.; Stehle, P.; Teta, D.; et al. Evidence-based recommendations for optimal dietary protein intake in older people: A position paper from the PROT-AGE Study Group. *J. Am. Med. Dir. Assoc.* **2013**, *14*, 542–559. [CrossRef] [PubMed]
18. Paddon-Jones, D.; Short, K.R.; Campbell, W.W.; Volpi, E.; Wolfe, R.R. Role of dietary protein in the Sarcopenia of aging. *Am. J. Clin. Nutr.* **2008**, *87*, 1562S–1566S. [CrossRef] [PubMed]
19. Tremblay, F.; Lavigne, C.; Jacques, H.; Marette, A. Role of Dietary Proteins and Amino Acids in the Pathogenesis of Insulin Resistance. *Annu. Rev. Nutr.* **2007**, *27*, 293–310. [CrossRef] [PubMed]
20. Guigoz, Y. The mini nutritional assessment review of the literature: What does it tell us? *J. Nutr. Health Aging* **2006**, *10*, 466–485. [PubMed]
21. Liu, M.; Chan, C.P.; Yan, B.P.; Zhang, Q.; Lam, Y.Y.; Li, R.J.; Sanderson, J.E.; Coats, A.J.; Sun, J.P.; Yip, G.W.; Yu, C.M. Albumin levels predict survival in patients with heart failure and preserved ejection fraction. *Eur. J. Heart Fail.* **2012**, *14*, 39–44. [CrossRef] [PubMed]
22. Anker, S.D.; Ponikowski, P.; Varney, S.; Chua, T.P.; Clark, A.L.; Webb-Peploe, K.M.; Harrington, D.; Kox, W.J.; Poole-Wilson, P.A.; Coats, A.J. Wasting as independent risk factor for mortality in chronic heart failure. *Lancet* **1997**, *349*, 1050–1053. [CrossRef]

23. Wolfe, E.W. The underappreciated role of muscle in health and diseases. *Am. J. Clin. Nutr.* **2006**, *84*, 475–482. [CrossRef] [PubMed]
24. Lainscak, M.; von Haehling, S.; Doehner, W.; Anker, S.D. The obesity paradox in chronic disease: Facts and numbers. *J. Cachexia Sarcopenia Muscle* **2012**, *3*, 1–4. [CrossRef] [PubMed]
25. Aquilani, R.; Opasich, C.; Viglio, S.; Iadarola, P.; Pasini, E. Nutrition in acute decompensation of patients with acute heart failure syndrome. In *Acute Heart Failure*; Springer: London, UK, 2008; pp. 876–882.
26. Pasini, E.; Aquilani, R.; Dioguardi, F.S. The enemy within. How to identify chronic diseases induced-protein metabolism impairment and its possible pharmacological treatment. *Pharmacol. Res.* **2013**, *76*, 28–33. [CrossRef] [PubMed]
27. Magnani, R. Sampling guide. In *Food and Nutrition Technical Assistance (FANTA) Project*; Academy for Educational Development: Washington, DC, USA, 1997.
28. Cogil, B. Anthropometric indicators measurement guide. In *Food and Nutrition Technical Assistance (FANTA) Project*; Academy for Educational Development: Washington, DC, USA, 2003.
29. Frisancho, R. *Anthropometric Standards for the Assessment of Growth and Nutritional Status*; The University of Michigan Press: Ann Arbor, MI, USA, 1990.
30. Watson, R.R. Nutritional stresses: Levels of complement proteins and their functions. In *Nutrition, Disease Resistance and Immune Function*; Watson, R.R., Ed.; Marcel Dekker: New York, NY, USA, 1984; pp. 175–188.
31. Ferrari, F.; Fumagalli, M.; Viglio, S.; Aquilani, R.; Pasini, E.; Iadarola, P. A rapid method for simultaneous determination of creatine, 1-and 3 methyhistidine in human urine. *Electrophoresis* **2009**, *30*, 1–3. [CrossRef] [PubMed]
32. Aquilani, R.; Opasic, C.; Gualco, A.; Bairdi, P.; Pasini, E.; Testa, A.; Viglio, S.; Iadarola, P.; Verri, M.; D'Agostino, L.; Boschi, F. A practical method to diagnose muscle degradation in normo-nourished patient with chronic heart failure. *Int. J. Med.* **2009**, *2*, 226–230.
33. Acanfora, D.; Gheorghiade, M.; Trojano, L.; Furgi, G.; Pasini, E.; Picone, C.; Papa, A.; Iannuzzi, G.L.; Bonow, R.O.; Rengo, F. Relative lymphocyte count: A prognostic indicator of mortality in elderly patients with congestive heart failure. *Am. Heart J.* **2001**, *142*, 167–173. [CrossRef] [PubMed]
34. Pasini, E.; Aquilani, R.; Testa, C.; Baiardi, P.; Angioletti, S.; Boschi, F.; Verri, M.; Dioguardi, F.S. Pathogenic Gut Flora in Patients with Chronic Heart Failure. *JACC Heart Fail.* **2016**, *4*, 220–227. [CrossRef] [PubMed]
35. Rondanelli, M.; Aquilani, R.; Verri, M.; Boschi, F.; Pasini, E.; Perna, S.; Faliva, A.; Condino, A.M. Plasma kinetics of essential amino acids following their ingestion as free formula or as dietary protein components. *Aging Clin. Exp. Res.* **2017**, *29*, 801–805. [CrossRef] [PubMed]
36. Volpi, E.; Kobayashi, H.; Sheffield-Moore, M.; Mittendorfer, B.; Wolfe, R.R. Essential amino acids are primarily responsible for the amino acid stimulation of muscle protein anabolism in healthy elderly adults. *Am. J. Clin. Nutr.* **2003**, *78*, 250–258. [CrossRef] [PubMed]
37. Nisoli, E.; Cozzi, V.; Carruba, M. Amino Acids and mitochondrial biogenesis. *Am. J. Cardiol.* **2008**, *101*, 22E–25E. [CrossRef] [PubMed]
38. D'Antona, G.; Ragni, M.; Cardile, A.; Tedesco, L.; Dossena, M.; Bruttini, F.; Caliaro, F.; Corsetti, G.; Bottinelli, R.; Carruba, M.O.; et al. Branched-chain amino acid supplementation promotes survival and supports cardiac and skeletal muscle mitochondrial biogenesis in middle-aged mice. *Cell Metab.* **2010**, *12*, 362–372. [CrossRef] [PubMed]
39. Fujita, S.; Dreyer, H.C.; Drummond, M.J.; Glynn, E.L.; Cadenas, J.G.; Yoshizawa, F.; Volpi, E.; Rasmussen, B.B. Nutrient signalling in the regulation of human muscle protein synthesis. *J. Physiol.* **2007**, *582*, 813–823. [CrossRef] [PubMed]
40. Aquilani, R.; Viglio, S.; Iadarola, P.; Opasich, C.; Testa, A.; Dioguardi, F.S.; Pasini, E. Oral amino acid supplementation improve exercise capacities in elderly patients with heart failure. *Am. J. Cardiol.* **2008**, *101*, 104E–110E. [CrossRef] [PubMed]
41. Scognamiglio, R.; Testa, A.; Aquilani, R.; Dioguardi, F.S.; Pasini, E. Impairment in walking capacity and myocardial function in the elderly: It is a role for non-pharmacologic therapy with nutritional amino acid supplementation? *Am. J. Cardiol.* **2008**, *101*, 78E–81E. [CrossRef] [PubMed]
42. Aquilani, R.; Opasich, C.; Gualco, C.; Veiir, M.; Testa, A.; Pasini, E.; Viglio, C.; Iadarola, P.; Pastoris, O.; Dossena, M.; et al. Adequate energy-protein intake is not enough to improve nutritional and metabolic status in muscle-depleted patients with chronic heart failure. *Eur. J. Heart Fail.* **2008**, *10*, 1127–1135. [CrossRef] [PubMed]

43. Solerte, S.B.; Gazzaruso, C.; Bonacasa, R.; Rondanelli, M.; Zamboni, M.; Basso, C.; Locatelli, E.; Schifino, N.; Giustina, A.; Fioravanti, M. Nutritional supplements with oral amino acid mixture increases whole body lean mass and insulin sensitivity in elderly subjects with Sarcopenia. *Am. J. Cardiol.* **2008**, *101*, 69E–77E. [CrossRef] [PubMed]
44. Corsetti, G.; Pasini, E.; D'Antona, G.; Nisoli, E.; Flati, V.; Assanelli, D.; Dioguardi, S.F.; Bianchi, R. Morphometric changes induced by amino acid supplementation in skeletal and cardiac muscles of old mice. *Am. J. Cardiol.* **2008**, *101*, 26E–34E. [CrossRef] [PubMed]
45. Broqvist, M.; Dahlstrom, U.; Larsson, J.; Larsson, J.; Nylander, E.; Permert, J. Nutritional assessment and muscle energy metabolism in severe chronic congestive heart failure: Effects of long-term dietary supplementation. *Eur. Heart J.* **1994**, *15*, 1641–1650. [CrossRef] [PubMed]
46. Layman, D.K. Dietary Guidelines should reflect new understandings about adult protein needs. *Nutr. Metab.* **2009**, *6*, 12. [CrossRef] [PubMed]

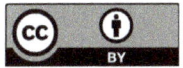

© 2018 by the authors. Licensee MDPI, Basel, Switzerland. This article is an open access article distributed under the terms and conditions of the Creative Commons Attribution (CC BY) license (http://creativecommons.org/licenses/by/4.0/).

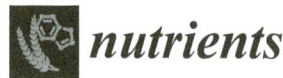

Review

Resistance Training Prevents Muscle Loss Induced by Caloric Restriction in Obese Elderly Individuals: A Systematic Review and Meta-Analysis

Amanda V. Sardeli [1,2,*], Tiemy R. Komatsu [2], Marcelo A. Mori [3,4], Arthur F. Gáspari [1] and Mara Patrícia T. Chacon-Mikahil [1,2]

1. Laboratory of Exercise Physiology—FISEX, Faculty of Physical Education, University of Campinas (UNICAMP), Campinas, Sao Paulo 13083-851, Brazil; arthur.fg@hotmail.com (A.F.G.); marapatricia@fef.unicamp.br (M.P.T.C.-M.)
2. Gerontology Program—Faculty of Medical Sciences, UNICAMP, Campinas, Sao Paulo 13083-887, Brazil; tiemy.komatsu@gmail.com
3. Laboratory of Aging Biology (LaBE), Department of Biochemistry and Tissue Biology, Institute of Biology, University of Campinas (UNICAMP), Campinas, Sao Paulo 13083-862, Brazil; morima@unicamp.br
4. Graduate Program in Genetics and Molecular Biology, Institute of Biology University of Campinas (UNICAMP), Campinas, Sao Paulo 13083-862, Brazil
* Correspondence: amandaveigasardeli@yahoo.com.br; Tel.: +55-19-3521-6625

Received: 22 December 2017; Accepted: 14 February 2018; Published: 29 March 2018

Abstract: It remains unclear as to what extent resistance training (RT) can attenuate muscle loss during caloric restriction (CR) interventions in humans. The objective here is to address if RT could attenuate muscle loss induced by CR in obese elderly individuals, through summarized effects of previous studies. Databases MEDLINE, Embase and Web of Science were used to perform a systematic search between July and August 2017. Were included in the review randomized clinical trials (RCT) comparing the effects of CR with (CRRT) or without RT on lean body mass (LBM), fat body mass (FBM), and total body mass (BM), measured by dual-energy X-ray absorptiometry, on obese elderly individuals. The six RCTs included in the review applied RT three times per week, for 12 to 24 weeks, and most CR interventions followed diets of 55% carbohydrate, 15% protein, and 30% fat. RT reduced 93.5% of CR-induced LBM loss (0.819 kg [0.364 to 1.273]), with similar reduction in FBM and BM, compared with CR. Furthermore, to address muscle quality, the change in strength/LBM ratio tended to be different ($p = 0.07$) following CRRT (20.9 ± 23.1%) and CR interventions (−7.5 ± 9.9%). Our conclusion is that CRRT is able to prevent almost 100% of CR-induced muscle loss, while resulting in FBM and BM reductions that do not significantly differ from CR.

Keywords: exercise; training; aging; sarcopenia; muscle mass; strength training; caloric restriction; diet

1. Introduction

Caloric restriction (CR) has been shown to increase lifespans and attenuate the harmful effects of aging across the evolutionary spectrum [1,2]. Retrospective studies also demonstrate an association between CR and health span in humans [3]. The exact mechanism underlying the benefits of CR remains unknown, but it involves changes in nutrient-sensing pathways, metabolic homeostasis, and body composition [1,4–6]. Weight loss is a normal feature of CR, and some groups claim that it is necessary for beneficial effects, including a reduction of chronic inflammation, which is an important trigger of non-communicable diseases [7–9]. However, weight loss via CR is accompanied by a significant decrease in lean body mass (LBM) [10], which may be deleterious to elderly individuals suffering from sarcopenia. Sarcopenia is often associated with frailty and increased mortality at advanced ages, and is a challenge for successful aging [11].

Resistance training (RT), associated or not with a high protein intake, has been shown to increase LBM, promote strength, and attenuate sarcopenia in elderly individuals [12,13]. However, it is unclear whether RT represents a good strategy to prevent muscle loss during CR (which includes dietary protein restriction). Some studies have reported no change or even reduced LBM following CR when RT is included in the intervention program [7,14–18]. On the other hand, randomized clinical trials (RCT) comparing CR with and without RT have shown the preservation of LBM with RT [19,20]. This inconsistency could be due to different protocols, populations, methods of analysis, lack of statistic power, or methodological rigor (i.e., control group, randomization, and weight stabilization periods). Here, we performed a meta-analysis, based on data from RCTs, in order to determine the level of LBM that can be preserved when RT is associated with CR interventions in elderly obese humans. We hypothesized that elderly individuals treated with CRRT will lose less LBM compared to elderly treated with only CR.

2. Materials and Methods

2.1. Data Source

A systematic search was conducted between July and August 2017 using MEDLINE, Embase and Web of Science. There was no restriction on the publication's date, and the terms were searched within all words in titles and abstracts. The following terms were searched: "caloric restriction", "resistance training" (including "weight training", "weight lifting", "strength training", "resistance exercise", "strength exercise", "resistance program" and "strength program"), and "muscle mass" (including "muscle body mass", "lean mass" and "lean body mass"). Two reviewers selected the studies independently, and the disagreements were solved with further discussion. The data extraction was also made independently, and further compared to avoid errors. To isolate the effects of RT over CR, only RCTs comparing the CR with (CRRT) or without RT (CR) were included. Details of the data selection process are described in Figure 1. Non-original studies, non-human studies, and studies without a control intervention were the only exclusion criteria. Considering that only one study assessed body composition by hydrostatic weighing in young adults [21] (instead of the DEXA in older adults), and another one prescribed RT only for abdomen muscles [22] (instead of the whole body), they were not included in the meta-analyses. Six RCTs were included for the final meta-analysis [7,15,16,20,23]. One of these studies [24] reported part of its data from a previous publication [25], so both studies were included as one.

2.2. Study Selection

The RCTs included strictly similar samples, RT protocols, and CR protocols (Table 1). In summary, the samples were composed of older adults or elderly people (mean > 57 years old), including men, women, obese, sedentary, healthy, dyslipidemic, hyperglycemic, and diabetic individuals. Most CR diets were nutritionally balanced (55% carbohydrate, 15% protein, 30% fat) [15,16,19,20], while others had increased protein [7] or reduced fat intake [24]. Percentages of CR varied among studies, as shown in Table 1. RT protocols lasted from 12 to 24 weeks, and applied a general warm-up on a treadmill or cycle ergometer, followed by two or three trials of 8 to 15 repetitions, with a minimum of 65% of one repetition maximum (1RM) for each exercise, three times per week.

2.3. Assessment of Risk of Bias

The researchers assessed the studies' qualities using the PEDro scale [26]. As patients and care providers could not be blinded in exercise interventions, these questions were nullified. Thus, scores on the PEDro scale ranged from 0 (very low methodological quality) to 9 (high methodological quality). The risk of publication bias was assessed through the Egger test.

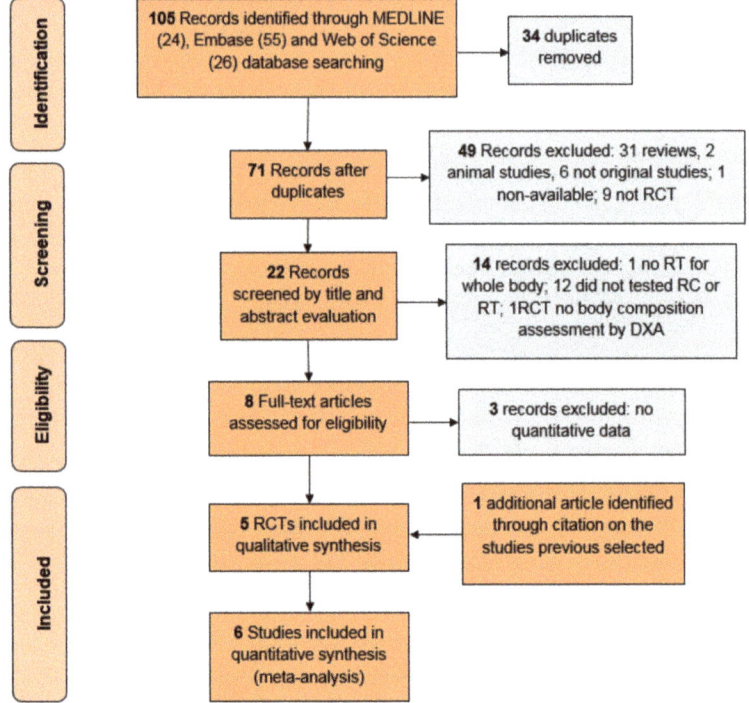

Figure 1. Flowchart of study selection. RCT: randomized control trials; RT: Resistance training; DXA: Dual X-ray Absorbance; CRRT: caloric restriction with resistance training group.

2.4. Statistical Analysis

The meta-analyses were performed using Comprehensive Meta-Analysis (CMA) software, version 3.3.070. We performed three meta-analyses: lean body mass (LBM), fat body mass (FBM), and total body mass (BM). The effect size was calculated based on the raw mean difference (RMD) of the delta (pre- to post-intervention) between CRRT and control groups (CR). As the studies tested were significantly homogeneous ($p < 0.05$), the authors used the fixed effect model in all three meta-analyses. Despite the existence of particular differences between the samples studied and RT and CR protocols deserving comparisons, the absence of between-studies variance precluded further subgroup analysis. A conservative pre–post correlation of 0.5 was assumed [27]. In addition to the main results, an analysis of whole-body muscle quality was performed. The percent delta of muscle quality (strength/LBM ratio) following CRRT and CR was calculated, excluding only one study that did not report strength values [7], by the following equation: percent delta of muscle quality = (average strength/average LBM pre-intervention) − (average strength/average LBM post-intervention) × (100)/(average strength/average LBM pre-intervention). The ratio was calculated from whole-body LBM and muscle group strength presented by each original study, which count six lower limb measurements and two upper limb measurements. The Mann Whitney test was used to compare the mean differences between groups.

Table 1. Studies features.

First Author, Year	Weight Stabilization	Age (Years Mean ± SD)	Sex	Health Status	CR or BM Reduction	Diet (CARBOHYDRATE/ Protein/fat%)	RT Load	RT Volume	CRRT Duration (Weeks)
Amamou, 2016 [6]	4 weeks stabilization	65.8 ± 3.1	both	dyslipidemic and diabetics	472.74 ± 52.5/day	25–30 g protein supplementation (45–50/25–30/25–30)	65 to 80% 1RM	2 × (8 to 15)	16
Bouchard, 2009 [18]	no	63 ± 4	women	health	0.5 to 1 kg/week	balanced (55/15/30)	80% 1RM	3 × 8	12
Brochu, 2009 [15]	2 kg stabilization	57.2 ± 5	women	health	624 ± 133/day (33.4 ± 4.9%)	balanced (55/15/30)	65 to 75% 1RM	(2 to 3) × (15 to 10)	24
Dunstan, 2005 [21]	not reported	67.6 ± 5.2	both	diabetics	0.25 kg/week	balanced (70% carbohydrate and protein/30%fat)	75 to 85% 1RM	3 × (8 to 10)	24
Sénéchal, 2012 [14]	no	62.6 ± 4.1	women	health	0.5 to 1 kg/week	balanced (55/15/30)	not reported	3 × 8	12
St-Onge, 2012 [19]	4 weeks stabilization	57.6 ± 4	women	health	500 to 800 kcal/day	balanced (55/15/30)	8 to 15RM	(1 to 3) × (8 to 12)	24

CR: caloric restriction; BM: body mass; 1RM: one repetition maximum; RM: range of repetition maximum; HRmax: maximum heart rate predicted by age equations; BM: body mass.

3. Results

3.1. Studies' Features

The quality of studies were homogeneous, as observed by their scores of 5 [7,16,20], 6 [19,24], and 7 [15] on the PEDro scale. Egger tests ($p > 0.1$ for all) for the different analyses did not indicate any publication bias. The studies' main features are detailed in Table 1. Some studies reported using a weight stabilization period to ensure that subjects were maintaining their weight before the intervention. All studies selected included sedentary and obese individuals, and prescribed resistance exercise for the main muscle groups, including upper and lower limbs, three times per week. LBM, FBM, and BM in kg were assessed by dual-energy X-ray absorptiometry.

3.2. Evidence Synthesis

Figure 2 shows the forest plot comparing the different reductions of LBM, FBM and BM for CRRT and CR. Although the reduction of BM and FBM in the CRRT group was not different from the CR group, the LBM loss in the CRRT group was 93.5% less than the CR group (RMD = 0.819 kg, 95% CI = 0.364 to 1.273, $p < 0.001$). The means standard deviations (SD) of deltas for LBM, FBM, and BM were 0.05 ± 0.3 kg, -3.86 ± 1.3 kg, and -4.16 ± 1.2 kg for CRRT, and -0.76 ± 0.1 kg, -3.73 ± 1.2 kg, and -4.73 ± 1.2 kg for CR, respectively (Figure 3a). The percentage of muscle quality changes, defined as force production per unit of muscle tissue [23], was calculated as strength divided by LBM following CRRT ($20.9 \pm 23.1\%$) and CR ($-7.5 \pm 9.9\%$), and there was a tendency for a significant difference between the groups ($p = 0.07$) (Figure 3b).

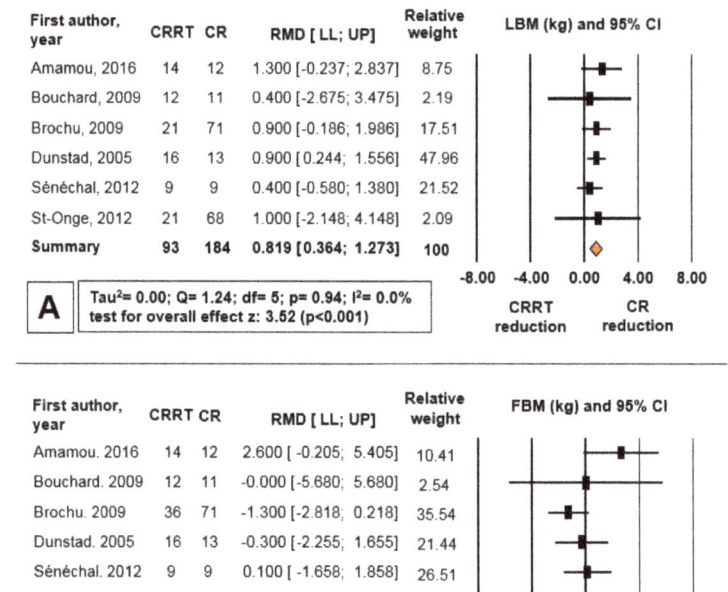

Figure 2. Cont.

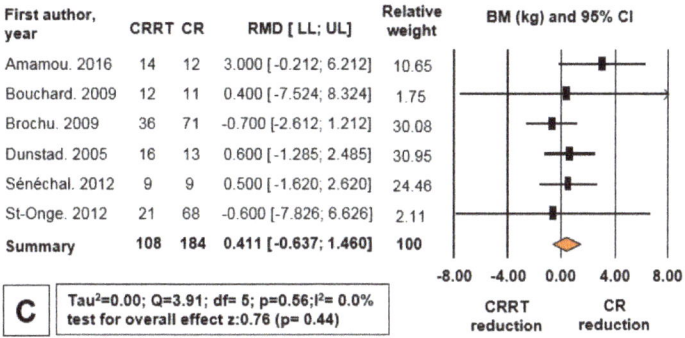

Figure 2. Forest plot for differences between caloric restriction plus resistance training (CRRT) and caloric restriction (CR) reductions of LBM (**A**); FBM (**B**); and BM (**C**). RMD: raw mean difference (kg); LL: lower limit of 95% CI; UP: upper limit of 95% CI; CI: confidence interval.

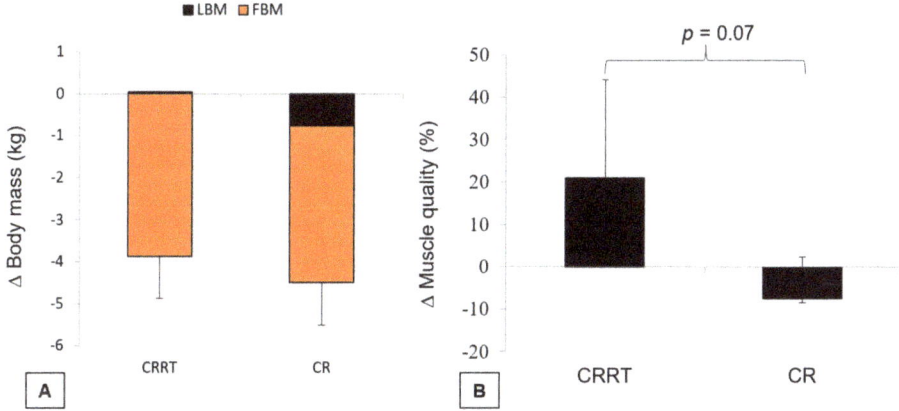

Figure 3. (**A**) Illustrative change in body mass after CRRT and CR; (**B**) percentage of muscle quality change after CRRT and CR. Data is presented in mean and standard deviation. P: *p*-value for difference between groups (Mann Whitney test).

4. Discussion

The main finding of the present meta-analyses was that CRRT prevents 93% of the LBM loss induced by CR, although it does not affect BM and FBM reductions as compared to CR without RT. A previous meta-analysis showed only 50% LBM loss attenuation when different types of exercise were added to CR in sarcopenic obese individuals over 50 years old [10]. However, since endurance, resistance, and combined types of training were included in this analysis, it was not possible to identify which type of exercise led to the preventive effect. Endurance exercise is the most efficient type to increase energy expenditure and induce weight loss, mainly when associated with CR [28–31]. On the other hand, we propose that RT is an excellent alternative to prevent CR-induced LBM loss in elderly individuals. Furthermore, future studies should compare the preventive effect of different modalities of exercise training on CR-induced LBM loss.

A proposed mechanism to explain such protection relies on the energy costs of protein synthesis. During CR without RT, the blunted muscle protein synthesis with elevated proteolysis might allow energy maintenance [32]. Alternatively, CRRT induces muscle protein synthesis [33], likely shifting energy towards LBM maintenance while stimulating fat depletion, to allow for fuel availability to cope with the increased energy demand. Indeed, Murphy and colleagues have shown that RT restores the depressed rates of myofibrillar protein synthesis induced by CR [33].

Preservation of LBM with CR could also be obtained by additional protein intake. Longland and colleagues [34] have shown that CRRT with high protein consumption induces an increase in LBM and promotes larger fat loss, if compared to CRRT with low protein consumption. The only study that has investigated the CR effects in combination with higher protein intake (30% compared to 15% of the rest) found lower LBM loss than the others (RMD 1.3 kg compared to the main effect of RMD 0.6 kg) [7]. However, whether or ot the beneficial effects of CR are dependent on protein restriction is not clear, and deserves further attention. Although the evidence towards a longer lifespan in humans is still unclear [35], decreased protein intake is often beneficial and increases lifespan in other animals [36]. Moreover, the mammalian target of rapamycin (mTOR) pathway, which is induced by amino acids, growth factors, and RT, is often inhibited during CR, and mediates CR-induced health benefits in model organisms [37]. However, while chronic mTOR activation during obesity or aging might be deleterious [37], like in CRRT, mTOR activation concurrent with decreased energy balance may preserve protein synthesis, while stimulating fat depletion.

Cross-sectional studies have shown potential detrimental effects of higher muscle mass on insulin sensitivity in sedentary older adults [38], which oppose the well-known beneficial effects of exercise on glucose metabolism [39,40]. However, it is likely that the exercise-induced LBM increase may not lead to such impairments in insulin sensitivity [41]. While reduced glucose disposal, total cholesterol, and LDL were maintained or even improved upon implementing CRRT [7,15,16,24], in two studies blood triglyceride levels were reduced after CR, but not after CRRT [15,16]. In one of them, HDL was decreased following CRRT [15], and fasting insulin was reduced only in the CR group [16]. The authors suggest these controversial findings may be due to the presence of a varied pool of diabetic, dyslipidemic, or hypertensive patients among the study populations. These observations reinforce the need for further comparisons of CR effects and exercise training on overall health markers in healthy and diseased populations.

It goes beyond the scope of this study to determine whether CR-induced LBM reduction can be as harmful to muscle function as aging-induced LBM reduction. Sarcopenia is characterized not only by an LBM reduction, but also a reduction in muscle function [11]. Despite the fact that larger muscle areas are associated with higher muscle strength, LBM is not the only determinant [42,43]. Thus, despite the marked LBM reduction following CR in some species, CR delays age-associated muscle dysfunction in *D. melanogaster* [44] and rhesus monkeys [45], and delays the onset of sarcopenia in the latter [46].

CR intervention in elderly humans results in a reduction [18,19] or maintenance [15,16,20,24] of muscle strength. Even though the present study was not designed to test muscle function, we showed a trend towards the increase in whole body muscle quality when RT was added to CR ($p = 0.07$), suggesting that in humans, RT improves muscle function regardless of muscle mass changes during CR. It is noteworthy that muscle group strength was related to whole LBM, instead of local muscle mass, which is a limitation of the method. In agreement with our findings, in a study with elderly individuals, when CRRT was compared to RT alone, the addition of CR to RT improved mobility (400 m of walk time) without compromising other functional adaptations of RT alone [14].

Another concern regarding body composition following CR interventions is the bone mass loss, which exercise is shown to prevent, at least in rodent models of male senile osteoporosis [47]. RT is known to be highly effective to increase bone mineral density after long-term interventions in humans [48]. However, the only intervention that assessed bone mass in this review was too short to address either positive or negative effects from CRRT or CR [20]. In this sense, despite the anti-aging potential of CR to humans, future studies are required to test its long-term effects in a comprehensive health perspective.

5. Conclusions

CRRT almost stopped CR-induced LBM loss completely, while resulting in similar FBM and BM reductions as seen with CR alone. The confidence intervals showed there was a wide range of responsivity among individuals; therefore, future studies should investigate which factors are different between groups of responders and non-responders for LBM prevention after CRRT, in order to address the possible mediators of this process.

Author Contributions: A.V.S. developed the experimental design. A.V.S. and T.R.K. carried out the data collection and data analysis. A.V.S. and T.R.K. conceived the manuscript that was reviewed for A.F.G., M.A.M. and M.P.T.C.-M.

Conflicts of Interest: The authors declare no conflict of interest.

References

1. Fontana, L.; Partridge, L. Promoting health and longevity through diet: From model organisms to humans. *Cell* **2015**, *161*, 106–118. [CrossRef] [PubMed]
2. Mitchell, S.J.; Madrigal-Matute, J.; Scheibye-Knudsen, M.; Fang, E.; Aon, M.; Gonzalez-Reyes, J.A.; Cortassa, S.; Kaushik, S.; Gonzalez-Freire, M.; Petel, B.; et al. Effects of Sex, Strain, and Energy Intake on Hallmarks of Aging in Mice. *Cell Metab.* **2016**, *23*, 1093–1112. [CrossRef] [PubMed]
3. Balasubramanian, P.; Howell, P.R.; Anderson, R.M. Aging and Caloric Restriction Research: A Biological Perspective with Translational Potential. *EBioMedicine* **2017**, *21*, 37–44. [CrossRef] [PubMed]
4. Brestoff, J.R.; Artis, D. Immune regulation of metabolic homeostasis in health and disease. *Cell* **2015**, *161*, 146–160. [CrossRef] [PubMed]
5. Thomou, T.; Mori, M.A.; Dreyfuss, J.M.; Konishi, M.; Sakaguchi, M.; Wolfrum, C.; Rao, T.N.; Winnay, J.N.; Garcia-Martin, R.; Grinspon, S.K.; et al. Adipose-derived circulating miRNAs regulate gene expression in other tissues. *Nature* **2017**, *542*, 450–455. [CrossRef] [PubMed]
6. Reis, F.C.; Branquinho, J.L.; Brandao, B.B.; Guerra, B.A.; Silva, I.D.; Frontini, A.; Thomou, T.; Sartini, L.; Cinti, S.; Kahan, C.R.; et al. Fat-specific Dicer deficiency accelerates aging and mitigates several effects of dietary restriction in mice. *Aging (Albany NY)* **2016**, *8*, 1201–1222. [CrossRef] [PubMed]
7. Amamou, T.; Normandin, E.; Pouliot, J.; Dionne, I.J.; Brochu, M.; Riesco, E. Effect of a High-Protein Energy-Restricted Diet Combined with Resistance Training on Metabolic Profile in Older Individuals with Metabolic Impairments. *J. Nutr. Health Aging* **2017**, *21*, 67–74. [CrossRef] [PubMed]
8. Giannopoulou, I.; Fernhall, B.; Carhart, R.; Weinstock, R.S.; Baynard, T.; Figueroa, A.; Kanaley, J.A. Effects of diet and/or exercise on the adipocytokine and inflammatory cytokine levels of postmenopausal women with type 2 diabetes. *Metabolism* **2005**, *54*, 866–875. [CrossRef] [PubMed]
9. Madsen, E.L.; Rissanen, A.; Bruun, J.M.; Skogstrand, K.; Tonstad, S.; Hougaard, D.M.; Richelsen, B. Weight loss larger than 10% is needed for general improvement of levels of circulating adiponectin and markers of inflammation in obese subjects: A 3-year weight loss study. *Eur. J. Endocrinol.* **2008**, *158*, 179–187. [CrossRef] [PubMed]
10. Weinheimer, E.M.; Sands, L.P.; Campbell, W.W. A systematic review of the separate and combined effects of energy restriction and exercise on fat-free mass in middle-aged and older adults: Implications for sarcopenic obesity. *Nutr. Rev.* **2010**, *68*, 375–388. [CrossRef] [PubMed]
11. Fielding, R.A.; Vellas, B.; Evans, W.J.; Bhasin, S.; Morley, J.E.; Newman, A.B.; Abellan van Kan, G.; Andrieu, S.; Bauer, J.; Breuille, D.; et al. Sarcopenia: An undiagnosed condition in older adults. Current consensus definition: Prevalence, etiology, and consequences. International working group on sarcopenia. *J. Am. Med. Dir. Assoc.* **2011**, *12*, 249–256. [CrossRef] [PubMed]
12. Cermak, N.M.; Res, P.T.; de Groot, L.C.; Saris, W.H.; van Loon, L.J. Protein supplementation augments the adaptive response of skeletal muscle to resistance-type exercise training: A meta-analysis. *Am. J. Clin. Nutr.* **2012**, *96*, 1454–1464. [CrossRef] [PubMed]
13. Thomas, D.K.; Quinn, M.A.; Saunders, D.H.; Greig, C.A. Protein Supplementation Does Not Significantly Augment the Effects of Resistance Exercise Training in Older Adults: A Systematic Review. *J. Am. Med. Dir. Assoc.* **2016**, *17*, 959.e1–959.e9. [CrossRef] [PubMed]

14. Nicklas, B.J.; Chmelo, E.; Delbono, O.; Carr, J.J.; Lyles, M.F.; Marsh, A.P. Effects of resistance training with and without caloric restriction on physical function and mobility in overweight and obese older adults: A randomized controlled trial. *Am. J. Clin. Nutr.* **2015**, *101*, 991–999. [CrossRef] [PubMed]
15. Senechal, M.; Bouchard, D.R.; Dionne, I.J.; Brochu, M. The effects of lifestyle interventions in dynapenic-obese postmenopausal women. *Menopause* **2012**, *19*, 1015–1021. [CrossRef] [PubMed]
16. Brochu, M.; Malita, M.F.; Messier, V.; Doucet, E.; Strychar, I.; Lavoie, J.M.; Prud'homme, D.; Rabasa-Lhoret, R. Resistance training does not contribute to improving the metabolic profile after a 6-month weight loss program in overweight and obese postmenopausal women. *J. Clin. Endocrinol. Metable* **2009**, *94*, 3226–3233. [CrossRef] [PubMed]
17. Chmelo, E.A.; Beavers, D.P.; Lyles, M.F.; Marsh, A.P.; Nicklas, B.J.; Beavers, K.M. Legacy effects of short-term intentional weight loss on total body and thigh composition in overweight and obese older adults. *Nutr. Diabetes* **2016**, *6*, e203. [CrossRef] [PubMed]
18. Kim, B.; Tsujimoto, T.; So, R.; Tanaka, K. Changes in lower extremity muscle mass and muscle strength after weight loss in obese men: A prospective study. *Obes. Res. Clin. Pract.* **2015**, *9*, 365–373. [CrossRef] [PubMed]
19. Bouchard, D.R.; Soucy, L.; Senechal, M.; Dionne, I.J.; Brochu, M. Impact of resistance training with or without caloric restriction on physical capacity in obese older women. *Menopause* **2009**, *16*, 66–72. [CrossRef]
20. St-Onge, M.; Rabasa-Lhoret, R.; Strychar, I.; Faraj, M.; Doucet, E.; Lavoie, J.M. Impact of energy restriction with or without resistance training on energy metabolism in overweight and obese postmenopausal women: A Montreal Ottawa New Emerging Team group study. *Menopause* **2013**, *20*, 194–201. [CrossRef] [PubMed]
21. Ballor, D.L.; Katch, V.L.; Becque, M.D.; Marks, C.R. Resistance weight training during caloric restriction enhances lean body weight maintenance. *Am. J. Clin. Nutr.* **1988**, *47*, 19–25. [CrossRef] [PubMed]
22. Kordi, R.; Dehghani, S.; Noormohammadpour, P.; Rostami, M.; Mansournia, M.A. Effect of abdominal resistance exercise on abdominal subcutaneous fat of obese women: A randomized controlled trial using ultrasound imaging assessments. *J. Manipul. Physiol. Therap.* **2015**, *38*, 203–209. [CrossRef] [PubMed]
23. Bouchard, C.; An, P.; Rice, T.; Skinner, J.S.; Wilmore, J.H.; Gagnon, J.; Leon, A.S.; Rao, D.C. Familial aggregation of VO(2max) response to exercise training: Results from the HERITAGE Family Study. *J. Appl. Physiol.* **1999**, *87*, 1003–1008. [CrossRef] [PubMed]
24. Dunstan, D.W.; Daly, R.M.; Owen, N.; Jolley, D.; Vulikh, E.; Shaw, J.; Zimmet, P. Home-based resistance training is not sufficient to maintain improved glycemic control following supervised training in older individuals with type 2 diabetes. *Diabetes Care* **2005**, *28*, 3–9. [CrossRef] [PubMed]
25. Dunstan, D.W.; Daly, R.M.; Owen, N.; Jolley, D.; De Courten, M.; Shaw, J.; Zimmet, P. High-intensity resistance training improves glycemic control in older patients with type 2 diabetes. *Diabetes Care* **2002**, *25*, 1729–1736. [CrossRef] [PubMed]
26. Maher, C.G.; Sherrington, C.; Herbert, R.D.; Moseley, A.M.; Elkins, M. Reliability of the PEDro scale for rating quality of randomized controlled trials. *Phys. Ther.* **2003**, *83*, 713–721. [PubMed]
27. Boreinstein, M.; Hedges, L.; Higgins, J.; Rothstein, H.R. *Introduction to Meta-Analysis*; Wiley: Chichester, UK, 2009.
28. Csapo, R.; Alegre, L.M. Effects of resistance training with moderate vs heavy loads on muscle mass and strength in the elderly: A meta-analysis. *Scand. J. Med. Sci. Sports* **2016**, *26*, 995–1006. [CrossRef] [PubMed]
29. Hall, K.S.; Morey, M.C.; Dutta, C.; Manini, T.M.; Weltman, A.L.; Nelson, M.E.; Morgan, A.L.; Senior, J.G.; Seyffarth, C.; Buchner, D.M. Activity-related energy expenditure in older adults: A call for more research. *Med. Sci. Sports Exerc.* **2014**, *46*, 2335–2340. [CrossRef] [PubMed]
30. Donnelly, J.E.; Blair, S.N.; Jakicic, J.M.; Manore, M.M.; Rankin, J.W.; Smith, B.K. American College of Sports Medicine Position Stand. Appropriate physical activity intervention strategies for weight loss and prevention of weight regain for adults. *Med. Sci. Sports Exerc.* **2009**, *41*, 459–471. [CrossRef] [PubMed]
31. Chodzko-Zajko, W.J.; Proctor, D.N.; Fiatarone Singh, M.A.; Minson, C.T.; Nigg, C.R.; Salem, G.J.; Skinner, J.S. American College of Sports Medicine position stand. Exercise and physical activity for older adults. *Med. Sci. Sports Exerc.* **2009**, *41*, 1510–1530. [CrossRef] [PubMed]
32. Lu, Y.; Bradley, J.S.; McCoski, S.R.; Gonzalez, J.M.; Ealy, A.D.; Johnson, S.E. Reduced skeletal muscle fiber size following caloric restriction is associated with calpain-mediated proteolysis and attenuation of IGF-1 signaling. *Am. J. Physiol. Regul. Integr. Comp. Physiol.* **2017**, *312*, R806–R815. [CrossRef] [PubMed]

33. Murphy, C.H.; Churchward-Venne, T.A.; Mitchell, C.J.; Kolar, N.M.; Kassis, A.; Karagounis, L.G.; Burke, L.M.; Hawley, J.A.; Phillips, S.M. Hypoenergetic diet-induced reductions in myofibrillar protein synthesis are restored with resistance training and balanced daily protein ingestion in older men. *Am. J. Physiol. Endocrinol. Metable* **2015**, *308*, E734–E743. [CrossRef] [PubMed]
34. Longland, T.M.; Oikawa, S.Y.; Mitchell, C.J.; Devries, M.C.; Phillips, S.M. Higher compared with lower dietary protein during an energy deficit combined with intense exercise promotes greater lean mass gain and fat mass loss: A randomized trial. *Am. J. Clin. Nutr.* **2016**, *103*, 738–746. [CrossRef] [PubMed]
35. Levine, M.E.; Suarez, J.A.; Brandhorst, S.; Balasubramanian, P.; Cheng, C.W.; Madia, F.; Fontana, L.; Mirisola, M.G.; Guevara-Aguirre, J.; Wan, J.; et al. Low protein intake is associated with a major reduction in IGF-1, cancer, and overall mortality in the 65 and younger but not older population. *Cell Metab.* **2014**, *19*, 407–417. [CrossRef] [PubMed]
36. Solon-Biet, S.M.; Mitchell, S.J.; Coogan, S.C.; Cogger, V.C.; Gokarn, R.; McMahon, A.C.; Raubenheimer, D.; de Cabo, R.; Simpson, S.J.; Le Couteur, D.G. Dietary Protein to Carbohydrate Ratio and Caloric Restriction: Comparing Metabolic Outcomes in Mice. *Cell Rep.* **2015**, *11*, 1529–1534. [CrossRef] [PubMed]
37. Johnson, S.C.; Rabinovitch, P.S.; Kaeberlein, M. mTOR is a key modulator of ageing and age-related disease. *Nature* **2013**, *493*, 338–345. [CrossRef] [PubMed]
38. Barsalani, R.; Brochu, M.; Dionne, I.J. Is there a skeletal muscle mass threshold associated with the deterioration of insulin sensitivity in sedentary lean to obese postmenopausal women? *Diabetes Res. Clin. Pract.* **2013**, *102*, 123–128. [CrossRef] [PubMed]
39. Shiroma, E.J.; Cook, N.R.; Manson, J.E.; Moorthy, M.V.; Buring, J.E.; Rimm, E.B.; Lee, I.M. Strength Training and the Risk of Type 2 Diabetes and Cardiovascular Disease. *Med. Sci. Sports Exerc.* **2017**, *49*, 40–46. [CrossRef] [PubMed]
40. Sylow, L.; Kleinert, M.; Richter, E.A.; Jensen, T.E. Exercise-stimulated glucose uptake-regulation and implications for glycaemic control. *Nat. Rev. Endocrinol.* **2017**, *13*, 133–148. [CrossRef] [PubMed]
41. Pesta, D.H.; Goncalves, R.L.S.; Madiraju, A.K.; Strasser, B.; Sparks, L.M. Resistance training to improve type 2 diabetes: Working toward a prescription for the future. *Nutr. Metab.* **2017**, *14*. [CrossRef] [PubMed]
42. Delmonico, M.J.; Harris, T.B.; Visser, M.; Park, S.W.; Conroy, M.B.; Velasquez-Mieyer, P.; Boudreau, R.; Manini, T.M.; Nevitt, M.; Newman, A.B.; et al. Longitudinal study of muscle strength, quality, and adipose tissue infiltration. *Am. J. Clin. Nutr.* **2009**, *90*, 1579–1585. [CrossRef] [PubMed]
43. Dam, T.T.; Peters, K.W.; Fragala, M.; Cawthon, P.M.; Harris, T.B.; McLean, R.; Shardell, M.; Alley, D.E.; Kenny, A.; Ferrucci, L.; et al. An evidence-based comparison of operational criteria for the presence of sarcopenia. *J. Gerontol. A Biol. Sci. Med. Sci.* **2014**, *69*, 584–590. [CrossRef] [PubMed]
44. Gill, S.; Le, H.D.; Melkani, G.C.; Panda, S. Time-restricted feeding attenuates age-related cardiac decline in Drosophila. *Science* **2015**, *347*, 1265–1269. [CrossRef] [PubMed]
45. Kastman, E.K.; Willette, A.A.; Coe, C.L.; Bendlin, B.B.; Kosmatka, K.J.; McLaren, D.G.; Xu, G.; Canu, E.; Field, A.S.; Alexander, A.L. A calorie-restricted diet decreases brain iron accumulation and preserves motor performance in old rhesus monkeys. *J. Neurosci.* **2010**, *30*, 7940–7947. [CrossRef] [PubMed]
46. Colman, R.J.; Beasley, T.M.; Allison, D.B.; Weindruch, R. Attenuation of sarcopenia by dietary restriction in rhesus monkeys. *J. Gerontol. A Biol. Sci. Med. Sci.* **2008**, *63*, 556–559. [CrossRef] [PubMed]
47. Bodnar, M.; Skalicky, M.; Viidik, A.; Erben, R.G. Interaction between exercise, dietary restriction and age-related bone loss in a rodent model of male senile osteoporosis. *Gerontology* **2012**, *58*, 139–149. [CrossRef] [PubMed]
48. Moreira, L.D.; Oliveira, M.L.; Lirani-Galvao, A.P.; Marin-Mio, R.V.; Santos, R.N.; Lazaretti-Castro, M. Physical exercise and osteoporosis: Effects of different types of exercises on bone and physical function of postmenopausal women. *Arq. Bras. Endocrinol. Metabol.* **2014**, *58*, 514–522. [CrossRef] [PubMed]

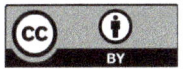

© 2018 by the authors. Licensee MDPI, Basel, Switzerland. This article is an open access article distributed under the terms and conditions of the Creative Commons Attribution (CC BY) license (http://creativecommons.org/licenses/by/4.0/).

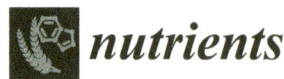

Review

Dietary Protein and Muscle in Aging People: The Potential Role of the Gut Microbiome

Mary Ni Lochlainn [1,2,*], Ruth C. E. Bowyer [1] and Claire J. Steves [1,2]

1. The Department of Twin Research, Kings College London, 3-4th Floor South Wing Block D, St Thomas' Hospital, Westminster Bridge Road, London SE1 7EH, UK; ruth.c.bowyer@kcl.ac.uk (R.C.E.B.); claire.j.steves@kcl.ac.uk (C.J.S.)
2. Clinical Age Research Unit, Kings College Hospital Foundation Trust, London SE5 9RS, UK
* Correspondence: marynilochlainn@gmail.com

Received: 8 June 2018; Accepted: 18 July 2018; Published: 20 July 2018

Abstract: Muscle mass, strength, and physical function are known to decline with age. This is associated with the development of geriatric syndromes including sarcopenia and frailty. Dietary protein is essential for skeletal muscle function. Resistance exercise appears to be the most beneficial form of physical activity for preserving skeletal muscle and a synergistic effect has been noted when this is combined with dietary protein. However, older adults have shown evidence of anabolic resistance, where greater amounts of protein are required to stimulate muscle protein synthesis, and response is variable. Thus, the recommended daily amount of protein is greater for older people. The aetiologies and mechanisms responsible for anabolic resistance are not fully understood. The gut microbiota is implicated in many of the postulated mechanisms for anabolic resistance, either directly or indirectly. The gut microbiota change with age, and are influenced by dietary protein. Research also implies a role for the gut microbiome in skeletal muscle function. This leads to the hypothesis that the gut microbiome might modulate individual response to protein in the diet. We summarise the existing evidence for the role of the gut microbiota in anabolic resistance and skeletal muscle in aging people, and introduce the metabolome as a tool to probe this relationship in the future.

Keywords: protein; skeletal muscle; sarcopenia; gut microbiome; metabolome; diet; supplementation

1. Introduction

Skeletal muscle has several important functions beyond locomotion, including insulin-stimulated glucose uptake, influence on bone density via mechanical force on bones, and whole-body protein metabolism [1]. Age associated loss of muscle mass starts as early as age thirty, and is a gradual process [1]. Older people lose more skeletal muscle with bedrest and show an attenuated response to retraining after immobilisation, in comparison to younger individuals [2–4]. Sarcopenia is a geriatric syndrome defined as the age-related loss of skeletal mass and function, quantified by objective measures of muscle mass, strength, and physical function [5]. One major risk factor for the development of sarcopenia is protein-energy malnutrition [6]. A number of factors can lead to reduced protein intake in older age, as summarised in Figure 1 [7–18]. Patients with sarcopenia are often frail (vulnerable to minor stressors) and the two concepts (frailty and sarcopenia) share an increased risk of adverse outcomes [19]. As life expectancy worldwide has more than doubled over the past two centuries, the importance of understanding and optimising muscle function in older age is paramount.

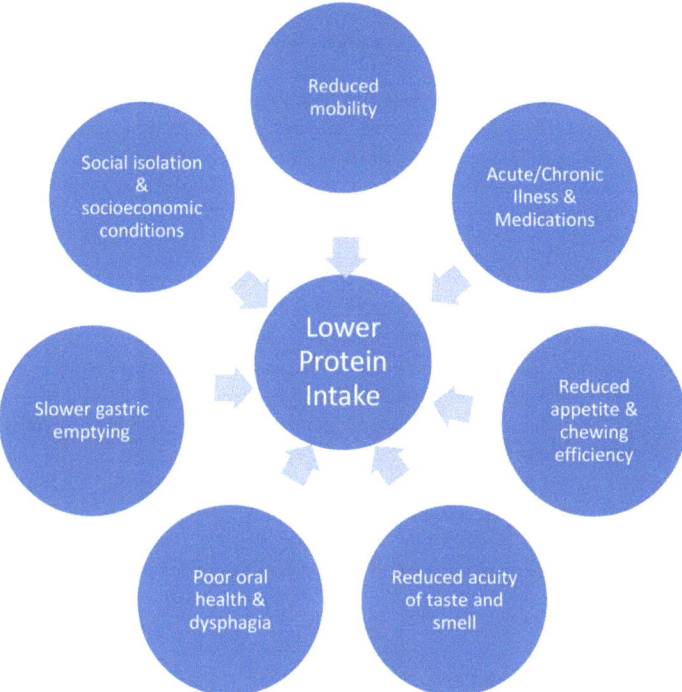

Figure 1. Factors leading to lower protein intake in older adults.

Three large observational studies have supported an association between protein intake and muscle strength and mass [20–22], but multiple trials carried out in healthy, replete, older adults, without an exercise intervention, have been negative [23–25]. In those with suboptimal protein intake, the most promising results are for specific essential amino acids, particularly leucine, but also its metabolite β-hydroxy β-methylbutyric acid (HMB) [25–29]. Supplementation with these more targeted regulators of muscle protein synthesis (MPS) may be most effective for overcoming anabolic resistance in this cohort, especially if combined with exercise, a potent stimulator of anabolic response in muscle at all ages [28,30–32]. Anabolic resistance refers to the phenomenon whereby older adults require a higher dose of protein to achieve the same response in MPS as a younger adult [1]. The aetiologies and mechanisms for this are not understood, but we propose that the gut microbiome may be implicated in one or many of those suggested in the literature.

The gut microbiome is composed of bacteria, archaea, viruses, and eukaryotic microbes that reside in the gut. Its role in maintaining a healthy physiology and contributing to disease is a rapidly evolving field of enquiry. The gut microbiome has a collective genome size that may be as much as 150-fold that of the human host [33], and it has been argued that the metabolic capacity of microbiota merits its consideration as an organ of the human body in its own right, with its own intrinsic functions and metabolic needs [34]. With age and frailty in particular, the resilience of the gut microbiome is reduced, as it becomes more vulnerable to medications, disease, and changes in lifestyle, with changed species richness and increased inter-individual variability [35–37]. The potential of the gut microbiota to alter physiology has been shown by landmark animal studies assessing faecal transplant, which have demonstrated body composition changes in the recipient reflective of the phenotype of the donor [38]. This highlights the role of microbiota in characterising metabolic phenotypes, which we are only now beginning to understand.

Ageing is associated with chronic inflammation [39], often referred to as 'inflammaging'. Here we suggest that this 'inflammaging', in combination with altered gut microbiome composition and/or diversity [40], leads to changes in protein metabolism, absorption and availability; ultimately contributing to anabolic resistance and therefore to reduced MPS and the development of sarcopenia. Proposed interventions such as protein supplementation, probiotics or faecal transplants should address this rationale. This review summarises the available literature on anabolic resistance in older adults, with a particular focus on the role of the gut microbiome and its metabolome.

2. Anabolic Resistance

Skeletal muscle mass is regulated by the processes of muscle protein synthesis and breakdown (MPS and MPB). MPS rates are largely controlled by responsiveness to anabolic stimuli, such as consumption of food, and physical activity. Catabolic stressors include illness, physical inactivity, and inflammation, of which the older population tend to have higher rates (Figure 2). Ageing does not seem to influence MPB to the same degree as MPS, and so much of the focus of the aging literature is on MPS [27,41–43]. Older adults have shown evidence of 'anabolic resistance', whereby a higher dose of protein is required to achieve the same MPS response as a younger person [1,28,39,40,44]. While this concept has been questioned, especially in the context of healthy older adults [45], it is now considered consensus that a higher recommended daily amount of 1–1.3 g/kg/day should be consumed by older people to offset catabolic conditions [1,46–49]. In the context of illness or injury, older adults may require as much as 2 g/kg/day, as recommended by the PROT-AGE Study Group [50].

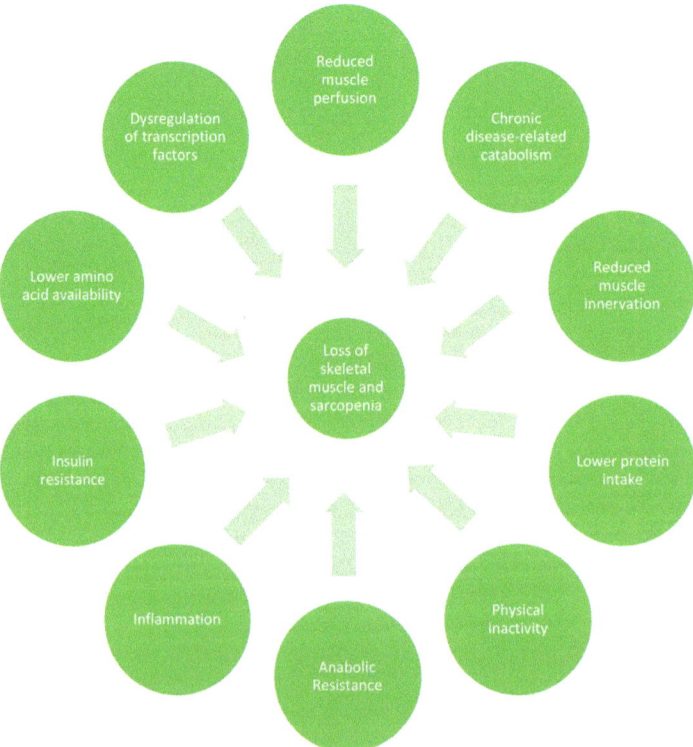

Figure 2. Factors leading to loss of skeletal muscle and sarcopenia in older adults.

The aetiology of anabolic resistance is complex, involving aging physiology, accumulation of chronic disease, and changes in physical inactivity (see Table 1). The multiple mechanisms postulated involve impairments at most levels of protein metabolism (see Table 2). There may also be sex-differences in anabolic resistance [51–54], which has received little attention in the literature.

Table 1. Factors influencing anabolic resistance.

Anabolic Resistance Aetiology	References
Declining activity levels	[1,6,55–57]
Protracted disuse events	[6,58–61]
Chronic inflammation	[31,41,56,62,63]
Insulin resistance	[1,27,41,62,64,65]
Higher circulating oxidative and inflammatory stressors	[1,27,56]
Obesity	[62,66]
Reduced oestrogen/testosterone	[1,67]
Increased production of catabolic hormones such as cortisol	[27]
Alcohol	[68]
Smoking	[1]
Poor vitamin D status	[56]
Reduced food intake	[56]
Metabolic acidosis	[1]
More chronic & acute disease in older adults (increased catabolic conditions)	[50]

Table 2. Molecular mechanisms implicated in anabolic resistance.

Anabolic Resistance Mechanisms	References
Differences in gene expression of proteins involved in MPS	[69–73]
Dysregulation of key signalling proteins in the mTOR pathway	[1,41,70,71,74,75]
Decreased phosphorylation of mTORC1	[41,74,76–79]
Impaired transport of amino acids into muscle/peripheral tissues	[56,75,80,81]
Diminished mRNA translational signalling	[74,78,82,83]
Inflammation (raised TNFα/IL-6/hs-CRP/NFkB)	[1,41,74,84,85]
Decreased phosphorylation of transcription factors (e.g., p70S6K, S6K1)	[41,74,75,82]
Dysregulation of nutritive blood flow to skeletal muscle	[56,65,86]
Attenuated protein digestion & absorption	[56,87–89]
Mitochondrial dysfunction	[1,35,72]
Autophagy/mitophagy dysfunction	[1,72]
Denervation of muscle fibres	[56,90]
Higher splanchnic extraction of protein	[50,88]
Lipid-induced muscle insulin resistance	[35,91]
Increased AMPKα phosphorylation (leads to increased MPB)	[70]
Increased cortisol generation within muscle by 11bHSD1	[92]
Loss of skeletal muscle stem cells	[93]

3. The Role of the Gut Microbiome

The composition of the human gut microbiome is dependent on, amongst other things, age, diet, health, and geographical location, with significant individual variability [94,95]. It is dynamic across the lifespan, changing rapidly between birth and early childhood, and then becoming more stable [36]. In older life, however, research shows that the propensity for compositional change accelerates once again [36,96,97]. Multiple cross-sectional studies have found associations between gut microbiome composition and frailty [98–100], while the ELDERMET study showed significant loss of diversity amongst people in a care-home setting versus community dwellers [95]. Among older hospitalised patients, polypharmacy has been associated with gut microbiota dysbiosis [99]. It is well established that antibiotics cause significant changes in microbiota composition [101], and older adults tend to have more frequent antibiotic therapy.

Age-related chronic inflammation ('inflammaging'), is implicated in the development of sarcopenia [102,103]. Changes in the gut microbiota have been suggested to contribute to inflammaging [37,103–105]. A recent animal study showed that transferring gut microbes of young killifish to older ones ameliorates ageing conditions, and extends the lifespan of the older fish [106]. Notably, the transplanted older fish also displayed increased 'spontaneous exploratory behaviour' [106], essentially physical activity. Few studies to date have had the ability to delve into the operational capacity and functional readout of the gut microbiome in relation to aging, but this is likely to shed more light on possible mechanisms of the interaction between dietary intake and host utilisation of protein in skeletal muscle.

3.1. Gut Microbiota and Skeletal Muscle

The influence of the gut microbiome in metabolic health has been one of the primary focuses of research in this area thus far, particularly in the context of obesity and insulin resistance [107]. Studies have used faecal transplants in germ-free mice to demonstrate changes in body fat, insulin resistance and glucose tolerance [108], highlighting the key role of the microbiome in these metabolic pathways. Considering the role of skeletal muscle in glucose metabolism, animal studies have investigated the relationship between gut microbiota and skeletal muscle metabolism. For example, skeletal muscle from colonised versus germ free mice appears to have altered metabolic efficiency, with higher levels of the enzyme adenosine monophosphate (AMP)-activated protein kinase, a central regulator of metabolism at both a cellular and organismal level, found in the skeletal muscle of germ-free mice [109]. CD-14 mutant mice, who lack an endotoxin receptor on their innate immune cells, have increased levels of circulating lipopolysaccharide (LPS), and this LPS was found to induce skeletal muscle inflammation, as well as insulin resistance [36]. This is important because the healthy gut microbiome is considered to contribute to gut barrier function (Section 3.3 below), providing gut enterocytes with essential nutrition [110] and reducing LPS levels in the blood. Lastly, Yan et al. (2016) carried out a study in which gut microbiota was transferred from obese pigs to germ free mice [111]. Fibre characteristics and the metabolic profile of the skeletal muscle were replicated in the recipients [111], again implicating the gut microbiome in skeletal muscle composition and metabolism. Some of the fibre changes noted were similar to those seen in aging skeletal muscle (e.g., increased proportion of slower contracting fibres). This raises the possibility that faecal microbial transplantation could be used as a means to transmit muscle fibre characteristics between humans, perhaps even from young to old, as a means of improving skeletal muscle function.

Gut microbiota modulation in animal models has also produced preliminary supportive data for effect on skeletal muscle. This includes lower intestinal permeability and lower plasma LPS and cytokines noted in prebiotic-treated mice [112], reduced expression of muscle atrophy markers in mice models of leukaemia supplemented with a *Lactobacillus* species [113], and increased muscle mass and function (measured by grip strength and swim time) in healthy mice supplemented with *L. plantarum* [114]. These studies and others [115,116], suggest that targeting the gut microbiota may be used as a tool to modulate muscle mass.

In terms of human data, two probiotic trials have shown improvements in athletic performance amongst elite athletes. A small, four week trial of probiotic capsules in male runners reported increased run time to fatigue in the probiotic group [117], while a trial of probiotic yoghurt in teenage female endurance swimmers reported improved aerobic performance, measured by maximal oxygen consumption (VO2 max) [118]. Dietary standardisation was carried out in the male runner study, however in the swimmer study participants continued their regular diet which may have confounded results. These studies build on evidence from observational studies for an association between exercise and gut microbiota [119–124]. Clark et al. (2014) compared the gut microbial diversity of professional male athletes to healthy controls and reported significantly higher diversity amongst the athletes [125]. Furthermore, moderate exercise has been shown to increase intestinal mobility [126], which is known to affect gut microbiota [127,128]. These changes in gut health with exercise implicate skeletal muscle as a potential regulator of gut microbiota composition and suggest a bi-directional relationship between skeletal muscle and the gut microbiome.

Amongst older adults, a single randomised controlled trial has explored the effect of modulating the gut microbiota on muscle function and frailty. Here, 60 older adults received a prebiotic (F-GOS) or placebo for 13 weeks. While the study remains to be replicated, promisingly, both exhaustion and handgrip strength were significantly improved in the treatment arm [129], highlighting the potential role for the gut microbiome in future interventions. The science of pre- and probiotic use is in its infancy, as are studies of faecal transplantation, with much scope for further investigation of these therapeutic options.

3.2. Gut Microbiota and Dietary Protein

The digestive system consists of a complex interaction between digestive secretions, intestinal conditions, and the gut microbiome. Nutrients, especially dietary proteins, provide energy sources for the host, as well as substrates for the gut microbiota [130]. A significant proportion of undigested peptides and proteins can reach the colon, and this is increased in the context of a high protein diet [131]. Consumption of proteins with high digestibility, or a low protein diet, results in less protein reaching the colon, limiting the amount available for protein-fermenting bacteria [130]. Furthermore, changes in the gut microbiota can impact the bioavailability of dietary amino acids [104,132].

Studies carried out in mice, rats, and hamsters have shown higher microbial diversity in those fed soy protein versus animal protein [133,134] and increased abundance of *Bacteroidales* family S24-7 in those fed soy protein versus other diets [79]. Li et al. (2017) assessed high protein, low carbohydrate diets in dogs and found decreased *Bacteroidetes* to *Firmicutes* ratio, increased *Bacteroides* to *Prevotella* ratio and increased abundance of *Clostridium hiranonis*, *Clostridium perfringens*, and *Ruminococcus gnavus*, the latter of which has been proposed to have beneficial effects in the human gut [135].

It has been reported that protein consumption is correlated positively with gut microbiota diversity [136]. This is based on studies carried out on healthy volunteers [137], elite athletes [125], and obese/overweight individuals [138]. The source of protein appears influential, with plant protein associated with more *Bifidofacterium*, *Lactobacillus*, *Roseburia*, *Eubacterium rectale*, and *Ruminococcus bromii*; and less *Bacteroides* and *Clostridium perfringens* [136,137]. Meanwhile animal protein was associated with higher levels of *Bacteroides*, *Alistipes*, *Bilophila* and *Ruminococcus*, and lower levels of *Bifidobacterium* [136,137]. High levels of *Bacteroides* have also been reported with Western diets, which are high in protein and animal fat [33], although it has been suggested that differences in fat content, rather than protein, is the major influencing factor here [139]. Significant associations have been reported between increased levels of faecal short chain fatty acids (SCFAs), *Prevotella* and some *Firmicutes*, with consumption of a Mediterranean diet [35,140], which is typically lower in protein than animal-based diets, although may contain high levels of plant-source protein. Dietary fibre is an important factor in gut microbiome diversity and composition and it is important to note that most plant sources of protein are also high in fibre, whereas animal source protein are not. This is likely to be an influential factor in the findings of these studies.

The gut microbiomes of critically ill patients on average display enrichment of virulent pathogens, and loss of health-promoting microbes [141]. Protein supplementation has shown some benefits for muscle parameters in this population [142,143], but whether this effect is modulated by the gut microbiome remains to be tested. Evidently dietary protein has a significant effect on gut microbiota composition and vice versa, however more research is needed to further characterise this relationship. It is notable that almost exclusively, studies to date have focused on composition of the microbiota rather than functional capacity of the microbiome. Investigation into the differences in microbial genes involved in protein metabolism between individuals differing in anabolic response to protein could lead to the engineering of new probiotics with specific capacity to influence MPS.

3.3. Gut Microbiota and Anabolic Resistance

A healthy gut microbiome plays a role in many of the physiological processes implicated in the various mechanisms proposed for the development of anabolic resistance (see Table 2 and Figure 3). These include suppression of chronic inflammation, prevention of insulin resistance, modulation of host gene expression, enhancement of antioxidant activity, and maintenance of gut barrier function [35,104].

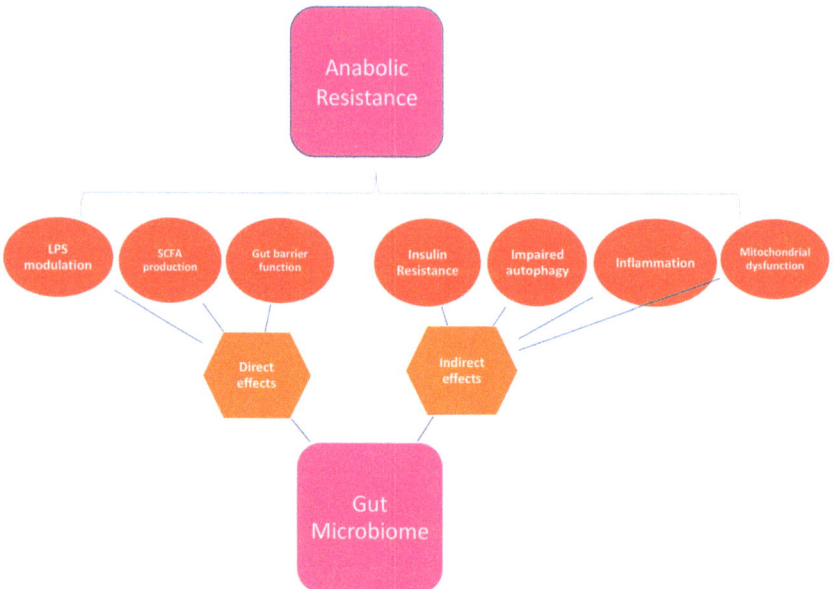

Figure 3. Mechanisms by which the gut microbiome may influence anabolic resistance. LPS: Lipopolysaccharide; SCFA: Short chain fatty acids.

Inflammation has been proposed as a contributing factor to anabolic resistance in aging, and indeed inflammaging has been suggested as a major aetiological factor in the development of sarcopenia. Biagi et al. (2010) studied age-related differences in both the gut microbiota and the inflammatory status among different stages of the whole adult life, including centenarians, and reported dysbiosis in the older population, which correlated with increased inflammatory status, as determined by peripheral blood inflammatory markers [37].

Work in animal models has shown evidence of increased intestinal permeability in association with age-associated microbial dysbiosis [36,104,144]. This can facilitate translocation of microbial byproducts into the circulation, including endotoxins, and may influence a number of the mechanisms listed in Table 2, such as protein digestion and absorption. It has been suggested that pathogenic drivers of inflammation and muscle atrophy may enter the system via this process [132]. Within humans, a randomised controlled trial of probiotic use in athletic men reported reduced zonulin in faeces, a surrogate marker of enhanced gut permeability [145], suggesting that modulation of the gut microbiota can affect the gut's barrier function.

Older adults tend to have reduced intestinal motility, which may unfavourably affect the utilisation of dietary protein by the gut [104]. Indeed it has been reported that the proteolytic potential of the gut microbiota appeared to be enhanced in older age [146], and may therefore contribute to anabolic resistance to ingested protein. There is also some evidence that probiotics may improve amino acid absorption from protein [147,148], which adds weight to the suggestion that targeting the gut microbiota may ameliorate anabolic resistance in older adults. Production of SCFAs by the gut microbiota has been associated with anabolism itself [110] and depletion of taxa producing SCFAs may promote anabolic resistance [149]. Of note, an age-related reduction of the abundance of genes in pathways that are involved in SCFA production has been reported [146]. SCFAs are mainly produced by the fermentation of dietary fibre, so the fibre content of dietary protein sources is likely too, to influence protein metabolism.

Treatment with butyrate (a SCFA), which is associated with *Bifidobacterium*, was found to be protective of muscle atrophy in mice [116]. Notably, studies showing correlation between frailty and gut microbiota composition have also reported dysbiotic shifts in higher functioning older adults towards a greater abundance of butyrate-producing bacteria such as *Faecalibacterium prausnitzii* [95,150], which suggests these microbes may have a positive role in protection against muscle loss and frailty. Butyrate also has a role in intestinal barrier function [151], and therefore may be implicated in intestinal permeability. Notably, a randomised controlled trial of symbiotic (a combination of pre- and probiotic) use in older people noted an increase in butyrate production in those given the synbiotic [152].

Mitochondrial dysfunction and impaired autophagy have both been suggested as possible mechanisms for anabolic resistance (see Table 2). Interestingly, they have also been implicated in animal models of aging [153] and in the development of sarcopenia and cachexia [154,155]. A recent paper has postulated that dysfunctional mitochondria may represent a key link between chronic inflammation and age-related muscle loss, and that dysbiosis of the gut microbiota may be a key mediator in this gut-muscle crosstalk [104].

Evidently, there are multiple mechanisms by which the gut microbiome may influence anabolic resistance in older adults (see Figure 3), and it is likely to be a complex interaction between a number of, if not all, of these postulated processes. The hypothesis that the dysbiotic gut plays a role in the loss of skeletal muscle and response to protein is yet to be tested. If supported, the gut microbiota could represent a target for interventions aiming to overcome anabolic resistance, to maintain muscle mass and strength in older adults, with the aim of ultimately preventing the development of sarcopenia and/or frailty.

3.4. The Metabolome

Studies use multiple ways of estimating dietary protein intake. The validity and reliability of these dietary measures has usually been verified in younger populations and may not be relevant to older people. Indeed reduced reliability coefficients of the Food Frequency Questionnaire have been reported with increasing age [156]. In order to overcome this, researchers have sought objective estimates of dietary intakes. Protein is the major nitrogen-containing substance in the body, and therefore urinary excretion of nitrogen is used as a marker of protein loss [23,40]. Urinary [31,131] and blood urea concentration [131], and urinary HMB levels [157] have also been used with the aim of objectively verifying compliance. These methods are not without limitations, as they may not consider subtle changes with protein metabolism that occur with age, such as increased splanchnic uptake [50]. The amount of fermentation metabolites detectable in the urine depends on the digestibility of the protein [130], so this too needs to be considered. Another way to study gut microbiota composition is altered fermentation products. Promisingly, the faecal metabolome has been shown to be largely reflective of gut microbial composition [158]. Trials using ^{1}H-nuclear magnetic resonance (NMR) technology have shown a shift in bacterial metabolism with different metabolite profiles according to the source of protein [131]. A growing number of studies are using ^{1}H-NMR technology to assess faecal, urinary, and plasma metabolomes as measures of metabolic health (e.g., [159]). More research is needed into the use of the metabolome in the context of dietary protein intake, and the significance of metabolome changes for skeletal muscle mass and function.

4. Discussion

As the world's population ages, it has become imperative to gain more understanding of the aging process. Declines in muscle mass and function with age have significant associated morbidity and mortality, and the prevalence of both sarcopenia and frailty is increasing. The care of older people is complex, and a multitude of factors influence lower protein intake and loss of skeletal muscle with age (see Figure 1). Studies show that supplementing protein, particularly in combination with resistance exercise, is beneficial for aging muscle. However, trials have had conflicting results. Perhaps a more personalised approach is warranted? Attempting to answer this question is a large randomised controlled trial, currently being carried out, on personalised dietary recommendations as part of a multi-component intervention in the management of sarcopenia [160].

Anabolic resistance is likely to result from cumulative declines across multiple physiological systems, with effects on both MPS and MPB, a dynamic interaction of multiple factors (see Figure 2). Current thinking must not be limited to one or two mechanisms but focus on anabolic resistance as a complex and multidimensional construct. The aetiologies and mechanisms involved are not understood and may be different for each aging individual, again suggesting a potential need for personalised medicine within this population to guide future interventions. The potential role of the gut microbiota in a substantial number of postulated mechanisms for anabolic resistance warrants further investigation (Figure 3). Targeting the gut microbiota to overcome anabolic resistance holds promise in maximising responses in participants who can undertake exercise programs, but where resources and time limit such programs. Moreover, the potential ability to influence skeletal muscle function via gut microbiota in the context of those who cannot feasibly carry out vigorous exercise programs is also an attractive idea.

Few human studies have evaluated the effects of the gut microbiome on dietary protein metabolism, and the ensuing metabolome or vice versa. Studies addressing the role of the gut microbiota in skeletal muscle function are also limited in number. Animal studies have shown promise, and one human trial in older adults showed positive improvements in muscle function with prebiotic gut microbiome modulation [129]. Furthermore, in light of difficulties in accurately capturing an individual's dietary intake from questionnaire data [161], the use of the metabolome may represent an objective and reliable way of assessing compliance with dietary interventions going forward [162], and provide a functional readout for the gut microbiome.

To date there is some supporting evidence for a hypothesis that the gut microbiome may influence the health of skeletal muscle and vice versa [35,36,104], however this remains to be formally tested. In particular, processes such as muscle metabolism and inflammation may be susceptible to modulation. Research is needed to establish whether deleterious changes in the gut microbiome contribute to skeletal muscle loss in the context of acute or chronic illness, or changes detected in apparently healthy aging. The plasticity and diversity of the gut microbiome and its metabolome, represent exciting prospects to individualise the response of skeletal muscle in older adults to dietary protein.

Author Contributions: M.N.L. and C.J.S. conceived the idea for the manuscript. M.N.L. undertook the majority of the drafting of the manuscript, under the supervision of C.J.S., R.C.E.B. assisted in the drafting and critique of the work.

Funding: This research was funded by the Chronic Disease Research Foundation grant number [WT081878MA].

Acknowledgments: M.N.L. is an Academic Clinical Fellow in Geriatric Medicine, this fellowship is funded by the National Institute of Health Research (NIHR). TwinsUK is funded by the Wellcome Trust, Medical Research Council, European Union, the NIHR-funded BioResource, Clinical Research Facility and Biomedical Research Centre based at Guy's and St Thomas' NHS Foundation Trust in partnership with King's College London. C.J.S. acknowledges funding from the Chronic Disease Research Foundation (which receives funding from The Denise Coates Foundation), the Wellcome Trust (grant WT081878MA) and the Medical Research Council (grant MR/N01183X/1).

Conflicts of Interest: The authors declare no conflict of interest.

References

1. Welch, A.A. Nutritional influences on age-related skeletal muscle loss. *Proc. Nutr. Soc.* **2014**, *73*, 16–33. [CrossRef] [PubMed]
2. Suetta, C.; Hvid, L.G.; Justesen, L.; Christensen, U.; Neergaard, K.; Simonsen, L.; Ortenblad, N.; Magnusson, S.P.; Kjaer, M.; Aagaard, P. Effects of aging on human skeletal muscle after immobilization and retraining. *J. Appl. Physiol.* **2009**, *107*, 1172–1180. [CrossRef] [PubMed]
3. Rejc, E.; Floreani, M.; Taboga, P.; Botter, A.; Toniolo, L.; Cancellara, L.; Narici, M.; Šimunič, B.; Pišot, R.; Biolo, G.; et al. Loss of maximal explosive power of lower limbs after 2 weeks of disuse and incomplete recovery after retraining in older adults. *J. Physiol.* **2018**, *596*, 647–665. [CrossRef] [PubMed]
4. Kortebein, P.; Ferrando, A.; Lombeida, J.; Wolfe, R.; Evans, W.J. Effect of 10 Days of Bed Rest on Skeletal Muscle in Healthy Older Adults. *JAMA* **2007**, *297*, 1769. [CrossRef] [PubMed]
5. Fielding, R.A.; Vellas, B.; Evans, W.J.; Bhasin, S.; Morley, J.E.; Newman, A.B.; van Kan, G.A.; Andrieu, S.; Bauer, J.; Breuille, D.; et al. Sarcopenia: An undiagnosed condition in older adults. Consensus Definition: Prevalence, Etiology, and Consequences. *J. Am. Med. Dir. Assoc.* **2011**, *12*, 249–256. [CrossRef] [PubMed]
6. Landi, F.; Calvani, R.; Tosato, M.; Martone, A.M.; Ortolani, E.; Savera, G.; D'Angelo, E.; Sisto, A.; Marzetti, E. Protein intake and muscle health in old age: From biological plausibility to clinical evidence. *Nutrients* **2016**, *8*, 295. [CrossRef] [PubMed]
7. Pilgrim, A.; Robinson, S.; Sayer, A.A.; Roberts, H. An overview of appetite decline in older people. *Nurs. Older People* **2015**, *27*, 29–35. [CrossRef] [PubMed]
8. Whitelock, E.; Ensaff, H. On Your Own: Older Adults' Food Choice and Dietary Habits. *Nutrients* **2018**, *10*. [CrossRef] [PubMed]
9. Parry, S.W.; Finch, T.; Deary, V. How should we manage fear of falling in older adults living in the community? *BMJ* **2013**, *346*, f2933. [CrossRef] [PubMed]
10. Evans, J.R.; Fletcher, A.E.; Wormald, R.P.L.; Ng, E.S.-W.; Stirling, S.; Smeeth, L.; Breeze, E.; Bulpitt, C.J.; Nunes, M.; Jones, D.; et al. Prevalence of visual impairment in people aged 75 years and older in Britain: Results from the MRC trial of assessment and management of older people in the community. *Br. J. Ophthalmol.* **2002**, *86*, 795–800. [CrossRef] [PubMed]
11. Kremer, S.; Bult, J.H.F.; Mojet, J.; Kroeze, J.H.A. Food Perception with Age and Its Relationship to Pleasantness. *Chem. Senses* **2007**, *32*, 591–602. [CrossRef] [PubMed]
12. Malagelada, J.; Bazzoli, F.; Boeckxstaens, G.; De Loose, D.; Fried, M.; Kahrilas, P.; Lindberg, G.; Maltertheiner, P.; Salis, G.; Sharma, P.; et al. World Gastroenterology Organisation Global Guidelines: Dysphagia. *J. Clin. Gastroenterol.* **2014**, *49*, 370–378. [CrossRef] [PubMed]
13. Sura, L.; Madhavan, A.; Carnaby, G.; Crary, M.A. Dysphagia in the elderly: Management and nutritional considerations. *Clin. Interv. Aging* **2012**, *7*, 287–298. [CrossRef] [PubMed]
14. Delaney, M.; McCarthy, M. Food Choice and Health across the Life Course: A Qualitative Study Examining Food Choice in Older Irish Adults. *J. Food Prod. Mark.* **2011**, *17*, 114–140. [CrossRef]
15. Age UK Later Life in the United Kingdom. 2018. Available online: https://www.ageuk.org.uk/globalassets/age-uk/documents/reports-and-publications/later_life_uk_factsheet.pdf (accessed on 2 June 2018).
16. Barnett, A.M.; Roy, N.C.; McNabb, W.C.; Cookson, A.L. The interactions between endogenous bacteria, dietary components and the mucus layer of the large bowel. *Food Funct.* **2012**, *3*, 690. [CrossRef] [PubMed]
17. Payne, R.A.; Avery, A.J.; Duerden, M.; Saunders, C.L.; Simpson, C.R.; Abel, G.A. Prevalence of polypharmacy in a Scottish primary care population. *Eur. J. Clin. Pharmacol.* **2014**, *70*, 575–581. [CrossRef] [PubMed]
18. Kamphuis, C.B.; de Bekker-Grob, E.W.; van Lenthe, F.J. Factors affecting food choices of older adults from high and low socioeconomic groups: A discrete choice experiment. *Am. J. Clin. Nutr.* **2015**, *101*, 768–774. [CrossRef] [PubMed]
19. Clegg, A.; Young, J.; Iliffe, S.; Rikkert, M.O.; Rockwood, K. Frailty in elderly people. *Lancet* **2013**, *381*, 752–762. [CrossRef]
20. Houston, D.K.; Nicklas, B.J.; Ding, J.; Harris, T.B.; Tylavsky, F.A.; Newman, A.B.; Lee, J.S.; Sahyoun, N.R.; Visser, M.; Kritchevsky, S.B. Dietary protein intake is associated with lean mass change in older, community-dwelling adults: The Health, Aging, and Body Composition (Health ABC) Study. *Am. J. Clin. Nutr.* **2008**, *87*, 150–155. [CrossRef] [PubMed]

21. Isanejad, M.; Mursu, J.; Sirola, J.; Kröger, H.; Rikkonen, T.; Tuppurainen, M.; Erkkilä, A.T. Dietary protein intake is associated with better physical function and muscle strength among elderly women. *Br. J. Nutr.* **2016**, *115*, 1281–1291. [CrossRef] [PubMed]
22. Landi, F.; Calvani, R.; Tosato, M.; Martone, A.M.; Picca, A.; Ortolani, E.; Savera, G.; Salini, S.; Ramaschi, M.; Bernabei, R.; et al. Animal-derived protein consumption is associated with muscle mass and strength in community-dwellers: Results from the Milan EXPO Survey. *J. Nutr. Health Aging* **2017**, *21*, 1050–1056. [CrossRef] [PubMed]
23. Zhu, K.; Kerr, D.A.; Meng, X.; Devine, A.; Solah, V.; Binns, C.W.; Prince, R.L. Two-Year Whey Protein Supplementation Did Not Enhance Muscle Mass and Physical Function in Well-Nourished Healthy Older Postmenopausal Women. *J. Nutr.* **2015**, *145*, 2520–2526. [CrossRef] [PubMed]
24. Tieland, M.; Franssen, R.; Dullemeijer, C.; van Dronkelaar, C.; Kim, H.K.; Ispoglou, T.; Zhu, K.; Prince, R.L.; van Loon, L.J.C.; de Groot, L.C.P.G.M. The impact of dietary protein or amino acid supplementation on muscle mass and strength in elderly people: Individual participant data and meta-analysis of RCT's. *J. Nutr. Health Aging* **2017**, *21*, 994–1001. [CrossRef] [PubMed]
25. Beaudart, C.; Rabenda, V.; Simmons, M.; Geerinck, A.; Araujo de Carvalho, I.; Reginster, J.-Y.; Amuthavalli Thiyagarajan, J.; Bruyère, O. Effects of protein, essential amino acids, B-hydroxy B-methylbutyrate, creatine, dehydroepiandrosterone and fatty acid supplementation on muscle mass, muscle strength and physical performance in older people aged 60 years and over. A systematic review of the literature. *J. Nutr. Health Aging* **2017**, 1–14. [CrossRef]
26. Cruz-Jentoft, A.J.; Landi, F.; Schneider, S.M.; Zúñiga, C.; Arai, H.; Boirie, Y.; Chen, L.K.; Fielding, R.A.; Martin, F.C.; Michel, J.; et al. Prevalence of and interventions for sarcopenia in ageing adults: A systematic review. Report of the International Sarcopenia Initiative (EWGSOP and IWGS). *Age Ageing* **2014**, *43*, 748–759. [CrossRef] [PubMed]
27. Cholewa, J.M.; Dardevet, D.; Lima-Soares, F.; de Araújo Pessôa, K.; Oliveira, P.H.; dos Santos Pinho, J.R.; Nicastro, H.; Xia, Z.; Cabido, C.E.T.; Zanchi, N.E. Dietary proteins and amino acids in the control of the muscle mass during immobilization and aging: Role of the MPS response. *Amino Acids* **2017**, *49*, 811–820. [CrossRef] [PubMed]
28. Deutz, N.E.P.; Bauer, J.M.; Barazzoni, R.; Biolo, G.; Boirie, Y.; Bosy-Westphal, A.; Cederholm, T.; Cruz-Jentoft, A.J.; Krznaric, Z.; Sreekumaran Nair, K.; et al. Protein intake and exercise for optimal muscle function with aging: Recommendations from the ESPEN Expert Group. *Clin. Nutr.* **2014**, *33*, 929–936. [CrossRef] [PubMed]
29. Murphy, C.H.; Saddler, N.I.; Devries, M.C.; McGlory, C.; Baker, S.K.; Phillips, S.M. Leucine supplementation enhances integrative myofibrillar protein synthesis in free-living older men consuming lower- and higher-protein diets: A parallel-group crossover study. *Am. J. Clin. Nutr.* **2016**, *104*, 1594–1606. [CrossRef] [PubMed]
30. Daly, R.; Formica, M.B.; Gianoudis, J.; Ellis, K.; O'Connell, S. Does lean red meat enhance the effetcs of exercise on muscle health and function in the elderly? *Innov. Aging* **2017**, *1*, 3–4. [CrossRef]
31. Daly, R.M.; O'Connell, S.L.; Mundell, N.L.; Grimes, C.A.; Dunstan, D.W.; Nowson, C.A. Protein-enriched diet, with the use of lean red meat, combined with progressive resistance training enhances lean tissue mass and muscle strength and reduces circulating IL-6 concentrations in elderly women: A cluster randomized controlled trial. *Am. J. Clin. Nutr.* **2014**, 899–910. [CrossRef] [PubMed]
32. Cermak, N.M.; Res, P.T.; De Groot, L.C.; Saris, W.H.M.; Loon, L.J.C. Van Protein supplementation augments the adaptive response of skeletal muscle to resistance type exercise training a meta analysis. *Am. J. Clin. Nutr.* **2012**, *96*, 1454–1464. [CrossRef] [PubMed]
33. Wu, G.D.; Bushmanc, F.D.; Lewis, J.D. Diet, the human gut microbiota, and IBD. *Anaerobe* **2013**, *24*, 117–120. [CrossRef] [PubMed]
34. O'Keefe, S.J.D. Towards the determination of the nutritional needs of the body and its microbiome in sickness and in health. *Curr. Opin. Gastroenterol.* **2014**, *30*, 175–177. [CrossRef] [PubMed]
35. Ticinesi, A.; Lauretani, F.; Milani, C.; Nouvenne, A.; Tana, C.; Del Rio, D.; Maggio, M.; Ventura, M.; Meschi, T. Aging Gut Microbiota at the Cross-Road between Nutrition, Physical Frailty, and Sarcopenia: Is There a Gut-Muscle Axis? *Nutrients* **2017**, *9*. [CrossRef] [PubMed]

36. Grosicki, G.J.; Fielding, R.A.; Lustgarten, M.S. Gut Microbiota Contribute to Age-Related Changes in Skeletal Muscle Size, Composition, and Function: Biological Basis for a Gut-Muscle Axis. *Calcif. Tissue Int.* **2018**, *102*, 433–442. [CrossRef] [PubMed]
37. Biagi, E.; Nylund, L.; Candela, M.; Ostan, R.; Bucci, L.; Pini, E.; Nikkïla, J.; Monti, D.; Satokari, R.; Franceschi, C.; et al. Through Ageing, and Beyond: Gut Microbiota and Inflammatory Status in Seniors and Centenarians. *PLoS ONE* **2010**, *5*, e10667. [CrossRef]
38. Ridaura, V.K.; Faith, J.J.; Rey, F.E.; Cheng, J.; Alexis, E.; Kau, A.L.; Griffin, N.W.; Lombard, V.; Henrissat, B.; Bain, J.R.; et al. Gut microbiota from twins discordant for obesity modulate metabolism in mice. *Science* **2013**, *341*, 1241214. [CrossRef] [PubMed]
39. Dillon, E.L. Nutritionally essential amino acids and metabolic signaling in aging. *Amino Acids* **2013**, *45*, 431–441. [CrossRef] [PubMed]
40. Mitchell, C.J.; Milan, A.M.; Mitchell, S.M.; Zeng, N.; Ramzan, F.; Sharma, P.; Knowles, S.O.; Roy, N.C.; Sjödin, A.; Wagner, K.H.; et al. The effects of dietary protein intake on appendicular lean mass and muscle function in elderly men: A 10-wk randomized controlled trial. *Am. J. Clin. Nutr.* **2017**, *106*, 1375–1383. [CrossRef] [PubMed]
41. Haran, P.H.; Rivas, D.A.; Fielding, R.A. Role and potential mechanisms of anabolic resistance in sarcopenia. *J. Cachexia. Sarcopenia Muscle* **2012**, *3*, 157–162. [CrossRef] [PubMed]
42. Breen, L.; Phillips, S.M. Skeletal Muscle Protein Metabolism in the Elderly: Interventions to Counteract the "Anabolic Resistance" of Ageing. Available online: http://www.ncbi.nlm.nih.gov/pubmed/21975196 (accessed on 13 July 2018).
43. Stefanetti, R.J.; Zacharewicz, E.; Della Gatta, P.; Garnham, A.; Russell, A.P.; Lamon, S. Ageing Has No Effect on the Regulation of the Ubiquitin Proteasome-Related Genes and Proteins Following Resistance Exercise. Available online: http://www.ncbi.nlm.nih.gov/pubmed/24550841 (accessed on 13 July 2018).
44. Moore, D.R.; Churchward-Venne, T.A.; Witard, O.; Breen, L.; Burd, N.A.; Tipton, K.D.; Phillips, S.M. Protein ingestion to stimulate myofibrillar protein synthesis requires greater relative protein intakes in healthy older versus younger men. *J. Gerontol. Ser. A Biol. Sci. Med. Sci.* **2015**, *70*, 57–62. [CrossRef] [PubMed]
45. Shad, B.J.; Thompson, J.L.; Breen, L. Does the muscle protein synthetic response to exercise and amino acid-based nutrition diminish with advancing age? A systematic review. *Am. J. Physiol. Endocrinol. Metab.* **2016**, *311*, E803–E817. [CrossRef] [PubMed]
46. Wolfe, R.R. The role of dietary protein in optimizing muscle mass, function and health outcomes in older individuals. *Br. J. Nutr.* **2012**, *108*, 88–93. [CrossRef] [PubMed]
47. Malafarina, V.; Uriz-Otano, F.; Iniesta, R.; Gil-Guerrero, L. Effectiveness of Nutritional Supplementation on Muscle Mass in Treatment of Sarcopenia in Old Age: A Systematic Review. *J. Am. Med. Dir. Assoc.* **2013**, *14*, 10–17. [CrossRef] [PubMed]
48. Dulac, M.C.; Pion, C.H.; Lemieux, F.; Boutros El Hajj, G.; Belanger, M.; Gaudreau, P.; Chevalier, S.; Morais, J.A.; Gouspillou, G.; Aubertin-Leheudre, M. Differences in muscle adaptation to a 12-week mixed power training in elderly men, depending on usual protein intake. *Exp. Gerontol.* **2018**. [CrossRef] [PubMed]
49. Nowson, C.; O'Connell, S. Protein requirements and recommendations for older people: A review. *Nutrients* **2015**, *7*, 6874–6899. [CrossRef] [PubMed]
50. Bauer, J.; Biolo, G.; Cederholm, T.; Cesari, M.; Cruz-Jentoft, A.J.; Morley, J.E.; Phillips, S.; Sieber, C.; Stehle, P.; Teta, D.; et al. Evidence-Based Recommendations for Optimal Dietary Protein Intake in Older People: A Position Paper From the PROT-AGE Study Group. *J. Am. Med. Dir. Assoc.* **2013**, 542–559. [CrossRef] [PubMed]
51. Churchward-Venne, T.A.; Breen, L.; Phillips, S.M. Alterations in human muscle protein metabolism with aging: Protein and exercise as countermeasures to offset sarcopenia. *BioFactors* **2014**, *40*, 199–205. [CrossRef] [PubMed]
52. Markofski, M.M.; Volpi, E. Protein metabolism in women and men: Similarities and disparities. *Curr. Opin. Clin. Nutr. Metab. Care* **2011**, *14*, 93–97. [CrossRef] [PubMed]
53. Smith, G.I.; Villareal, D.T.; Sinacore, D.R.; Shah, K.; Mittendorfer, B. Muscle Protein Synthesis Response to Exercise Training in Obese, Older Men and Women. Available online: http://www.ncbi.nlm.nih.gov/pubmed/22246218 (accessed on 4 July 2018).

54. Karastergiou, K.; Smith, S.R.; Greenberg, A.S.; Fried, S.K. Sex Differences in Human Adipose Tissues—The Biology of Pear Shape. Available online: http://www.ncbi.nlm.nih.gov/pubmed/22651247 (accessed on 4 July 2018).
55. Burd, N.A.; Gorissen, S.H.; Van Loon, L.J.C. Anabolic Resistance of Muscle Protein Synthesis with Aging. *Exerc. Sport Sci. Rev.* **2013**, *41*, 169–173. [CrossRef] [PubMed]
56. Murton, A.J. Muscle protein turnover in the elderly and its potential contribution to the development of sarcopenia. *Proc. Nutr. Soc.* **2015**, *74*, 387–396. [CrossRef] [PubMed]
57. Breen, L.; Stokes, K.A.; Churchward-Venne, T.A.; Moore, D.R.; Baker, S.K.; Smith, K.; Atherton, P.J.; Phillips, S.M. Two weeks of reduced activity decreases leg lean mass and induces "anabolic resistance" of myofibrillar protein synthesis in healthy elderly. *J. Clin. Endocrinol. Metab.* **2013**, *98*, 2604–2612. [CrossRef] [PubMed]
58. Wall, B.T.; van Loon, L.J. Nutritional strategies to attenuate muscle disuse atrophy. *Nutr. Rev.* **2013**, *71*, 195–208. [CrossRef] [PubMed]
59. Biolo, G.; Ciocchi, B.; Lebenstedt, M.; Barazzoni, R.; Zanetti, M.; Platen, P.; Heer, M.; Guarnieri, G. Short-term bed rest impairs amino acid-induced protein anabolism in humans. *J. Physiol.* **2004**, *558*, 381–388. [CrossRef] [PubMed]
60. Glover, E.I.; Phillips, S.M.; Oates, B.R.; Tang, J.E.; Tarnopolsky, M.A.; Selby, A.; Smith, K.; Rennie, M.J. Immobilization induces anabolic resistance in human myofibrillar protein synthesis with low and high dose amino acid infusion. Supplementary Data. *J. Physiol.* **2008**, *586*, 6049–6061. [CrossRef] [PubMed]
61. Wall, B.T.; Snijders, T.; Senden, J.M.G.; Ottenbros, C.L.P.; Gijsen, A.P.; Verdijk, L.B.; van Loon, L.J.C. Disuse Impairs the Muscle Protein Synthetic Response to Protein Ingestion in Healthy Men. *J. Clin. Endocrinol. Metab.* **2013**, *98*, 4872–4881. [CrossRef] [PubMed]
62. Guillet, C.; Masgrau, A.; Walrand, S.; Boirie, Y. Impaired protein metabolism: Interlinks between obesity, insulin resistance and inflammation. *Obes. Rev.* **2012**, *13*, 51–57. [CrossRef] [PubMed]
63. Balage, M.; Averous, J.; Rémond, D.; Bos, C.; Pujos-Guillot, E.; Papet, I.; Mosoni, L.; Combaret, L.; Dardevet, D. Presence of low-grade inflammation impaired postprandial stimulation of muscle protein synthesis in old rats. *J. Nutr. Biochem.* **2010**, *21*, 325–331. [CrossRef] [PubMed]
64. Volpi, E.; Mittendorfer, B.; Rasmussen, B.B.; Wolfe, R.R. The response of muscle protein anabolism to combined hyperaminoacidemia and glucose-induced hyperinsulinemia is impaired in the elderly. *J. Clin. Endocrinol. Metab.* **2000**, *85*, 4481–4490. [CrossRef] [PubMed]
65. Meneilly, G.S.; Elliot, T.; Bryer-Ash, M.; Floras, J.S. Insulin-mediated increase in blood flow is impaired in the elderly. *J. Clin. Endocrinol. Metab.* **1995**, *80*, 1899–1903. [CrossRef] [PubMed]
66. Murton, A.J.; Marimuthu, K.; Mallinson, J.E.; Selby, A.L.; Smith, K.; Rennie, M.J.; Greenhaff, P.L. Obesity Appears to Be Associated With Altered Muscle Protein Synthetic and Breakdown Responses to Increased Nutrient Delivery in Older Men, but Not Reduced Muscle Mass or Contractile Function. *Diabetes* **2015**, *64*, 3160–3171. [CrossRef] [PubMed]
67. Volpato, S.; Bianchi, L.; Cherubini, A.; Landi, F.; Maggio, M.; Savino, E.; Bandinelli, S.; Ceda, G.P.; Guralnik, J.M.; Zuliani, G.; et al. Prevalence and clinical correlates of sarcopenia in community-dwelling older people: Application of the EWGSOP definition and diagnostic algorithm. *J. Gerontol. A. Biol. Sci. Med. Sci.* **2014**, *69*, 438–446. [CrossRef] [PubMed]
68. Parr, E.B.; Camera, D.M.; Areta, J.L.; Burke, L.M.; Phillips, S.M.; Hawley, J.A.; Coffey, V.G. Alcohol Ingestion Impairs Maximal Post-Exercise Rates of Myofibrillar Protein Synthesis following a Single Bout of Concurrent Training. *PLoS ONE* **2014**, *9*, e88384. [CrossRef] [PubMed]
69. Drummond, M.J.; Miyazaki, M.; Dreyer, H.C.; Pennings, B.; Dhanani, S.; Volpi, E.; Esser, K.A.; Rasmussen, B.B. Expression of growth-related genes in young and older human skeletal muscle following an acute stimulation of protein synthesis. *J. Appl. Physiol.* **2009**, *106*, 1403–1411. [CrossRef] [PubMed]
70. Tanner, R.E.; Brunker, L.B.; Agergaard, J.; Barrows, K.M.; Briggs, R.A.; Kwon, O.S.; Young, L.M.; Hopkins, P.N.; Volpi, E.; Marcus, R.L.; et al. Age-related differences in lean mass, protein synthesis and skeletal muscle markers of proteolysis after bed rest and exercise rehabilitation. *J. Physiol.* **2015**, *593*, 4259–4273. [CrossRef] [PubMed]
71. Greig, C.A.; Gray, C.; Rankin, D.; Young, A.; Mann, V.; Noble, B.; Atherton, P.J. Blunting of adaptive responses to resistance exercise training in women over 75 y. *Exp. Gerontol.* **2011**, *46*, 884–890. [CrossRef] [PubMed]

72. Drummond, M.J.; Addison, O.; Brunker, L.; Hopkins, P.N.; McClain, D.A.; Lastayo, P.C.; Marcus, R.L. Downregulation of E3 ubiquitin ligases and mitophagy-related genes in skeletal muscle of physically inactive, frail older women: A cross-sectional comparison. *J. Gerontol. Ser. A Biol. Sci. Med. Sci.* **2014**, *69*, 1040–1048. [CrossRef] [PubMed]
73. Lecker, S.H.; Jagoe, R.T.; Gilbert, A.; Gomes, M.; Baracos, V.; Bailey, J.; Price, S.R.; Mitch, W.E.; Goldberg, A.L. Multiple types of skeletal muscle atrophy involve a common program of changes in gene expression. *FASEB J.* **2004**, *18*, 39–51. [CrossRef] [PubMed]
74. Cuthbertson, D.; Smith, K.; Babraj, J.; Leese, G.; Waddell, T.; Atherton, P.; Wackerhage, H.; Taylor, P.M.; Rennie, M.J. Anabolic signaling deficits underlie amino acid resistance of wasting, aging muscle. *FASEB J.* **2005**, *19*, 422–424. [CrossRef] [PubMed]
75. Drummond, M.J.; Dickinson, J.M.; Fry, C.S.; Walker, D.K.; Gundermann, D.M.; Reidy, P.T.; Timmerman, K.L.; Markofski, M.M.; Paddon-Jones, D.; Rasmussen, B.B.; et al. Bed rest impairs skeletal muscle amino acid transporter expression, mTORC1 signaling, and protein synthesis in response to essential amino acids in older adults. *Am. J. Physiol. Endocrinol. Metab.* **2012**, *302*, E1113–E1122. [CrossRef] [PubMed]
76. Fry, C.S.; Drummond, M.J.; Glynn, E.L.; Dickinson, J.M.; Gundermann, D.M.; Timmerman, K.L.; Walker, D.K.; Volpi, E.; Rasmussen, B.B. Skeletal muscle autophagy and protein breakdown following resistance exercise are similar in younger and older adults. *J. Gerontol. A Biol. Sci. Med. Sci.* **2013**, *68*, 599–607. [CrossRef] [PubMed]
77. Dickinson, J.M.; Fry, C.S.; Drummond, M.J.; Gundermann, D.M.; Walker, D.K.; Glynn, E.L.; Timmerman, K.L.; Dhanani, S.; Volpi, E.; Rasmussen, B.B. Mammalian target of rapamycin complex 1 activation is required for the stimulation of human skeletal muscle protein synthesis by essential amino acids. *J. Nutr.* **2011**, *141*, 856–862. [CrossRef] [PubMed]
78. Fry, C.S.; Drummond, M.J.; Glynn, E.L.; Dickinson, J.M.; Gundermann, D.M.; Timmerman, K.L.; Walker, D.K.; Dhanani, S.; Volpi, E.; Rasmussen, B.B. Aging impairs contraction-induced human skeletal muscle mTORC1 signaling and protein synthesis. *Skelet. Muscle* **2011**, *1*, 11. [CrossRef] [PubMed]
79. Kar, S.K.; Jansman, A.J.M.; Benis, N.; Ramiro-Garcia, J.; Schokker, D.; Kruijt, L.; Stolte, E.H.; Taverne-Thiele, J.J.; Smits, M.A.; Wells, J.M. Dietary protein sources differentially affect microbiota, mTOR activity and transcription of mTOR signaling pathways in the small intestine. *PLoS ONE* **2017**, *12*, e0188282. [CrossRef] [PubMed]
80. Dickinson, J.M.; Gundermann, D.M.; Walker, D.K.; Reidy, P.T.; Borack, M.S.; Drummond, M.J.; Arora, M.; Volpi, E.; Rasmussen, B.B. Leucine-enriched amino acid ingestion after resistance exercise prolongs myofibrillar protein synthesis and amino acid transporter expression in older men. *J. Nutr.* **2014**, *144*, 1694–1702. [CrossRef] [PubMed]
81. Dickinson, J.M.; Drummond, M.J.; Coben, J.R.; Volpi, E.; Rasmussen, B.B. Aging differentially affects human skeletal muscle amino acid transporter expression when essential amino acids are ingested after exercise. *Clin. Nutr.* **2013**, *32*, 273–280. [CrossRef] [PubMed]
82. Guillet, C.; Prod'homme, M.; Balage, M.; Gachon, P.; Giraudet, C.; MORIN, L.; Grizard, J.; Boirie, Y. Impaired anabolic response of muscle protein synthesis is associated with S6K1 dysregulation in elderly humans. *FASEB J.* **2004**, *18*, 1586–1587. [CrossRef] [PubMed]
83. Markofski, M.M.; Dickinson, J.M.; Drummond, M.J.; Fry, C.S.; Fujita, S.; Gundermann, D.M.; Glynn, E.L.; Jennings, K.; Paddon-Jones, D.; Reidy, P.T.; et al. Effect of age on basal muscle protein synthesis and mTORC1 signaling in a large cohort of young and older men and women. *Exp. Gerontol.* **2015**, *65*, 1–7. [CrossRef] [PubMed]
84. Welch, A.A.; Kelaiditi, E.; Jennings, A.; Steves, C.J.; Spector, T.D.; MacGregor, A. Dietary Magnesium Is Positively Associated With Skeletal Muscle Power and Indices of Muscle Mass and May Attenuate the Association Between Circulating C-Reactive Protein and Muscle Mass in Women. *J. Bone Min. Res.* **2016**, *31*, 317–325. [CrossRef] [PubMed]
85. Schaap, L.A.; Pluijm, S.M.F.; Deeg, D.J.H.; Harris, T.B.; Kritchevsky, S.B.; Newman, A.B.; Colbert, L.H.; Pahor, M.; Rubin, S.M.; Tylavsky, F.A.; et al. Higher inflammatory marker levels in older persons: Associations with 5-year change in muscle mass and muscle strength. *J. Gerontol. A Biol. Sci. Med. Sci.* **2009**, *64*, 1183–1189. [CrossRef] [PubMed]

86. Dillon, E.L.; Casperson, S.L.; Durham, W.J.; Randolph, K.M.; Urban, R.J.; Volpi, E.; Ahmad, M.; Kinsky, M.P.; Sheffield-Moore, M. Muscle protein metabolism responds similarly to exogenous amino acids in healthy younger and older adults during NO-induced hyperemia. *Am. J. Physiol. Integr. Comp. Physiol.* **2011**, *301*, R1408–R1417. [CrossRef] [PubMed]
87. Saffrey, M.J. Aging of the mammalian gastrointestinal tract: A complex organ system. *Age* **2014**, *36*, 9603. [CrossRef] [PubMed]
88. Boirie, Y.; Gachon, P.; Beaufrère, B. Splanchnic and whole-body leucine kinetics in young and elderly men. *Am. J. Clin. Nutr.* **1997**, *65*, 489–495. [CrossRef] [PubMed]
89. Gorissen, S.H.M.; Witard, O.C. Characterising the muscle anabolic potential of dairy, meat and plant-based protein sources in older adults. *Proc. Nutr. Soc.* **2018**, *77*, 20–30. [CrossRef] [PubMed]
90. Piasecki, M.; Ireland, A.; Piasecki, J.; Stashuk, D.W.; Swiecicka, A.; Rutter, M.K.; Jones, D.A.; McPhee, J.S. Failure to expand the motor unit size to compensate for declining motor unit numbers distinguishes sarcopenic from non-sarcopenic older men. *J. Physiol.* **2018**, *596*, 1627–1637. [CrossRef] [PubMed]
91. Stephens, F.B.; Chee, C.; Wall, B.T.; Murton, A.J.; Shannon, C.E.; van Loon, L.J.C.; Tsintzas, K. Lipid-induced insulin resistance is associated with an impaired skeletal muscle protein synthetic response to amino acid ingestion in healthy young men. *Diabetes* **2015**, *64*, 1615–1620. [CrossRef] [PubMed]
92. Kilgour, A.H.M.; Gallagher, I.J.; MacLullich, A.M.J.; Andrew, R.; Gray, C.D.; Hyde, P.; Wackerhage, H.; Husi, H.; Ross, J.A.; Starr, J.M.; et al. Increased skeletal muscle 11βHSD1 mRNA is associated with lower muscle strength in ageing. *PLoS ONE* **2013**, *8*, e84057. [CrossRef] [PubMed]
93. Liu, W.; Klose, A.; Forman, S.; Paris, N.D.; Wei-LaPierre, L.; Cortés-Lopéz, M.; Tan, A.; Flaherty, M.; Miura, P.; Dirksen, R.T.; et al. Loss of adult skeletal muscle stem cells drives age-related neuromuscular junction degeneration. *Elife* **2017**, *6*, e26464. [CrossRef] [PubMed]
94. Jeffery, I.B.; O'Toole, P.W. Diet-microbiota interactions and their implications for healthy living. *Nutrients* **2013**, *5*, 234–252. [CrossRef] [PubMed]
95. Claesson, M.J.; Jeffery, I.B.; Conde, S.; Power, S.E.; O'Connor, E.M.; Cusack, S.; Harris, H.M.B.; Coakley, M.; Lakshminarayanan, B.; O'Sullivan, O.; et al. Gut microbiota composition correlates with diet and health in the elderly. *Nature* **2012**, *488*, 178–184. [CrossRef] [PubMed]
96. Gi Langille, M.; Meehan, C.J.; Koenig, J.E.; Dhanani, A.S.; Rose, R.A.; Howlett, S.E.; Beiko, R.G. Microbial shifts in the aging mouse gut. *Microbiome* **2014**. [CrossRef] [PubMed]
97. Rampelli, S.; Candela, M.; Turroni, S.; Biagi, E.; Pflueger, M.; Wolters, M.; Ahrens, W.; Brigidi, P. Microbiota and lifestyle interactions through the lifespan. *Trends Food Sci. Technol.* **2016**, *57*, 265–272. [CrossRef]
98. Jackson, M.A.; Jeffery, I.B.; Beaumont, M.; Bell, J.T.; Clark, A.G.; Ley, R.E.; O'Toole, P.W.; Spector, T.D.; Steves, C.J. Signatures of early frailty in the gut microbiota. *Genome Med.* **2016**, *8*, 8. [CrossRef] [PubMed]
99. Ticinesi, A.; Milani, C.; Lauretani, F.; Nouvenne, A.; Mancabelli, L.; Lugli, G.A.; Turroni, F.; Duranti, S.; Mangifesta, M.; Viappiani, A.; et al. Gut microbiota composition is associated with polypharmacy in elderly hospitalized patients. *Sci. Rep.* **2017**, *7*, 11102. [CrossRef] [PubMed]
100. Jeffery, I.B.; Lynch, D.B.; O'Toole, P.W. Composition and temporal stability of the gut microbiota in older persons. *ISME J.* **2016**, *10*, 170–182. [CrossRef] [PubMed]
101. Pérez-Cobas, A.E.; Gosalbes, M.J.; Friedrichs, A.; Knecht, H.; Artacho, A.; Eismann, K.; Otto, W.; Rojo, D.; Bargiela, R.; von Bergen, M.; et al. Gut microbiota disturbance during antibiotic therapy: A multi-omic approach. *Gut* **2013**, *62*, 1591–1601. [CrossRef] [PubMed]
102. Boirie, Y. Physiopathological mechanism of sarcopenia. *J. Nutr. Health Aging* **2009**, *13*, 717–723. [CrossRef] [PubMed]
103. Steves, C.J.; Bird, S.; Williams, F.M.; Spector, T.D. The Microbiome and Musculoskeletal Conditions of Aging: A Review of Evidence for Impact and Potential Therapeutics. *J. Bone Min. Res.* **2016**, *31*, 261–269. [CrossRef] [PubMed]
104. Picca, A.; Fanelli, F.; Calvani, R.; Mulè, G.; Pesce, V.; Sisto, A.; Pantanelli, C.; Bernabei, R.; Landi, F.; Marzetti, E. Gut Dysbiosis and Muscle Aging: Searching for Novel Targets against Sarcopenia. *Mediat. Inflamm.* **2018**, 7026198. [CrossRef] [PubMed]
105. Quigley, E.M.M. Commentary: Synbiotics and gut microbiota in older people—A microbial guide to healthy ageing. *Aliment. Pharmacol. Ther.* **2013**, *38*, 1141–1142. [CrossRef] [PubMed]

106. Smith, P.; Willemsen, D.; Popkes, M.L.; Metge, F.; Gandiwa, E.; Reichard, M.; Valenzano, D.R. Regulation of Life Span by the Gut Microbiota in The Short-Lived African Turquoise Killifish. Available online: https://www.biorxiv.org/content/early/2017/03/27/120980 (accessed on 8 June 2018).
107. Power, S.E.; O'Toole, P.W.; Stanton, C.; Ross, R.P.; Fitzgerald, G.F. Intestinal microbiota, diet and health. *Br. J. Nutr.* **2014**, *111*, 387–402. [CrossRef] [PubMed]
108. Bäckhed, F.; Ding, H.; Wang, T.; Hooper, L.V.; Koh, G.Y.; Nagy, A.; Semenkovich, C.F.; Gordon, J.I. The gut microbiota as an environmental factor that regulates fat storage. *Proc. Natl. Acad. Sci. USA* **2004**, *101*, 15718–15723. [CrossRef] [PubMed]
109. Bäckhed, F.; Manchester, J.K.; Semenkovich, C.F.; Gordon, J.I. Mechanisms underlying the resistance to diet-induced obesity in germ-free mice. *Proc. Natl. Acad. Sci. USA* **2007**, *104*, 979–984. [CrossRef] [PubMed]
110. Den Besten, G.; Lange, K.; Havinga, R.; Van Dijk, T.H.; Gerding, A.; Van Eunen, K.; Müller, M.; Groen, A.K.; Hooiveld, G.J.; Bakker, B.M.; et al. Gut-derived short-chain fatty acids are vividly assimilated into host carbohydrates and lipids. *Am. J. Physiol. Gastrointest. Liver Physiol.* **2013**, *305*, G900–G910. [CrossRef] [PubMed]
111. Yan, H.; Diao, H.; Xiao, Y.; Li, W.; Yu, B.; He, J.; Yu, J.; Zheng, P.; Mao, X.; Luo, Y.; et al. Gut microbiota can transfer fiber characteristics and lipid metabolic profiles of skeletal muscle from pigs to germ-free mice. *Sci. Rep.* **2016**, *6*, 31786. [CrossRef] [PubMed]
112. Cani, P.D.; Possemiers, S.; Van de Wiele, T.; Guiot, Y.; Everard, A.; Rottier, O.; Geurts, L.; Naslain, D.; Neyrinck, A.; Lambert, D.M.; et al. Changes in gut microbiota control inflammation in obese mice through a mechanism involving GLP-2-driven improvement of gut permeability. *Gut* **2009**, *58*, 1091–1103. [CrossRef] [PubMed]
113. Bindels, L.B.; Beck, R.; Schakman, O.; Martin, J.C.; De Backer, F.; Sohet, F.M.; Dewulf, E.M.; Pachikian, B.D.; Neyrinck, A.M.; Thissen, J.-P.; et al. Restoring Specific Lactobacilli Levels Decreases Inflammation and Muscle Atrophy Markers in an Acute Leukemia Mouse Model. *PLoS ONE* **2012**, *7*, e37971. [CrossRef] [PubMed]
114. Chen, Y.-M.; Wei, L.; Chiu, Y.-S.; Hsu, Y.-J.; Tsai, T.-Y.; Wang, M.-F.; Huang, C.-C. Lactobacillus plantarum TWK10 Supplementation Improves Exercise Performance and Increases Muscle Mass in Mice. *Nutrients* **2016**, *8*, 205. [CrossRef] [PubMed]
115. Bindels, L.B.; Neyrinck, A.M.; Claus, S.P.; Le Roy, C.I.; Grangette, C.; Pot, B.; Martinez, I.; Walter, J.; Cani, P.D.; Delzenne, N.M. Synbiotic approach restores intestinal homeostasis and prolongs survival in leukaemic mice with cachexia. *ISME J.* **2016**, *10*, 1456–1470. [CrossRef] [PubMed]
116. Walsh, M.E.; Bhattacharya, A.; Sataranatarajan, K.; Qaisar, R.; Sloane, L.; Rahman, M.M.; Kinter, M.; Van Remmen, H. The histone deacetylase inhibitor butyrate improves metabolism and reduces muscle atrophy during aging. *Aging Cell* **2015**, *14*, 957–970. [CrossRef] [PubMed]
117. Shing, C.M.; Peake, J.M.; Lim, C.L.; Briskey, D.; Walsh, N.P.; Fortes, M.B.; Ahuja, K.D.K.; Vitetta, L. Effects of probiotics supplementation on gastrointestinal permeability, inflammation and exercise performance in the heat. *Eur. J. Appl. Physiol.* **2014**, *114*, 93–103. [CrossRef] [PubMed]
118. Salarkia, N.; Ghadamli, L.; Zaeri, F.; Sabaghian Rad, L. Effects of probiotic yogurt on performance, respiratory and digestive systems of young adult female endurance swimmers: A randomized controlled trial. *Med. J. Islam. Repub. Iran* **2013**, *27*, 141–146. [PubMed]
119. Cerdá, B.; Pérez, M.; Pérez-Santiago, J.D.; Tornero-Aguilera, J.F.; González-Soltero, R.; Larrosa, M. Gut Microbiota Modification: Another Piece in the Puzzle of the Benefits of Physical Exercise in Health? *Front. Physiol.* **2016**, *7*, 51. [CrossRef] [PubMed]
120. Clark, A.; Mach, N. The Crosstalk between the Gut Microbiota and Mitochondria during Exercise. *Front. Physiol.* **2017**, *8*, 319. [CrossRef] [PubMed]
121. Choi, J.J.; Eum, S.Y.; Rampersaud, E.; Daunert, S.; Abreu, M.T.; Toborek, M. Exercise attenuates PCB-induced changes in the mouse gut microbiome. *Environ. Health Perspect.* **2013**, *121*, 725–730. [CrossRef] [PubMed]
122. Queipo-Ortuño, M.I.; Seoane, L.M.; Murri, M.; Pardo, M.; Gomez-Zumaquero, J.M.; Cardona, F.; Casanueva, F.; Tinahones, F.J. Gut microbiota composition in male rat models under different nutritional status and physical activity and its association with serum leptin and ghrelin levels. *PLoS ONE* **2013**, *8*, e65465. [CrossRef] [PubMed]

123. Petriz, B.A.; Castro, A.P.; Almeida, J.A.; Gomes, C.P.; Fernandes, G.R.; Kruger, R.H.; Pereira, R.W.; Franco, O.L. Exercise induction of gut microbiota modifications in obese, non-obese and hypertensive rats. *BMC Genom.* **2014**, *15*, 511. [CrossRef] [PubMed]
124. Bilski, J.; Mazur-Bialy, A.; Hubalewska-Mazgaj, M.; Brzozowski, B.; Surmiak, M.; Wojcik, D.; Magierowski, M.; Chmura, A.; Magierowska, K.; Brzozowski, T. Role of Gut-Adipose-muscle Axis in Beneficial Effect of Voluntary Exercise on Experimental Colitis in Mice Fed a Diet-Induced Obesity. Involvement of Protective Irisin and Proinflammatory Biomarkers Released from Mesenteric Fat and Colonic Mucosa. *Gastroenterology* **2017**, *152*, S828. [CrossRef]
125. Clarke, S.F.; Murphy, E.F.; O'Sullivan, O.; Lucey, A.J.; Humphreys, M.; Hogan, A.; Hayes, P.; O'Reilly, M.; Jeffery, I.B.; Wood-Martin, R.; et al. Exercise and associated dietary extremes impact on gut microbial diversity. *Gut* **2014**, *63*, 1913–1920. [CrossRef] [PubMed]
126. Oettlé, G.J. Effect of moderate exercise on bowel habit. *Gut* **1991**, *32*, 941–944. [CrossRef] [PubMed]
127. Vandeputte, D.; Falony, G.; Vieira-Silva, S.; Tito, R.Y.; Joossens, M.; Raes, J. Stool consistency is strongly associated with gut microbiota richness and composition, enterotypes and bacterial growth rates. *Gut* **2015**. [CrossRef] [PubMed]
128. Zhu, L.; Liu, W.; Alkhouri, R.; Baker, R.D.; Bard, J.E.; Quigley, E.M.; Baker, S.S. Structural changes in the gut microbiome of constipated patients. *Physiol. Genom.* **2014**, *46*, 679–686. [CrossRef] [PubMed]
129. Buigues, C.; Fernández-Garrido, J.; Pruimboom, L.; Hoogland, A.J.; Navarro-Martínez, R.; Martínez-Martínez, M.; Verdejo, Y.; Mascarós, M.C.; Peris, C.; Cauli, O. Effect of a Prebiotic Formulation on Frailty Syndrome: A Randomized, Double-Blind Clinical Trial. *Int. J. Mol. Sci.* **2016**, *17*. [CrossRef] [PubMed]
130. Ma, N.; Tian, Y.; Wu, Y.; Ma, X. Contributions of the Interaction between Dietary Protein and Gut Microbiota to Intestinal Health. *Curr. Protein Pept. Sci.* **2017**, *18*. [CrossRef] [PubMed]
131. Beaumont, M.; Portune, K.J.; Steuer, N.; Lan, A.; Cerrudo, V.; Audebert, M.; Dumont, F.; Mancano, G.; Khodorova, N.; Andriamihaja, M.; et al. Quantity and source of dietary protein influence metabolite production by gut microbiota and rectal mucosa gene expression: A randomized, parallel, double-blind trial in overweight humans. *Am. J. Clin. Nutr.* **2017**, *106*, 1005–1019. [CrossRef] [PubMed]
132. Bindels, L.B.; Delzenne, N.M. Muscle wasting: The gut microbiota as a new therapeutic target? *Int. J. Biochem. Cell Biol.* **2013**, *45*, 2186–2190. [CrossRef] [PubMed]
133. Butteiger, D.N.; Hibberd, A.A.; Mcgraw, N.J.; Napawan, N.; Hall-porter, J.M.; Krul, E.S. Soy Protein Compared with Milk Protein in a Western Diet Increases Gut Microbial Diversity and Reduces Serum Lipids in Golden Syrian Hamsters. *J. Nutr.* **2016**, *146*, 697–705. [CrossRef] [PubMed]
134. An, C.; Kuda, T.; Yazaki, T.; Takahashi, H.; Kimura, B. Caecal fermentation, putrefaction and microbiotas in rats fed milk casein, soy protein or fish meal. *Appl. Microbiol. Biotechnol.* **2014**, *98*, 2779–2787. [CrossRef] [PubMed]
135. Li, Q.; Lauber, C.L.; Czarnecki-Maulden, G.; Pan, Y.; Hannah, S.S. Effects of the dietary protein and carbohydrate ratio on gut microbiomes in dogs of different body conditions. *MBio* **2017**, *8*, 1–14. [CrossRef] [PubMed]
136. Singh, R.K.; Chang, H.W.; Yan, D.; Lee, K.M.; Ucmak, D.; Wong, K.; Abrouk, M.; Farahnik, B.; Nakamura, M.; Zhu, T.H.; et al. Influence of diet on the gut microbiome and implications for human health. *J. Transl. Med.* **2017**, *15*, 1–17. [CrossRef] [PubMed]
137. David, L.A.; Maurice, C.F.; Carmody, R.N.; Gootenberg, D.B.; Button, J.E.; Wolfe, B.E.; Ling, A.V.; Devlin, A.S.; Varma, Y.; Fischbach, M.A.; et al. Diet rapidly and reproducibly alters the human gut microbiome. *Nature* **2014**, *505*, 559–563. [CrossRef] [PubMed]
138. Cotillard, A.; Kennedy, S.P.; Kong, L.C.; Prifti, E.; Pons, N.; Le Chatelier, E.; Almeida, M.; Quinquis, B.; Levenez, F.; Galleron, N.; et al. Dietary intervention impact on gut microbial gene richness. *Nature* **2013**, *500*, 585–588. [CrossRef] [PubMed]
139. Flint, H.J.; Duncan, S.H.; Scott, K.P.; Louis, P. Links between diet, gut microbiota composition and gut metabolism. *Proc. Nutr. Soc.* **2015**, *74*, 13–22. [CrossRef] [PubMed]
140. De Filippis, F.; Pellegrini, N.; Vannini, L.; Jeffery, I.B.; La Storia, A.; Laghi, L.; Serrazanetti, D.I.; Di Cagno, R.; Ferrocino, I.; Lazzi, C.; et al. High-level adherence to a Mediterranean diet beneficially impacts the gut microbiota and associated metabolome. *Gut* **2016**, *65*, 1812–1821. [CrossRef] [PubMed]
141. Krezalek, M.A.; Yeh, A.; Alverdy, J.C.; Morowitz, M. Influence of nutrition therapy on the intestinal microbiome. *Curr. Opin. Clin. Nutr. Metab. Care* **2017**, *20*, 131–137. [CrossRef] [PubMed]

142. Bear, D.E.; Wandrag, L.; Merriweather, J.L.; Connolly, B.; Hart, N.; Grocott, M.P.W. The role of nutritional support in the physical and functional recovery of critically ill patients: A narrative review. *Crit. Care* **2017**, *21*. [CrossRef] [PubMed]
143. Ferrie, S.; Allman-Farinelli, M.; Daley, M.; Smith, K. Protein Requirements in the Critically Ill: A Randomized Controlled Trial Using Parenteral Nutrition. *J. Parenter. Enter. Nutr.* **2016**, *40*, 795–805. [CrossRef] [PubMed]
144. Thevaranjan, N.; Puchta, A.; Schulz, C.; Naidoo, A.; Szamosi, J.C.; Verschoor, C.P.; Loukov, D.; Schenck, L.P.; Jury, J.; Foley, K.P.; et al. Age-Associated Microbial Dysbiosis Promotes Intestinal Permeability, Systemic Inflammation, and Macrophage Dysfunction. *Cell Host Microbe* **2017**, *21*, 455–466. [CrossRef] [PubMed]
145. Lamprecht, M.; Bogner, S.; Schippinger, G.; Steinbauer, K.; Fankhauser, F.; Hallstroem, S.; Schuetz, B.; Greilberger, J.F. Probiotic supplementation affects markers of intestinal barrier, oxidation, and inflammation in trained men; a randomized, double-blinded, placebo-controlled trial. *J. Int. Soc. Sports Nutr.* **2012**, *9*, 45. [CrossRef] [PubMed]
146. Rampelli, S.; Candela, M.; Turroni, S.; Biagi, E.; Collino, S.; Franceschi, C.; O'Toole, P.W.; Brigidi, P. Functional metagenomic profiling of intestinal microbiome in extreme ageing. *Aging* **2013**, *5*, 902–912. [CrossRef] [PubMed]
147. Maathuis, A.; Keller, D.; Farmer, S. Survival and metabolic activity of the GanedenBC^{30} strain of *Bacillus coagulans* in a dynamic *in vitro* model of the stomach and small intestine. *Benef. Microbes* **2010**, *1*, 31–36. [CrossRef] [PubMed]
148. Jäger, R.; Purpura, M.; Farmer, S.; Cash, H.A.; Keller, D. Probiotic Bacillus coagulans GBI-30, 6086 Improves Protein Absorption and Utilization. *Probiotics Antimicrob. Proteins* **2017**. [CrossRef] [PubMed]
149. Sonnenburg, J.L.; Bäckhed, F. Diet–microbiota interactions as moderators of human metabolism. *Nature* **2016**, *535*, 56–64. [CrossRef] [PubMed]
150. Van Tongeren, S.P.; Slaets, J.P.J.; Harmsen, H.J.M.; Welling, G.W. Fecal microbiota composition and frailty. *Appl. Environ. Microbiol.* **2005**, *71*, 6438–6442. [CrossRef] [PubMed]
151. Peng, L.; Li, Z.-R.; Green, R.S.; Holzman, I.R.; Lin, J. Butyrate enhances the intestinal barrier by facilitating tight junction assembly via activation of AMP-activated protein kinase in Caco-2 cell monolayers. *J. Nutr.* **2009**, *139*, 1619–1625. [CrossRef] [PubMed]
152. Macfarlane, S.; Cleary, S.; Bahrami, B.; Reynolds, N.; Macfarlane, G.T. Synbiotic consumption changes the metabolism and composition of the gut microbiota in older people and modifies inflammatory processes: A randomised, double-blind, placebo-controlled crossover study. *Aliment. Pharmacol. Ther.* **2013**, *38*, 804–816. [CrossRef] [PubMed]
153. Ko, F.; Abadir, P.; Marx, R.; Westbrook, R.; Cooke, C.; Yang, H.; Walston, J. Impaired mitochondrial degradation by autophagy in the skeletal muscle of the aged female interleukin 10 null mouse. *Exp. Gerontol.* **2016**, *73*, 23–27. [CrossRef] [PubMed]
154. Marzetti, E.; Calvani, R.; Lorenzi, M.; Tanganelli, F.; Picca, A.; Bossola, M.; Menghi, A.; Bernabei, R.; Landi, F. Association between myocyte quality control signaling and sarcopenia in old hip-fractured patients: Results from the Sarcopenia in HIp FracTure (SHIFT) exploratory study. *Exp. Gerontol.* **2016**, *80*, 1–5. [CrossRef] [PubMed]
155. Marzetti, E.; Lorenzi, M.; Landi, F.; Picca, A.; Rosa, F.; Tanganelli, F.; Galli, M.; Doglietto, G.B.; Pacelli, F.; Cesari, M.; et al. Altered mitochondrial quality control signaling in muscle of old gastric cancer patients with cachexia. *Exp. Gerontol.* **2017**, *87*, 92–99. [CrossRef] [PubMed]
156. Stevens, J.; Metcalf, P.A.; Dennis, B.H.; Tell, G.S.; Shimakawa, T.; Folsom, A.R. Reliability of a food frequency questionnaire by ethnicity, gender, age and education. *Nutr. Res.* **1996**, *16*, 735–745. [CrossRef]
157. Deutz, N.E.P.; Pereira, S.L.; Hays, N.P.; Oliver, J.S.; Edens, N.K.; Evans, C.M.; Wolfe, R.R. Effect of β-hydroxy-β-methylbutyrate (HMB) on lean body mass during 10 days of bed rest in older adults. *Clin. Nutr.* **2013**, *32*, 704–712. [CrossRef] [PubMed]
158. Zierer, J.; Jackson, M.A.; Kastenmüller, G.; Mangino, M.; Long, T.; Telenti, A.; Mohney, R.P.; Small, K.S.; Bell, J.T.; Steves, C.J.; et al. The fecal metabolome as a functional readout of the gut microbiome. *Nat. Genet.* **2018**, *50*, 790–795. [CrossRef] [PubMed]
159. Van de Rest, O.; Schutte, B.A.M.; Deelen, J.; Stassen, S.A.M.; van den Akker, E.B.; van Heemst, D.; Dibbets-Schneider, P.; van Dipten-van der Veen, R.A.; Kelderman, M.; Hankemeier, T.; et al. Metabolic effects of a 13-weeks lifestyle intervention in older adults: The Growing Old Together Study. *Aging* **2016**, *8*, 111–126. [CrossRef] [PubMed]

160. Marzetti, E.; Calvani, R.; Landi, F.; Hoogendijk, E.O.; Fougère, B.; Vellas, B.; Pahor, M.; Bernabei, R.; Cesari, M. SPRINTT Consortium, on behalf of the S. Innovative Medicines Initiative: The SPRINTT Project. *J. Frailty Aging* **2015**, *4*, 207–208. [PubMed]
161. Dhurandhar, N.V.; Schoeller, D.; Brown, A.W.; Heymsfield, S.B.; Thomas, D.; Sorensen, T.I.A.; Speakman, J.R.; Jeansonne, M.; Allison, D.B. Energy Balance Measurement: When Something is Not Better than Nothing. *Int. J. Obes.* **2015**, *39*, 1109–1113. [CrossRef] [PubMed]
162. Garcia-Perez, I.; Posma, J.M.; Gibson, R.; Chambers, E.S.; Hansen, T.H.; Vestergaard, H.; Hansen, T.; Beckmann, M.; Pedersen, O.; Elliott, P.; et al. Objective assessment of dietary patterns by use of metabolic phenotyping: A randomised, controlled, crossover trial. *Lancet Diabetes Endocrinol.* **2017**, *5*, 184–195. [CrossRef]

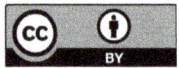

© 2018 by the authors. Licensee MDPI, Basel, Switzerland. This article is an open access article distributed under the terms and conditions of the Creative Commons Attribution (CC BY) license (http://creativecommons.org/licenses/by/4.0/).

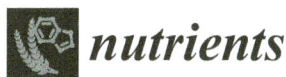

Review

Dietary Protein, Muscle and Physical Function in the Very Old

Bernhard Franzke [1,*,†], Oliver Neubauer [1,2,†], David Cameron-Smith [3] and Karl-Heinz Wagner [1]

1. Research Platform Active Ageing, University of Vienna, 1090 Vienna, Austria; oliver.neubauer@univie.ac.at (O.N.); karl-heinz.wagner@univie.ac.at (K.H.-W.)
2. School of Biomedical Sciences, Tissue Repair and Translational Physiology Program, Institute of Health and Biomedical Innovation, Queensland University of Technology, Brisbane, QLD 4059, Australia
3. Liggins Institute, University of Auckland, Private Bag 92019, Auckland, New Zealand; d.cameron-smith@auckland.ac.nz
* Correspondence: bernhard.franzke@univie.ac.at; Tel.: +43-676-955-94-46
† These authors contributed equally to this work.

Received: 2 July 2018; Accepted: 18 July 2018; Published: 20 July 2018

Abstract: There is an ongoing debate as to the optimal protein intake in older adults. An increasing body of experimental studies on skeletal muscle protein metabolism as well as epidemiological data suggest that protein requirements with ageing might be greater than many current dietary recommendations. Importantly, none of the intervention studies in this context specifically investigated very old individuals. Data on the fastest growing age group of the oldest old (aged 85 years and older) is very limited. In this review, we examine the current evidence on protein intake for preserving muscle mass, strength and function in older individuals, with emphasis on data in the very old. Available observational data suggest beneficial effects of a higher protein intake with physical function in the oldest old. Whilst, studies estimating protein requirements in old and very old individuals based on whole-body measurements, show no differences between these sub-populations of elderly. However, small sample sizes preclude drawing firm conclusions. Experimental studies that compared muscle protein synthetic (MPS) responses to protein ingestion in young and old adults suggest that a higher relative protein intake is required to maximally stimulate skeletal muscle MPS in the aged. Although, data on MPS responses to protein ingestion in the oldest old are currently lacking. Collectively, the data reviewed for this article support the concept that there is a close interaction of physical activity, diet, function and ageing. An attractive hypothesis is that regular physical activity may preserve and even enhance the responsiveness of ageing skeletal muscle to protein intake, until very advanced age. More research involving study participants particularly aged ≥85 years is warranted to better investigate and determine protein requirements in this specific growing population group.

Keywords: ageing; octogenarians; nonagenarians; centenarians; anabolic resistance; protein requirements; exercise; amino acids; skeletal muscle health

1. Introduction

The age-related loss of muscle mass, function and strength—termed either as sarcopenia or dynapenia—has a profound impact on mobility in the elderly. This loss of physical function capabilities compromises the ability to independently perform every-day activities [1–3]. Less immediately obvious but also of significance, is the link between the loss of muscle mass and function with increased risk of type 2 diabetes, cardiovascular diseases, some cancers and neuro-degenerative disorders, including Alzheimer's disease and dementia [4–6]. Most developed economies are experiencing rapid population ageing. Yet it is the oldest aged humans, individuals aged 80 years and older, which is the fastest growing of the age sectors [7]. The increasing number of exceptionally long-lived people and the fact that mortality rates beyond 105 years plateaus across these cohorts suggests that longevity is continuing to increase over time and that a limit has not been reached yet [8]. Therefore, it is important to consider the unique characteristics of the oldest old and develop potential strategies to sustain and enhance their quality of life.

Commencing from the mid-twenties muscle mass and muscle strength decline through middle-age, particularly in habitually sedentary individuals [9–11]. This is initially a slow process, with a strength loss of approximately 10% per decade. Strength loss further accelerates after the age of 60 to 70 years. Thus, the oldest in our society have only 30–40% of their peak adult strength. Putative cellular mechanisms of ageing include oxidative stress, chronic low-grade inflammation/impaired immune function, increased macromolecular damage and genomic instability, cellular senescence and reduced stress resistance [12–15]. However, malnutrition in the elderly is very common, with significant risk of micronutrient deficiencies [12–14,16]. It is likely then that malnutrition itself also exerts an impact on muscle loss.

Whilst all elements of dietary intake are critical for the maintenance of muscle mass, it is the regular adequate consumption of protein, that is essential to stimulate protein synthesis [17–19]. Current official nutritional recommendations for protein intake in the elderly vary between 0.8 g (see official WHO, US and UK guidelines) and 1.2 g/kg BW/day (e.g., guidelines from Nordic countries, Australia, New Zealand). However, there is recent evidence that in healthy elderly a higher intake of up to twice this amount could be beneficial, in the absence of side effects [17–20]. Studies to date have shown that a daily protein intake between 1.5 g up to 3 g (under special conditions)/kg BW/d is beneficial and safe in the elderly [21].

The purpose of this review is to analyse available evidence on protein intake for preserving muscle mass, strength and function in the very old. Further aims are to also identify opportunities to address knowledge gaps in this area. As yet, the exact protein needs for those aged 85 years and older has not been analysed in sufficient detail to allow formulation of nutritional guidelines. It then is important to review the current national and international recommendations for elderly (aged 70 years and above) and the position stands by varying expert groups, in order to identify if these recommendations are applicable to the very oldest in the community. Further, possible behavioural strategies that can be targeted to assist in successfully increasing protein intake in the oldest old will be examined.

2. Protein Recommendations for Elderly Humans

The global recommendations for daily protein intake, as proposed by the World Health Organization (WHO), is 0.8 g/kg BW/day, equally for all age groups and regardless of gender, physical activity or health status [22]. These recommendations were published in 2007 and have not been updated since. This position is then based on publications from the 1980s and 90s, with relatively small sample sizes, particularly in individuals aged over 70, with protein-balance methods likely underestimating protein requirements [23].

2.1. Global versus National Recommendations

Compared to the "one-for-all" recommendations for protein intake by the WHO, many countries have revised and increased protein intake recommendations for the elderly. Yet the guidelines of the US and the UK remain similar to the WHO, with the recommendation that a protein intake of 0.8 g/kg BW/d is sufficient for all age-groups [24]. This differs from what has now been adopted in many other countries. The Australian recommended dietary intake (RDI) for protein for people aged 65 years and older is about 25% higher, than the recommendations for younger adults. Their general recommendations for healthy elderly is to consume 1.1–1.2 g/kg BW/day of protein, with greater protein required during periods of increased physical activity (endurance and/or resistance exercise) and in the presence of acute or chronic diseases [24]. The recently updated

Nordic Nutrition Recommendations also suggest a slightly higher protein intake of 1.1–1.3 g/kg BW/day for healthy older adults [25]. Yet other countries, including the nutritional guidelines in German speaking countries (Austria, Germany, Switzerland), revised and only slightly increased protein recommendations from 0.8 g to 1.0 g/kg BW/day for healthy elderly [26]. There is therefore a wide range of protein recommendations for the elderly, from the lowest 0.83 g/kg BW/day to the highest of 1.3 g/kg BW/day (61% greater daily intake) highlighting the marked discrepancies that exist. Importantly, none of these national recommendations specifically address the possible protein requirements of the very old.

2.2. What Experts Are Saying

Over the last decade, a number of expert groups have reviewed available data and made recommendations for the nutritional needs of older persons. Most expert groupings broadly agree that existing official recommendations might underestimate the physiological protein needs of the elderly. These opinions are influenced by recent RCTs from elderly cohorts, combined with the data generated using the latest methods to determine protein requirements [23].

The nutritional recommendations for the treatment and/or prevention of sarcopenia, formulated by the Society for Sarcopenia, Cachexia and Wasting Disease (SCWD), recommend a protein intake of at least 1.0–1.5 g/kg BW/day in combination with adequate exercise as a key concept to prevent the loss of muscle mass and function with age [27]. Their multifactorial suggestions, including exercise, nutrition, specific nutrients, nutritional supplements and medical drugs, are based on a large literature review conducted and evaluated by experts.

The European Union Geriatric Medicine Society (EUGMS) invited experts from other groups/societies, including the International Association of Gerontology and Geriatrics-European Region (IAGG-ER), the International Association of Nutrition and Aging (IANA) and the Australian and New Zealand Society for Geriatric Medicine (ANZSGM), to establish the basis of the PROT-AGE study group [28]. In the context of increased emphasis on physical activity, the EUGMS recommend a protein intake of 1.2 g/kg BW/day or higher to enhance their physical function and health status and reduce risks for early mortality. This opinion is similarly shared by the European Society for Clinical Nutrition and Metabolism (ESPEN) Expert group which recommend the consumption of 1.0–1.2 g/kg BW/day of protein for healthy elderly (65+ years) and a further increased intake to 1.2–1.5 g/kg BW/day when people are chronically ill or malnourished [20].

As physical activity and therefore muscle strength and mass also contribute to the prevention of osteoporosis, the European Society for Clinical and Economic Aspects of Osteoporosis and Osteoarthritis (ESCEO) have also formulated a consensus statement regarding musculoskeletal health, including recommendations for protein intake. A dietary protein intake of 1.0–1.2 g/kg BW/day is recommended by ESCEO for the elderly. However, these suggestions were limited to postmenopausal women [29].

One of the major concerns against the adequacy of current protein recommendations is that these guidelines are based on the nitrogen-balance method, which has been shown to possibly drastically underestimate protein requirements [23,30]. The Indicator Amino Acid Oxidation (IAAO) approach and its variation, the 24h-IAAO and balance (24h-IAAO/IAAB) model, are minimally invasive methods to measure protein requirements in nearly all age-groups [23]. These techniques have demonstrated, that the current recommendations may be underestimating the actual requirements by 30–50%, especially in the elderly [19,23,30].

Although expert groupings have in the past few years focused on the possible protein needs of active, unwell and sarcopenic elderly, their considerations and recommendations to date have not differentiated between the old (65+ years) and the very old (85+ years).

2.3. Protein Consumption in Very Old Humans

Studies investigating dietary characteristics and nutrients intake of the very old (85+ years) are scarce and to date the limited evidence is only from Europe and Asia (Japan and China) [31–36]. The largest and most comprehensive study is the Newcastle 85+ Study, which has evaluated nutritional intake of over 700 individuals aged 85 years old. Overall dietary protein intake was reported to be approximately 1.0 g/kg BW/day, with men (1.04 g/kg BW/day) consuming more protein than the women (0.86 g/kg BW/day) [35]. Interestingly, however, 28% of the study participants had protein intakes below the WHO recommendation (<0.8 g/kg BW/day), which was associated with lower physical function and strength, in comparison to those consuming more protein (>1.0 g/kg BW/day) [34].

Similar conclusions have been established in studies examining well-being in China and Japan. Again, there was positive associations between frequent protein intake (fish, meat, egg, soybean derived products) and physical function, independent living, with higher survival rates and better self-rated health [31–33]. Interestingly, however, in one study a higher protein intake was associated with increased mortality [36]. Table 1 summarizes available studies linking protein intake with physical function and health parameters in elderly 80 years old or older.

In a recent review, Granic et al. [37] identified eight studies with data from nutritional surveys in elderly cohorts including very old participants aged 80 years and older. Collectively these studies showed comparable data regarding protein intake with about 15–16% of total energy from protein, which equals 0.8–1.0 g protein per kg bodyweight per day.

Table 1. Available studies on the oldest old with extracted results linking dietary protein intake with physical function and health parameter.

Study	Participants (N)	Age (years)	Nationality	Main Outcome for Protein
Newcastle 85+ Study [34,35]	793	85	UK	Protein intake over 1 g/kg adjusted BW/day was associated with better grip strength and timed-up-and-go performance compared to a lower intake; physically active elderly had higher protein intake than sedentary.
The Septuagenarians, Octogenarians, Nonagenarians Investigation with Centenarians Study [31]	629	80+	Japan	A slower walking speed was associated with a lower occlusion force and both linked to a lower protein intake.
The Japanese Centenarian Study [32]	1907	101.1 ± 1.5	Japan	A more frequent protein consumption was associated with autonomously living centenarians.
The Chinese Longitudinal Healthy Longevity Survey I [36]	8959	90.1 ± 6.9 (men) 93.8 ± 7.7 (women)	China	High frequency intake of protein rich foods (fish, bean and eggs) were associated with increased mortality. Physical activity was beneficial for preventing pre-mature death.
The Chinese Longitudinal Healthy Longevity Survey II [33]	7273	80+	China	Frequent consumption of meat, fish egg, soy products, fruit, vegetable, tea and garlic was linked to higher survival and better self-rated health

Acknowledging these data, as well as the steadily increasing age of the human population, it should be of general interest to review and critically challenge general recommendation regarding protein intake, requirements and factors influencing muscle metabolism in the ageing process.

3. Muscle Protein Synthetic Response to Protein Ingestion in Young and Older Adults

Evidence that protein requirements with ageing might be greater than many recommendations is largely based on experimental data on protein metabolism in skeletal muscle in young versus older individuals. Central for the notion of greater protein requirements in the elderly is the demonstration of impairments in the muscle protein synthesis (MPS) in response to protein intake in elderly as compared with young adults [19,38]. In this context, it is important to note that the progressive decline of muscle mass with ageing ultimately results from an imbalance between MPS and muscle protein breakdown (MPB), regardless of the mechanisms that are discussed to contribute to sarcopenia [39–41]. The proposed reduction in the muscle protein synthetic response to protein or amino acid ingestion in older adults, also known as age-related anabolic resistance, is therefore a critical aspect with wide-ranging implications for physiological function and health of older humans.

Protein/amino acid-based food intake and muscle contractions (i.e., resistance and endurance exercise) are the main physiological anabolic stimuli for MPS [39]. The ingestion of protein/amino acids increases MPS. While our understanding on MPB is limited due to methodological complexities, protein/amino acid ingestion also suppresses MPB in most studies [41]. This then results in a greater positive net protein balance. Furthermore, as discussed below, the combination of protein intake and exercise acts synergistically on skeletal muscle anabolism, thus improving net muscle protein accreditation [39,41].

Most of the experimental studies that compared MPS responses between young and old individuals involved only short-term dietary and/or exercise interventions (i.e., protein/amino acid ingestion, exercise, or both). Furthermore, none of these intervention studies have specifically investigated very old individuals. Nevertheless, these experimental trials provide important information on potential age-related differences in skeletal muscle anabolism. In a systematic review, Shad et al. [41] examined experimental studies that compared the muscle protein synthetic response to anabolic stimuli between young and older individuals by using tracer technology and calculation of the muscle fractional synthetic rate. Twenty-one studies were included for the data synthesis that investigated the MPS response to protein/amino acid intake as the only anabolic stimulus. Of these 21 studies, only eight provided sufficient evidence of age-related muscle anabolic resistance. However, when the studies used for this systematic review were pooled together, the authors noted that the magnitude of the MPS response was 28% lower in older compared with younger individuals.

Previous dose-response studies in healthy young individuals demonstrated that 20 g of high-quality protein is sufficient to maximize MPS rates during recovery from lower-body resistance exercise [42,43]. Moore et al. [40] retrospectively analysed data from their own studies that measured dose-dependent MPS responses to protein as single bolus in healthy older (~71 years) and younger adults (~22 years). These data suggest that the relative (to body weight) amount of protein required to maximally stimulate MPS is ~0.4 g/kg in older adults, as compared with ~0.24 g/kg in the young [40]. In support of this finding, Shad et al. [41] reported that four of five studies that provided ≥0.4 g/kg of amino acids/protein did not provide sufficient evidence of muscle anabolic resistance in older age. The picture that emerges from these findings is that skeletal muscle of older individuals does not lack the capacity for inducing a robust MPS response to protein ingestion but rather is less efficient. In other words, higher relative protein intake is required to maximally stimulate MPS in older adults [19,38,40].

To address the question of whether a higher protein intake is effective in maintaining muscle mass in older individuals, our own group has recently investigated the effects of a controlled diet containing either 0.8 or 1.6 g protein/kg BM/d on muscle mass and function [21]. The data from this 10-week parallel-group randomized trial involving 29 men aged >70 years, show that consuming a diet providing 1.6 as compared with 0.8 g protein/kg/d increased whole-body lean mass and improved leg power.

4. Estimated Protein Requirements in Old versus Very Old Individuals Based on Whole-Body Measurements

Importantly, however, the lack of intervention studies in very old individuals precludes us from drawing firm conclusions on whether MPS responses in the oldest old (aged ≥85 years) are different from than that of younger groups of older adults. A limited number of metabolic studies that used the minimally invasive indicator amino acid oxidation (IAAO) technique suggest that protein requirements for older women and men aged 65–87 years are in a range between 1.2–1.3 g protein/kg BM/d [30,44,45]. As compared with the studies that involved six men aged 71.3 ± 4.5 years [45] and 12 women aged 74.3 ± 7.4 [44] (for both, means ± SD), no substantial differences were observed in six women aged 82 ± 1 years (means ± SEM) [30]. An obvious limitation when comparing these studies is the relatively small sample sizes. Despite the complexities associated with muscle biopsies particularly in the vulnerable group of very old adults, muscle measurements may be required to examine MPS responses to protein ingestion in the oldest old.

5. Effect of Exercise on the Muscle Protein Synthetic Response to Protein Ingestion

A potential key strategy for improving the muscle protein synthetic response in the elderly is performing exercise in close temporal proximity to high-quality protein intake. It is a relatively consistent finding that the combined stimulus of acute exercise with protein/amino acid ingestion synergistically enhances MPS responses above rates observed to protein administration alone in young and older adults [41]. In agreement with this concept, Shad et al. [41] reported that eight of ten reviewed studies that investigated MPS responses to combined exercise and protein/amino acid provision did not provide evidence of muscle anabolic resistance in the older individuals.

In a study by Pennings et al. [46], 24 young (aged 21 ± 1 years) and 24 older individuals (aged 73 ± 1 years) were investigated after the ingestion of 20 g of protein at rest and during recovery from combined endurance and resistance-type exercise. In contrast to other studies suggesting that the muscle protein synthetic response to amino acid administration is reduced in older individuals [41], MPS did not differ between older and younger individuals. The authors observed a greater plasma insulin response and a more rapid increase in postprandial plasma amino acid concentration in the elderly that might represent a compensatory mechanism to preserve a robust postprandial MPS response and as such, could be regarded as an early indication of anabolic resistance at rest [46]. Importantly, postprandial MPS rates were higher after exercise than compared with resting conditions in both age groups [46]. This finding supports the notion that exercising before protein intake promotes postprandial muscle protein accretion independent of age [38,39,47]. While some data suggest that a certain "threshold" in exercise intensity and/or volume is required to overcome the age-related blunting of MPS [41], other findings have shown that even moderate exercise increases the muscle anabolic response to protein intake in older adults [48]. Another factor that might explain inconsistent results is the assessed time frame [41]. For example, Drummond et al. [49] reported that MPS following resistance exercise and ingestion of essential amino acids increased in young men at 1–3 h and at 3–6 h post exercise but only during the 3–6 h post exercise period in older men. This might suggest that the acute MPS response after exercise and essential amino acid ingestion is delayed rather than attenuated with advancing age [49,50].

Data on the long-term combined effects of regular exercise training and protein intake in older adults are limited and studies with very old individuals are lacking. There is some evidence suggesting that protein supplementation enhances adaptive responses of skeletal muscle to (resistance) training in healthy and frail older adults [51,52]. However, this does not automatically suggest that an additional protein intake cannot be achieved through the natural diet and protein-rich foods [38]. More long-term studies are warranted to determine the impact of exercise on protein requirements in older adults and in particular, in the very old.

Whilst anabolic sensitivity improves with physical activity, physical inactivity induces an anabolic resistance. In a relatively modest reduction in daily step-count for 14 days, in 10 healthy older men and women (aged 72 ± 1 years), the resulting reduction in postprandial MPS was a contributing factor to the significant loss of muscle mass [53]. With more severe immobilization, using a 7-day bed rest study in healthy older adults, the reduction in postprandial MPS was accompanied by attenuated anabolic cell signalling and muscle amino acid transporter expression [54].

The question that emerges in perspective of these findings is to which extent the proposed "age-related" muscle anabolic resistance is a consequence of the inherent biological ageing process. Rather it seems reasonable to suggest that impairments in the anabolic responsiveness of skeletal muscle of older adults, at least in part, are due to reduced levels of physical activity. Potential mechanisms underlying muscle anabolic resistance in old persons include impaired protein digestion and amino acid absorption resulting in a reduced availability of dietary protein-derived amino acids in the circulation, impaired muscle perfusion reducing amino acid delivery to the muscle, reduced uptake of amino acids by the muscle and impaired anabolic signalling in the muscle [19,39]. At least some of these mechanisms such as blood flow and oxygen/nutrient delivery in skeletal muscle in older adults can be preserved (or restored) through exercise training [55]. This further supports the hypothetical concept that physical inactivity, rather than the ageing process alone, contributes to muscle anabolic resistance with older age.

There is strong evidence that regular physical activity/exercise training contributes to maintaining function of different physiological systems, particularly of skeletal muscle, during ageing, even until very old age [56,57]. Hypothetically, regular physical activity might, to a certain extent, also preserve the sensitivity of skeletal muscle to anabolic stimuli with advancing age.

It is important to note that the adaptability of skeletal muscle in very advanced age differs from that of late middle-aged/older adults, partially due to impaired up-regulation of molecular pathways underlying metabolic and functional adaptations [58]. Studies in men aged 82 ± 1 years [59] and women aged 85 ± 1 years [60] show that skeletal muscle remodelling and plasticity in response to resistance training were limited. However, more recent comparative data from the same laboratory also suggest single muscle fibre quality improvements in octogenarians [61]. The authors concluded that the improved quality of remaining single muscle fibres may be a compensatory mechanism to help offset decrements in whole muscle function [61]. Another conclusion that might be drawn from these findings is that efforts to maintain skeletal muscle mass and function with ageing should begin before very old age. Whether specifically the anabolic sensitivity of skeletal muscle of the very old is different from groups of younger older adults and to which extent this is modulated by regular physical activity needs to be addressed in future research.

6. Effect of Protein Quality, Intake Patterns and the Protein Distribution Throughout the Day

In addition to the synergistic effects of exercise, the protein quality is a key determinant that contributes to the potential of dietary protein for skeletal muscle anabolism with ageing [38]. Important factors that have an impact on the quality and anabolic potential of dietary protein include the amino acid composition, digestibility and amino acid availability [38]. Similar as in young adults [62], whey protein stimulated postprandial protein accreditation in healthy older men more effectively than casein or casein hydrolysate [46]. This effect has been attributed to a combination of faster digestion, absorption kinetics, postprandial amino acid availability and higher leucine content of whey [46]. The leucine content of dietary protein has been shown to be a critical factor in this context, due to the role of leucine as a potent activator of anabolic signalling in skeletal muscle [63]. In many previous studies, isolated amino acids or protein were provided to assess postprandial MPS [41]. More recent investigations have adopted a more natural dietary approach by focusing on the potential of protein-rich whole foods to promote muscle protein anabolism in older individuals [38]. For example, it was shown that minced beef was more rapidly digested and absorbed than beefsteak in older men, which resulted in an increased amino acid availability and a greater whole-body protein balance [64]. This shows the relevance of the matrix of protein sources (such as the food texture) for postprandial protein metabolism and retention particularly in older adults. Furthermore, the consumption of a liquid protein-based meal elicited a more rapid and greater increase in plasma amino acid concentration compared with a solid macronutrient-matched test meal in older adults [65]. Liquid protein foods, such as milk and yoghurt, are therefore considered as effective sources of high quality protein for older and likely also, for very old adults [66]. While plant-based proteins are considered less anabolic, partly due to their lower content of essential amino acids and leucine, an adequate protein intake can still be achieved by consuming plant-based diets or a combination of plant and animal protein sources [19,38,66]. The consumption of multiple plant and animal protein whole-food sources provides a broad variety of macro- and micronutrients, fibre, plant bioactive compounds and so forth, all of which might be particularly important for individuals aged ≥85 years [37,66]. However, more research is needed to compare the anabolic effects of plant- versus animal-based protein in older and very old adults. Additional aspects concerning protein quality and the particular importance of leucine have been covered in other reviews [38,63,67].

In this review, we rather focus on the distribution of the daily protein intake that has recently received increased interest as an important factor in enhancing the potential for skeletal muscle anabolism in older adults. In accordance with the concept that a certain threshold of ingested protein is required to maximize the acute muscle protein synthetic response, recent studies have indicated that the amount of the protein intake with each of the main meals may play a significant role in counteracting sarcopenia [38,68–70].

In a crossover study in young adults, a greater 24-h muscle protein synthesis was observed after a 7-d diet with an even (i.e., 32, 30 and 33 g protein with breakfast, lunch and dinner, respectively) compared with a skewed intake (i.e., 11, 16 and 63 g protein/meal) [68]. Farsijani et al. [69,70] used data from older adults aged 67 to 84 years enrolled in a longitudinal study to examine whether this short-term result translate into preservation of lean mass and physical performance with ageing. The findings of these longitudinal studies suggest that an even protein intake distribution across meals was associated with higher muscle mass and greater muscle strength in older women and men [69,70]. While there are also conflicting results [71], the available data collectively suggest that a balanced distribution of adequate amounts of protein intake is the most favourable for muscle protein anabolism [68–70,72]. It is also important to note, that an optimal per-meal amount of dietary protein to maximally stimulate MPS in older adults (~0.4 g/kg/meal) can only be achieved at higher daily protein intakes (i.e., ca. 1.2 g/kg BW/day) [19].

There are no studies investigating the daily protein intake distribution in the very old (85+ years). Based on the limited data comparing old and very old adults by using the IAAO technique [30,44,45], we can only speculate that the oldest old would benefit from the same distribution and daily amount of protein as younger elderly.

7. Conclusions

The numbers of elderly and exceptionally long-lived people is steadily increasing. Based on a raising body of evidence from both epidemiological and experimental data, several expert groups have argued that higher protein intake of at least 1.0 g to 1.5 g/kg BW/day may be optimal for skeletal muscle and overall health in older adults [19,38]. Importantly, the age range of older participants in these physiological intervention studies was ~65 to 80 years [37]. There is a lack of data to conclude, whether for example the dose-dependent relationship between protein ingestion and MPS rates in very old differ from those observed in younger groups of older adults. More studies that include study participants aged ≥85 years are warranted to investigate and determine protein requirements in this population group.

Additional research is also required to verify the hypothetical concept that "age-related" anabolic resistance represents a combination of the ageing process interacting with the detrimental effects of inactivity. The metabolic and functional adaptability of skeletal muscle of older individuals aged between 65 and 75 years is different to individuals over 75 years [58]. Available data in octogenarians suggest that muscular adaptations to resistance training might be limited at a very old age [59,60]. However, the superior skeletal muscle and cardiovascular profiles of even octogenarian endurance athletes show that life-long exercise training provides a large functional reserve above the aerobic frailty threshold and is associated with lower risk for disability and mortality [56]. Furthermore, evidence from prospective exercise intervention trials in late middle-aged/older adults suggests that increasing physical activity later in life can preserve or even restore physiological function with ageing [15]. Regular exercise training may therefore also preserve the responsiveness of ageing skeletal muscle to protein intake, possibly up to a very advanced age. In this context, it should be noted that the proposed protein requirements for structural exercise training in young and middle-aged adults are in a similar range as those that are currently discussed for older adults, that is, $\geq$1.2 g protein/kg BW/d [20,73–75].

It is also important to note that many elderly could have difficulties in optimizing/increasing dietary protein intake and physical exercise. Dietary adherence might be negatively influenced by oral health problems, altered sensory function, reduced thirst sensation, as well as gastrointestinal malfunction [76]. Considering that adherence to fitness enhancing exercise is generally poor in people older than 80 years, previous and acute injuries might initially cause (more) pain when starting exercise programs, could be a large negative motivator and impede voluntary implementation of healthy ageing strategies [77]. It therefore remains critical to develop innovative, evidence-based, more effective and feasible lifestyle-behavioural approaches for old and very old adults to facilitate adopting and maintaining function- and health-preserving strategies [15].

The assertions about possible detrimental health effects of a diet high(er) in protein—for example, development of kidney dysfunction, impaired bone health—are, however, not supported by clinical data in humans [78]. Only in patients with pre-existing kidney dysfunction a high protein intake is associated with accelerated deterioration in renal health [19]. Moreover, an increased protein intake is positively associated with bone health [78], which is also supported by the guidelines of the ESCEO suggesting at least 1.0–1–2 g/kg BW/day to prevent osteopenia and osteoporosis [29]. A protein consumption of up to 2 g/kg BW/day and even higher seems to be safe for healthy adults and elderly [79]. Still there is a lack of data in very old humans.

Taken together, the data reviewed for this article support the notion that there is a close interaction of physical activity, diet, function and human ageing. Optimizing the timing and distribution of protein ingestion, with an intake of at least ~25–30 g protein per meal and in close temporal proximity to exercise/physical activity, appears to be a promising strategy for promoting healthy ageing of skeletal muscle in the elderly and likely also in the oldest old, aged 85 years and older.

Author Contributions: B.F. and O.N. equally contributed to conceptualizing and writing the manuscript. K.-H.W. and D.C.-S. edited and revised manuscript. B.F., O.N., K.-H.W. and D.C.-S. approved the final version of manuscript.

Funding: This research was funded by the European Regional Development Fund (INTERREG SK-AT, NutriAging) and the Open Access Publishing Fund of the University of Vienna.

Conflicts of Interest: The authors declare no conflict of interest.

References

1. Janssen, I.; Heymsfield, S.B.; Ross, R. Low relative skeletal muscle mass (sarcopenia) in older persons is associated with functional impairment and physical disability. *J. Am. Geriatr. Soc.* **2002**, *50*, 889–896. [CrossRef] [PubMed]
2. Mesquita, A.F.; Silva, E.C.D.; Eickemberg, M.; Roriz, A.K.C.; Barreto-Medeiros, J.M.; Ramos, L.B. Factors associated with sarcopenia in institutionalized elderly. *Nutr. Hosp.* **2017**, *34*, 345–351. [CrossRef] [PubMed]
3. Narici, M.V.; Maffulli, N. Sarcopenia. Characteristics, mechanisms and functional significance. *Br. Med. Bull.* **2010**, *95*, 139–159. [CrossRef] [PubMed]
4. Short, K.R.; Bigelow, M.L.; Kahl, J.; Singh, R.; Coenen-Schimke, J.; Raghavakaimal, S.; Nair, K.S. Decline in skeletal muscle mitochondrial function with aging in humans. *Proc. Natl. Acad. Sci. USA* **2005**, *102*, 5618–5623. [CrossRef] [PubMed]
5. Johnston, A.P.; De Lisio, M.; Parise, G. Resistance training, sarcopenia and the mitochondrial theory of aging. *Appl. Physiol. Nutr. Metab.* **2008**, *33*, 191–199. [CrossRef] [PubMed]

6. Christensen, K.; Doblhammer, G.; Rau, R.; Vaupel, J.W. Ageing populations: The challenges ahead. *Lancet.* **2009**, *374*, 1196–1208. [CrossRef]
7. Global Health and Aging. 2011. Available online: http://www.who.int/ageing/publications/global_health.pdf (accessed on 15 July 2018).
8. Barbi, E.; Lagona, F.; Marsili, M.; Vaupel, J.W.; Wachter, K.W. The plateau of human mortality: Demography of longevity pioneers. *Science* **2018**, *360*, 1459–1461. [CrossRef] [PubMed]
9. Lee, W.S.; Cheung, W.H.; Qin, L.; Tang, N.; Leung, K.S. Age-associated decrease of type iia/b human skeletal muscle fibres. *Clin. Orthop. Relat. Res.* **2006**, *450*, 231–237. [CrossRef] [PubMed]
10. Janssen, I.; Heymsfield, S.B.; Wang, Z.M.; Ross, R. Skeletal muscle mass and distribution in 468 men and women aged 18–88 yr. *J. Appl. Physiol. (1985)* **2000**, *89*, 81–88. [CrossRef] [PubMed]
11. Rogers, M.A.; Evans, W.J. Changes in skeletal muscle with aging: Effects of exercise training. *Exerc. Sport Sci. Rev.* **1993**, *21*, 65–102. [CrossRef] [PubMed]
12. Wagner, K.H.; Cameron-Smith, D.; Wessner, B.; Franzke, B. Biomarkers of aging: From function to molecular biology. *Nutrients* **2016**, *8*, 338. [CrossRef] [PubMed]
13. Song, Z.; von Figura, G.; Liu, Y.; Kraus, J.M.; Torrice, C.; Dillon, P.; Rudolph-Watabe, M.; Ju, Z.; Kestler, H.A.; Sanoff, H.; et al. Lifestyle impacts on the aging-associated expression of biomarkers of DNA damage and telomere dysfunction in human blood. *Aging Cell.* **2010**, *9*, 607–615. [CrossRef] [PubMed]
14. Ornish, D.; Lin, J.; Daubenmier, J.; Weidner, G.; Epel, E.; Kemp, C.; Magbanua, M.J.; Marlin, R.; Yglecias, L.; Carroll, P.R.; et al. Increased telomerase activity and comprehensive lifestyle changes: A pilot study. *Lancet Oncol.* **2008**, *9*, 1048–1057. [CrossRef]
15. Seals, D.R.; Justice, J.N.; LaRocca, T.J. Physiological geroscience: Targeting function to increase healthspan and achieve optimal longevity. *J. Physiol.* **2016**, *594*, 2001–2024. [CrossRef] [PubMed]
16. Smoliner, C.; Norman, K.; Wagner, K.H.; Hartig, W.; Lochs, H.; Pirlich, M. Malnutrition and depression in the institutionalised elderly. *Br. J. Nutr.* **2009**, *102*, 1663–1667. [CrossRef] [PubMed]
17. Phillips, S.M.; Chevalier, S.; Leidy, H.J. Protein "requirements" beyond the RDA: Implications for optimizing health. *Appl. Physiol. Nutr. Metab.* **2016**, *41*, 565–572. [CrossRef] [PubMed]
18. Lonnie, M.; Hooker, E.; Brunstrom, J.M.; Corfe, B.M.; Green, M.A.; Watson, A.W.; Williams, E.A.; Stevenson, E.J.; Penson, S.; Johnstone, A.M. Protein for life: Review of optimal protein intake, sustainable dietary sources and the effect on appetite in ageing adults. *Nutrients* **2018**, *10*, 360. [CrossRef] [PubMed]
19. Traylor, D.A.; Gorissen, S.H.M.; Phillips, S.M. Perspective: Protein requirements and optimal intakes in aging: Are we ready to recommend more than the recommended daily allowance? *Adv. Nutr.* **2018**, *9*, 171–182. [CrossRef] [PubMed]
20. Deutz, N.E.; Bauer, J.M.; Barazzoni, R.; Biolo, G.; Boirie, Y.; Bosy-Westphal, A.; Cederholm, T.; Cruz-Jentoft, A.; Krznariç, Z.; Nair, K.S.; et al. Protein intake and exercise for optimal muscle function with aging: Recommendations from the ESPEN Expert Group. *Clin. Nutr.* **2014**, *33*, 929–936. [CrossRef] [PubMed]
21. Mitchell, C.J.; Milan, A.M.; Mitchell, S.M.; Zeng, N.; Ramzan, F.; Sharma, P.; Knowles, S.; Roy, N.; Sjödin, A.; Wagner, K.-H.; et al. The effects of dietary protein intake on appendicular lean mass and muscle function in elderly men: A 10 week randomized controlled trial. *Am. J. Clin. Nutr.* **2017**, *106*, 1375–1383. [CrossRef] [PubMed]
22. World Health Organization. *Protein and Amino Acid Requirements in Human Nutrition*, 935th ed.; World Health Organization: Geneva, Switzerland, 2007.
23. Elango, R.; Ball, R.O.; Pencharz, P.B. Recent advances in determining protein and amino acid requirements in humans. *Br. J. Nutr.* **2012**, *108* (Suppl. 2), S22–S30. [CrossRef] [PubMed]
24. Nowson, C.; O'Connell, S. Protein requirements and recommendations for older people: A review. *Nutrients* **2015**, *7*, 6874–6899. [CrossRef] [PubMed]
25. *Nordic Nutrition Recommendations 2012: Integrating Nutrition and Physical Activity*, 5th ed.; Nordic Council of Ministers: Copenhagen, Denmark, 2014; Available online: https://books.google.com.hk/books?hl=zhTW&lr=&id=9_MblCPv5GcC&oi=fnd&pg=PA9&dq=Nordic+nutrition+recommendations+2012:+Integrating+nutrition+and+physical+activity%EF%BC%9B2014&ots=M7h_ndbEcZ&sig=5xbHmrVGfrkkYeerPXaw5cfcZT0&redir_esc=y#v=onepage&q&f=falseg (accessed on 15 July 2018).
26. *D-A-CH Referenzwerte für die Nährstoffzufuhr*; Deutsche Gesellschaft für Ernährung, Österreichische Gesellschaft für Ernährung, Schweizerische Gesellschaft für Ernährung: Bonn, Germany, 2017; Volume 2, ISBN 978-3-86528-148-7.

27. Morley, J.E.; Argiles, J.M.; Evans, W.J.; Bhasin, S.; Cella, D.; Deutz, N.E.; Doehner, W.; Fearon, K.C.; Ferrucci, L.; Hellerstein, M.K.; et al. Nutritional recommendations for the management of sarcopenia. *J. Am. Med. Dir. Assoc.* **2010**, *11*, 391–396. [CrossRef] [PubMed]
28. Bauer, J.; Biolo, G.; Cederholm, T.; Cesari, M.; Cruz-Jentoft, A.J.; Morley, J.E.; Phillips, S.; Sieber, C.; Stehle, P.; Teta, D.; et al. Evidence-based recommendations for optimal dietary protein intake in older people: A position paper from the PROT-AGE Study Group. *J. Am. Med. Dir. Assoc.* **2013**, *14*, 542–559. [CrossRef] [PubMed]
29. Rizzoli, R.; Stevenson, J.C.; Bauer, J.M.; van Loon, L.J.; Walrand, S.; Kanis, J.A.; Cooper, C.; Brandi, M.L.; Diez-Perez, A.; Reginster, J.Y.; et al. The role of dietary protein and vitamin d in maintaining musculoskeletal health in postmenopausal women: A consensus statement from the European society for clinical and economic aspects of osteoporosis and osteoarthritis (ESCEO). *Maturitas* **2014**, *79*, 122–132. [CrossRef] [PubMed]
30. Tang, M.; McCabe, G.P.; Elango, R.; Pencharz, P.B.; Ball, R.O.; Campbell, W.W. Assessment of protein requirement in octogenarian women with use of the indicator amino acid oxidation technique. *Am. J. Clin. Nutr.* **2014**, *99*, 891–898. [CrossRef] [PubMed]
31. Okada, T.; Ikebe, K.; Kagawa, R.; Inomata, C.; Takeshita, H.; Gondo, Y.; Ishioka, Y.; Okubo, H.; Kamide, K.; Masui, Y.; et al. Lower protein intake mediates association between lower occlusal force and slower walking speed: From the septuagenarians, octogenarians, nonagenarians investigation with centenarians study. *J. Am. Geriatr. Soc.* **2015**, *63*, 2382–2387. [CrossRef] [PubMed]
32. Ozaki, A.; Uchiyama, M.; Tagaya, H.; Ohida, T.; Ogihara, R. The japanese centenarian study: Autonomy was associated with health practices as well as physical status. *J. Am. Geriatr. Soc.* **2007**, *55*, 95–101. [CrossRef] [PubMed]
33. An, R.; Xiang, X.; Liu, J.; Guan, C. Diet and self-rated health among oldest-old Chinese. *Arch. Gerontol. Geriatr.* **2018**, *76*, 125–132. [CrossRef] [PubMed]
34. Granic, A.; Mendonça, N.; Sayer, A.A.; Hill, T.R.; Davies, K.; Adamson, A.; Siervo, M.; Mathers, J.C.; Jagger, C. Low protein intake, muscle strength and physical performance in the very old: The Newcastle 85+ study. *Clin. Nutr.* **2017**. [CrossRef] [PubMed]
35. Mendonça, N.; Hill, T.R.; Granic, A.; Davies, K.; Collerton, J.; Mathers, J.C.; Siervo, M.; Wrieden, W.L.; Seal, C.J.; Kirkwood, T.B.; et al. Macronutrient intake and food sources in the very old: Analysis of the Newcastle 85+ study. *Br. J. Nutr.* **2016**, *115*, 2170–2180. [CrossRef] [PubMed]
36. Shi, Z.; Zhang, T.; Byles, J.; Martin, S.; Avery, J.C.; Taylor, A.W. Food habits, lifestyle factors and mortality among oldest old Chinese: The Chinese longitudinal healthy longevity survey (CLHLS). *Nutrients* **2015**, *7*, 7562–7579. [CrossRef] [PubMed]
37. Granic, A.; Mendonça, N.; Hill, T.R.; Jagger, C.; Stevenson, E.J.; Mathers, J.C.; Sayer, A.A. Nutrition in the very old. *Nutrients* **2018**, *10*, 269. [CrossRef] [PubMed]
38. Paddon-Jones, D.; Campbell, W.W.; Jacques, P.F.; Kritchevsky, S.B.; Moore, L.L.; Rodriguez, N.R.; van Loon, L.J. Protein and healthy aging. *Am. J. Clin. Nutr.* **2015**. [CrossRef] [PubMed]
39. Burd, N.A.; Gorissen, S.H.; van Loon, L.J. Anabolic resistance of muscle protein synthesis with aging. *Exerc. Sport Sci. Rev.* **2013**, *41*, 169–173. [CrossRef] [PubMed]
40. Moore, D.R.; Churchward-Venne, T.A.; Witard, O.; Breen, L.; Burd, N.A.; Tipton, K.D.; Phillips, S.M. Protein ingestion to stimulate myofibrillar protein synthesis requires greater relative protein intakes in healthy older versus younger men. *J. Gerontol. A Biol. Sci. Med. Sci.* **2015**, *70*, 57–62. [CrossRef] [PubMed]
41. Shad, B.J.; Thompson, J.L.; Breen, L. Does the muscle protein synthetic response to exercise and amino acid-based nutrition diminish with advancing age? A systematic review. *Am. J. Physiol. Endocrinol. Metab.* **2016**, *311*, E803–E817. [CrossRef] [PubMed]
42. Moore, D.R.; Robinson, M.J.; Fry, J.L.; Tang, J.E.; Glover, E.I.; Wilkinson, S.B.; Prior, T.; Tarnopolsky, M.A.; Phillips, S.M. Ingested protein dose response of muscle and albumin protein synthesis after resistance exercise in young men. *Am. J. Clin. Nutr.* **2009**, *89*, 161–168. [CrossRef] [PubMed]
43. Witard, O.C.; Jackman, S.R.; Breen, L.; Smith, K.; Selby, A.; Tipton, K.D. Myofibrillar muscle protein synthesis rates subsequent to a meal in response to increasing doses of whey protein at rest and after resistance exercise. *Am. J. Clin. Nutr.* **2014**, *99*, 86–95. [CrossRef] [PubMed]
44. Rafii, M.; Chapman, K.; Owens, J.; Elango, R.; Campbell, W.W.; Ball, R.O.; Pencharz, P.B.; Courtney-Martin, G. Dietary protein requirement of female adults >65 years determined by the indicator amino acid oxidation technique is higher than current recommendations. *J. Nutr.* **2015**, *145*, 18–24. [CrossRef] [PubMed]

45. Rafii, M.; Chapman, K.; Elango, R.; Campbell, W.W.; Ball, R.O.; Pencharz, P.B.; Courtney-Martin, G. Dietary protein requirement of men >65 years old determined by the indicator amino acid oxidation technique is higher than the current estimated average requirement. *J. Nutr.* **2016**, *46*. [CrossRef] [PubMed]
46. Pennings, B.; Koopman, R.; Beelen, M.; Senden, J.M.; Saris, W.H.; van Loon, L.J. Exercising before protein intake allows for greater use of dietary protein-derived amino acids for de novo muscle protein synthesis in both young and elderly men. *Am. J. Clin. Nutr.* **2011**, *93*, 322–331. [CrossRef] [PubMed]
47. Burd, N.A.; Tang, J.E.; Moore, D.R.; Phillips, S.M. Exercise training and protein metabolism: Influences of contraction, protein intake and sex-based differences. *J. Appl. Physiol. (1985)* **2009**, *106*, 1692–1701. [CrossRef] [PubMed]
48. Timmerman, K.L.; Dhanani, S.; Glynn, E.L.; Fry, C.S.; Drummond, M.J.; Jennings, K.; Rasmussen, B.B.; Volpi, E. A moderate acute increase in physical activity enhances nutritive flow and the muscle protein anabolic response to mixed nutrient intake in older adults. *Am. J. Clin. Nutr.* **2012**, *95*, 1403–1412. [CrossRef] [PubMed]
49. Drummond, M.J.; Miyazaki, M.; Dreyer, H.C.; Pennings, B.; Dhanani, S.; Volpi, E.; Esser, K.A.; Rasmussen, B.B. Expression of growth-related genes in young and older human skeletal muscle following an acute stimulation of protein synthesis. *J. Appl. Physiol. (1985)* **2009**, *106*, 1403–1411. [CrossRef] [PubMed]
50. Drummond, M.J.; McCarthy, J.J.; Fry, C.S.; Esser, K.A.; Rasmussen, B.B. Aging differentially affects human skeletal muscle microRNA expression at rest and after an anabolic stimulus of resistance exercise and essential amino acids. *Am. J. Physiol. Endocrinol. Metab.* **2008**, *295*, E1333–1340. [CrossRef] [PubMed]
51. Cermak, N.M.; Res, P.T.; de Groot, L.C.; Saris, W.H.; van Loon, L.J. Protein supplementation augments the adaptive response of skeletal muscle to resistance-type exercise training: A meta-analysis. *Am. J. Clin. Nutr.* **2012**, *96*, 1454–1464. [CrossRef] [PubMed]
52. Tieland, M.; van de Rest, O.; Dirks, M.L.; van der Zwaluw, N.; Mensink, M.; van Loon, L.J.; de Groot, L.C. Protein supplementation improves physical performance in frail elderly people: A randomized, double-blind, placebo-controlled trial. *J. Am. Med. Dir. Assoc.* **2012**, *13*, 720–726. [CrossRef] [PubMed]
53. Breen, L.; Stokes, K.A.; Churchward-Venne, T.A.; Moore, D.R.; Baker, S.K.; Smith, K.; Atherton, P.J.; Phillips, S.M. Two weeks of reduced activity decreases leg lean mass and induces "anabolic resistance" of myofibrillar protein synthesis in healthy elderly. *J. Clin. Endocrinol. Metab.* **2013**, *98*, 2604–2612. [CrossRef] [PubMed]
54. Drummond, M.J.; Dickinson, J.M.; Fry, C.S.; Walker, D.K.; Gundermann, D.M.; Reidy, P.T.; Timmerman, K.L.; Markofski, M.M.; Paddon-Jones, D.; Rasmussen, B.B.; et al. Bed rest impairs skeletal muscle amino acid transporter expression, mTORC1 signaling and protein synthesis in response to essential amino acids in older adults. *Am. J. Physiol. Endocrinol. Metab.* **2012**, *302*, E1113–1122. [CrossRef] [PubMed]
55. Nyberg, M.; Hellsten, Y. Reduced blood flow to contracting skeletal muscle in ageing humans: Is it all an effect of sand through the hourglass? *J. Physiol.* **2016**, *594*, 2297–2305. [CrossRef] [PubMed]
56. Trappe, S.; Hayes, E.; Galpin, A.; Kaminsky, L.; Jemiolo, B.; Fink, W.; Trappe, T.; Jansson, A.; Gustafsson, T.; Tesch, P. New records in aerobic power among octogenarian lifelong endurance athletes. *J. Appl. Physiol.* **2013**, *114*, 3–10. [CrossRef] [PubMed]
57. Harridge, S.D.; Lazarus, N.R. Physical activity, aging and physiological function. *Physiology* **2017**, *32*, 152–161. [CrossRef] [PubMed]
58. Cartee, G.D.; Hepple, R.T.; Bamman, M.M.; Zierath, J.R. Exercise promotes healthy aging of skeletal muscle. *Cell Metab.* **2016**, *23*, 1034–1047. [CrossRef] [PubMed]
59. Raue, U.; Slivka, D.; Minchev, K.; Trappe, S. Improvements in whole muscle and myocellular function are limited with high-intensity resistance training in octogenarian women. *J. Appl. Physiol. (1985)* **2009**, *106*, 1611–1617. [CrossRef] [PubMed]
60. Slivka, D.; Raue, U.; Hollon, C.; Minchev, K.; Trappe, S. Single muscle fiber adaptations to resistance training in old (>80 yr) men: Evidence for limited skeletal muscle plasticity. *Am. J. Physiol. Regul. Integr. Comp. Physiol.* **2008**, *295*, R273–R280. [CrossRef] [PubMed]
61. Grosicki, G.J.; Standley, R.A.; Murach, K.A.; Raue, U.; Minchev, K.; Coen, P.M.; Newman, A.B.; Cummings, S.; Harris, T.; Kritchevsky, S.; et al. Improved single muscle fiber quality in the oldest-old. *J. Appl. Physiol. (1985)* **2016**, *121*, 878–884. [CrossRef] [PubMed]

62. Tang, J.E.; Moore, D.R.; Kujbida, G.W.; Tarnopolsky, M.A.; Phillips, S.M. Ingestion of whey hydrolysate, casein, or soy protein isolate: Effects on mixed muscle protein synthesis at rest and following resistance exercise in young men. *J. Appl. Physiol. (1985)* **2009**, *107*, 987–992. [CrossRef] [PubMed]
63. Van Loon, L.J. Leucine as a pharmaconutrient in health and disease. *Curr. Opin. Clin. Nutr. Metab. Care* **2012**, *15*, 71–77. [CrossRef] [PubMed]
64. Pennings, B.; Groen, B.B.; van Dijk, J.W.; de Lange, A.; Kiskini, A.; Kuklinski, M.; Senden, J.M.; van Loon, L.J. Minced beef is more rapidly digested and absorbed than beef steak, resulting in greater postprandial protein retention in older men. *Am. J. Clin. Nutr.* **2013**, *98*, 121–128. [CrossRef] [PubMed]
65. Conley, T.B.; Apolzan, J.W.; Leidy, H.J.; Greaves, K.A.; Lim, E.; Campbell, W.W. Effect of food form on postprandial plasma amino acid concentrations in older adults. *Br. J. Nutr.* **2011**, *106*, 203–207. [CrossRef] [PubMed]
66. Vliet, S.V.; Beals, J.W.; Martinez, I.G.; Skinner, S.K.; Burd, N.A. Achieving optimal post-exercise muscle protein remodeling in physically active adults through whole food consumption. *Nutrients.* **2018**, *10*, 224. [CrossRef] [PubMed]
67. Van Vliet, S.; Burd, N.A.; van Loon, L.J. The skeletal muscle anabolic response to plant- versus animal-based protein consumption. *J. Nutr.* **2015**, *145*, 1981–1991. [CrossRef] [PubMed]
68. Mamerow, M.M.; Mettler, J.A.; English, K.L.; Casperson, S.L.; Arentson-Lantz, E.; Sheffield-Moore, M.; Layman, D.K.; Paddon-Jones, D. Dietary protein distribution positively influences 24-h muscle protein synthesis in healthy adults. *J. Nutr.* **2014**, *144*, 876–880. [CrossRef] [PubMed]
69. Farsijani, S.; Morais, J.A.; Payette, H.; Gaudreau, P.; Shatenstein, B.; Gray-Donald, K.; Chevalier, S. Relation between mealtime distribution of protein intake and lean mass loss in free-living older adults of the NuAge study. *Am. J. Clin. Nutr.* **2016**, *104*, 694–703. [CrossRef] [PubMed]
70. Farsijani, S.; Payette, H.; Morais, J.A.; Shatenstein, B.; Gaudreau, P.; Chevalier, S. Even mealtime distribution of protein intake is associated with greater muscle strength but not with 3-y physical function decline, in free-living older adults: The Quebec longitudinal study on Nutrition as a Determinant of Successful Aging (NuAge study). *Am. J. Clin. Nutr.* **2017**, *106*, 113–124. [CrossRef] [PubMed]
71. Kim, I.Y.; Schutzler, S.; Schrader, A.; Spencer, H.; Kortebein, P.; Deutz, N.E.; Wolfe, R.R.; Ferrando, A.A. Quantity of dietary protein intake but not pattern of intake, affects net protein balance primarily through differences in protein synthesis in older adults. *Am. J. Physiol. Endocrinol. Metab.* **2015**, *308*, E21–28. [CrossRef] [PubMed]
72. Areta, J.L.; Burke, L.M.; Ross, M.L.; Camera, D.M.; West, D.W.; Broad, E.M.; Jeacocke, N.A.; Moore, D.R.; Stellingwerff, T.; Phillips, S.M.; et al. Timing and distribution of protein ingestion during prolonged recovery from resistance exercise alters myofibrillar protein synthesis. *J. Physiol.* **2013**, *591*, 2319–2331. [CrossRef] [PubMed]
73. Close, G.L.; Hamilton, D.L.; Philp, A.; Burke, L.M.; Morton, J.P. New strategies in sport nutrition to increase exercise performance. *Free. Radic. Biol. Med.* **2016**, *98*, 144–158. [CrossRef] [PubMed]
74. Phillips, S.M. A brief review of higher dietary protein diets in weight loss: A focus on athletes. *Sports Med.* **2014**, *44* (Suppl. 2), S149–S153. [CrossRef] [PubMed]
75. McGlory, C.; Devries, M.C.; Phillips, S.M. Skeletal muscle and resistance exercise training; the role of protein synthesis in recovery and remodeling. *J. Appl. Physiol. (1985)* **2017**, *122*, 541–548. [CrossRef] [PubMed]
76. Agarwal, E.; Miller, M.; Yaxley, A.; Isenring, E. Malnutrition in the elderly: A narrative review. *Maturitas* **2013**, *76*, 296–302. [CrossRef] [PubMed]
77. Rydwik, E.; Welmer, A.K.; Kåreholt, I.; Angleman, S.; Fratiglioni, L.; Wang, H.X. Adherence to physical exercise recommendations in people over 65—the SNAC-Kungsholmen study. *Eur. J. Public. Health* **2013**, *23*, 799–804. [CrossRef] [PubMed]

78. Calvez, J.; Poupin, N.; Chesneau, C.; Lassale, C.; Tomé, D. Protein intake, calcium balance and health consequences. *Eur. J. Clin. Nutr.* **2012**, *66*, 281–295. [CrossRef] [PubMed]
79. Aragon, A.A.; Schoenfeld, B.J.; Wildman, R.; Kleiner, S.; VanDusseldorp, T.; Taylor, L.; Earnest, C.P.; Arciero, P.J.; Wilborn, C.; Kalman, D.S.; et al. International society of sports nutrition position stand: Diets and body composition. *J. Int. Soc. Sports Nutr.* **2017**, *14*, 16. [CrossRef] [PubMed]

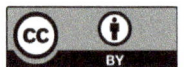

© 2018 by the authors. Licensee MDPI, Basel, Switzerland. This article is an open access article distributed under the terms and conditions of the Creative Commons Attribution (CC BY) license (http://creativecommons.org/licenses/by/4.0/).

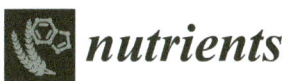

Article

Sensory-Driven Development of Protein-Enriched Rye Bread and Cream Cheese for the Nutritional Demands of Older Adults

Xiao Song *, Federico J. A. Perez-Cueto and Wender L. P. Bredie

FOOD Design and Consumer Behavior, Department of Food Science, Faculty of Science,
University of Copenhagen, Rolighedsvej 26, 1958 Frederiksberg, Denmark; apce@food.ku.dk (F.J.A.P.-C.);
wb@food.ku.dk (W.L.P.B.)
* Correspondence: xiao@food.ku.dk; Tel.: +45-353-36398

Received: 8 July 2018; Accepted: 30 July 2018; Published: 1 August 2018

Abstract: To promote healthy aging and minimize age-related loss of muscle mass and strength, adequate protein intake throughout the day is needed. Developing and commercializing protein-enriched foods holds great potential to help fulfill the nutritional demands of older consumers. However, innovation of appealing protein-enriched products is a challenging task since protein-enrichment often leads to reduced food palatability. In this study, rye bread and cream cheese prototypes fortified by whey protein hydrolysate (WPH), whey protein isolate (WPI), and/or soy protein isolate (SPI) were developed. Both sensory properties and consumer liking of prototypes were evaluated. Results showed that different proteins had various effects on the sensory characters of rye bread and cream cheese. The taste and texture modification strategies had positive effects in counteracting negative sensory changes caused by protein-enrichment. Consumers preferred 7% WPH and 4% WPH + 4% SPI-enriched breads with taste and texture modified. Sour taste and dry texture had considerable effects on consumer liking of rye bread. Addition of WPI and butter enhanced the flavor of cream cheese and increased consumer acceptance. Protein-enrichment doubled the protein content in the most liked prototypes, which have the potential to be incorporated into older consumers' diets and improve their protein intake substantially.

Keywords: whey protein; soy protein; older consumers; sensory; descriptive analysis; rye bread; cream cheese; protein-enrichment; muscle

---

1. Introduction

The aging of population is accelerating worldwide, creating a great challenge for societal health care systems [1]. Sufficient intake of a variety of dietary nutrients is required to promote active and healthy aging [2–4]. Protein is an essential nutrient to maintain muscle mass and strength during aging. Inadequate protein intake is associated with functional problems such as sarcopenia, which is the age-related loss of skeletal muscle mass, leading to functional decline or even a reduction in independence among 30% of individuals aged above 60 [5–8]. It has been repeatedly shown that physical exercise and adequate high-quality protein intake throughout the day are two of the most potent stimulators for counteracting the sarcopenic process [5,8–10]. Given this background, developing and commercializing appealing protein-enriched foods is a way by which the food industry can assist senior consumers in meeting their nutritional needs [11].

High-quality proteins, e.g., soy-based protein and milk-based whey protein, are popular protein supplements to sufficiently support muscle protein synthesis and accretion, since they are all nutritionally complete, highly digestible proteins with high contents and good composition of essential amino acids [12,13]. Consumption of foods enriched with high-quality proteins may not only increase the quantity of protein intake but also potentially improve the quality of protein in the consumer diet through e.g., modifying the amino acid composition of meals. However, the addition of different proteins alters sensory properties of food carriers in different ways, which might lead to reduced palatability for some products or be advantageous for some other products [11,14]. Wendin et al. [11] found that whey protein-fortified muffins were high in bitter taste and astringency mouthfeel and were perceived as very dry in texture. Höglund et al. [14] reported that off flavors were detected for muffins with extra whey protein. Tang and Liu [15] found that the addition of whey protein disrupted the gluten structure of wheat dough and affected cookie texture negatively. On the contrary, soy protein conferred a protective network on partial gluten structure which increased the overall acceptability of the cookies. Soy protein addition to gluten-free bread caused higher crumb hardness, while whey protein-fortified bread had higher crumb porosity [16]. In this context, to develop appealing protein-enriched products, exploring strategies to counteract the disadvantageous sensory influences of protein enrichment is a crucial task.

Moreover, selecting appropriate food carriers based on the "voice of target consumers" is of great importance for successful innovation of protein-enriched products. It was found that most older consumers perceived the healthy, traditional meal component food carriers as most appropriate for protein-enrichment, which they were most willing to trial purchase as well [17,18]. In the present study, rye bread and cream cheese were chosen for fortification with protein powder, since both rye bread and cream cheese are healthy, traditional foods in Denmark which play an important role in the diet of older Danish adults. Rye bread is one of the most commonly consumed staple foods on a daily basis, especially during breakfast and lunch, primarily among Danish adults. Cream cheese can be combined with meals and a variety of snacks. Through consumption of protein-enriched rye bread and cream cheese, senior consumers could gain a substantial increase in protein intake throughout the day without changing diet habits and meal frequency or size.

When developing protein-enriched food items for senior citizens, acceptability, which is normally measured in terms of product liking, is of great importance. The correlation between consumer liking and sensory properties could provide developers with a better understanding of product performance and optimization [19]. Consumer acceptance is assumed to be an indicator for prospective purchase intentions and intake as well [19,20]. Furthermore, product-evoked emotions and terms reflecting consumption desire and product satisfaction could be additional measures providing information on how the senior citizen would engage in consuming the product. For instance, product satisfaction could reflect the "confirmation" or "disconfirmation" between consumer expectation and actual food liking, which might influence the final acceptance due to the contrast effect [21]. Food-evoked desire might affect the subsequent food intake [20]. When developing nutrient-enriched products, such parameters may provide additional information beyond liking [19–24].

This study aims to: (1) compare the effects of whey protein hydrolysate (WPH), whey protein isolate (WPI), and/or soy protein isolate (SPI) enrichment on the sensory attributes of rye bread and cream cheese; and (2) develop protein-enriched rye bread and cream cheese with moderately high protein content and appealing sensory properties. Additionally, older consumers' liking and product-evoked emotion attributes, including satisfaction and desire, were evaluated to obtain a perspective on consumer experience and engagement in consuming the products.

2. Materials and Methods

2.1. Proteins

The following proteins were applied in this study: soy protein isolate (SPI, 90.0% protein content; Body-kraft, Hørning, Denmark), whey protein isolate (WPI, 87.0% protein content; Arla Foods Ingredients, Aarhus, Denmark), and whey protein hydrolysate (WPH, 86.4% protein content; Arla Foods Ingredients, Aarhus, Denmark).

2.2. Rye Bread

2.2.1. Preparation of Rye Bread Sample

In total, 15 rye bread prototypes were developed. Table 1 shows the details of the formulations per loaf of each prototype. The initial dough was prepared mainly according to the guidelines of Amo's rye bread mix, with additional sunflower seeds added. The amount of initial dough, additional proteins, and/or other ingredients to adjust the bread texture and taste can be seen in Table 1. Numbers in the sample labels indicate the amount of added whey or soy protein (4 = 4%, and 7 = 7%), while T means texture-modified samples and TS represents texture and taste-modified samples.

Wheat gluten, dried sourdough, and water were selected for texture and taste modifications, mainly because they are ingredients that rye bread already contains, thus avoiding too much taste or flavor interference in the bread. Moreover, wheat gluten contains 71.0% protein and sourdough contains 10.0% protein, thus also promoting the protein content of the prototypes. Blends of WPI/WPH and SPI were added in samples WPI 4 + SPI 4 and WPH 4 + SPI 4, respectively. This is because whey protein and soy protein have opposite effects on the texture of rye bread and could potentially counteract with each other's negative effects on bread texture. During the formula development period, pilot tasting tests were organized in order to investigate the optimal ratio of protein ingredients, wheat gluten, and dried sourdough. Besides, additional sunflower seeds were added to control and protein-enriched breads for improvement of flavor and texture properties, based on results of pilot tests. Moreover, the pH value of leavened bread dough was measured using a handheld pH meter (VWR pH 10, Malmö, Sweden). The heights of baked rye breads were also measured. The data were used to help optimize the addition of dried sourdough, water and wheat gluten for taste and texture modification.

The total weights of all bread dough before baking were the same. The bread dough was prepared and put in 1.2-liter silicone baking tins (length 22 cm/width 8 cm/height 7 cm) to rise at room temperature (around 22 °C) for two hours. Control bread and SPI-enriched breads were baked at 185 °C for 65 min. Breads enriched with WPI, WPH, and blends of whey protein and SPI were baked at 175 °C for 65 min. Breads were weighed before and after baking. The total protein contents per prototype (%) and per slice (g) after baking were calculated and shown in Table 1. Rye breads were cut into 0.85-cm-thick and approximately 2.0 cm × 2.0-cm-sized cubes and put into 60-mL-sized sample cups with lids. Each cup contained two pieces of bread cubes, and each cube had one side of crust.

Table 1. Recipes of rye bread samples (per loaf).

Sample [1]	Initial Dough [2] (g)	Protein Fortifier			Texture and Taste Modification			Total Weight before Baking (g)	Total Weight after Baking (g)	Total Protein Content (%)	Protein Content per Slice [5] (g)
		WPH (g)	WPI (g)	SPI (g)	Additional Water (g)	Wheat Gluten [3] (g)	Dried Sourdough [4] (g)				
Control	748	0	0	0	0	0	0	748	506.5	8.6	3.0
WPH 4	717.7	30.3	0	0	0	0	0	748	501.4	13.6	4.8
WPH 7	693.2	54.8	0	0	0	0	0	748	503.9	17.5	6.1
WPH 7-T	675.2	54.8	0	0	0	18	0	748	501.1	19.9	7.0
WPH 7-TS	660.2	54.8	0	0	0	18	15	748	500.9	20.0	7.0
WPI 4	717.7	0	30.3	0	0	0	0	748	498.4	13.7	4.8
WPI 7	693.2	0	54.8	0	0	0	0	748	503.9	17.5	6.1
WPI 7-T	675.2	0	54.8	0	0	18	0	748	504.5	19.8	6.9
WPI 7-TS	660.2	0	54.8	0	0	18	15	748	516.1	19.5	6.8
SPI 4	717.7	0	0	30.3	0	0	0	748	498.9	13.9	4.9
SPI 7	693.2	0	0	54.8	0	0	0	748	514.6	17.5	6.1
SPI7-T	623.2	0	0	54.8	70	0	0	748	501.5	17.7	6.2
SPI7-TS	612.7	0	0	54.8	70	0	10.5	748	515.2	17.3	6.1
WPI 4 + SPI 4	636.9	0	30.3	30.3	40	0	10.5	748	500.0	19.0	6.5
WPH 4 + SPI 4	636.9	30.3	0	30.3	40	0	10.5	748	502.7	18.8	6.6

[1] Labels of the sample: WPH = whey protein hydrolysate; WPI = whey protein isolate; SPI = soy protein isolate; TS = texture-modified samples; T = texture-modified samples. Numbers in the labels indicate amount of added whey or soy protein (4 = 4%, and 7 = 7%). [2] Preparation of initial dough: First, 20 g yeast was dissolved in 800 mL water, which was then mixed with 1000 g rye bread mix (Amo, Glostrup, Denmark) and 50 g sunflower seeds, using hand mixer in medium speed for 10 min. Amo's rye bread mix consists of rye flour, wheat flour, rye flakes, sunflower seeds, dried sourdough, salt, sugar, wheat starch, malt, and barley flour. It can also contain egg, milk, soy, and/or lupine. Amo's rye bread mix contains 9.9% protein. The additional sunflower seeds contain 21.0% protein. [3] Wheat gluten (Naturkost Engros, Odense, Denmark) contains 71.0% protein. [4] Dried sourdough powder (KageButikken, Albertslund, Denmark) is made from rye flour and wheat flour and contains 10.0% protein. [5] Bread weight per slice: 35 g.

2.2.2. Descriptive Analysis of Rye Bread

Panelists

The descriptive sensory analysis of rye bread was conducted in the sensory laboratory at the university. In total, 10 screened trained assessors, aged between 23 and 49 years of age, were recruited from the external panel at the Department of Food Science. They had more than one year of experience in sensory evaluation of foods and were familiar with consumption of rye bread. All panelists signed the informed consent of the study and were paid for their participation.

Training

Four 2-h training sessions were conducted. In the first session, panelists tasted samples and described odor, appearance, texture, mouthfeel, flavor, and taste of rye breads. They could select attributes from a list of rye bread sensory attributes provided to them, or they could generate new attributes. In the second and third sessions, reference standards of each attribute were presented or defined and discussed by the panelists to select the final sensory vocabulary. In the last session, a final list of odor, appearance, texture, mouthfeel, flavor, taste, and after-taste attributes of the crumb and crust were generated by the panel. Table 2 shows the list of sensory attributes and definitions. Trial assessments of rye breads were conducted in the last two training sessions to confirm that the training was sufficient to ensure clear understanding and proficient judgment of each attribute among panelists.

Table 2. Sensory attributes and corresponding definitions used in the descriptive analysis of rye breads.

Category	Attributes	Definitions
Odor	Yeasty	Odor associated with yeast fermentation in bread
	Malty	Odor associated with germinated cereal grains
	Burned	Odor associated with over-baked breads
Crumb		
Appearance	Brown	Degree of color brownness in the crumb, ranging from light brown to dark brown
	Compact	Appearance impression of the crumb density of the bread cross section
	Porosity	The extent of holes and cracks in the crumb of the bread cross section
Mouthfeel	Stickiness	The force needed to remove bread particles stuck to the palate completely
	Floury	Degree to which the crumb contains small grainy particles
	Astringent	The drying and puckering sensation evoked by strong black tea
Texture	Soft	Degree of yielding readily to pressure between palate and tongue
	Dry	Amount of saliva absorbed by sample crumbs during mastication
	Elasticity	The ability to resist force between palate and tongue and return to its original shape
	Crumbly	The force with which the sample crumbles
	Coarse	Degree to which particles abrade palate and tongue during mastication
Flavor	Buttermilk	Flavor impression of cultured buttermilk
	Beany	The off-flavor associated with soaked beans
	Grainy	Flavor impression of cereal derived rye grains, wheat grains etc.

Table 2. Cont.

Category	Attributes	Definitions
Taste	Sweet	Basic taste evoked by sucrose
	Salty	Basic taste elicited by sodium chloride
	Bitter	Basic taste of quinine
	Sour	Basic taste evoked by citric acid
	Umami	Basic taste elicited by monosodium glutamate
	Balance	The perceived overall balance of five basic tastes
After-taste	Sour	Taste sensation evoked by citric acid
	Bitter	Taste sensation of quinine
Crust		
Appearance	Brown	Degree of color brownness in the crust, ranging from light brown to dark brown
Texture	Hardness	The force needed to bite through the bread crust completely between molars
Taste	Sour	Basic taste evoked by citric acid
After-taste	Bitter	Taste sensation of quinine

Assessment

The 15 rye bread samples were evaluated in quadruplicate in four separate assessment sessions. All assessments were conducted in individual sensory booths at a temperature of 22 °C. Rye bread samples were served at room temperature in a randomized order. Panelists used a 15-cm line scale to rate the perceived intensities of the sensory attributes. Water, cucumber, and plain white bread cubes were provided for mouth cleansing between samples. Two short breaks were held during each assessment session. Photos of the rye bread cross-sections are shown in Figure 1.

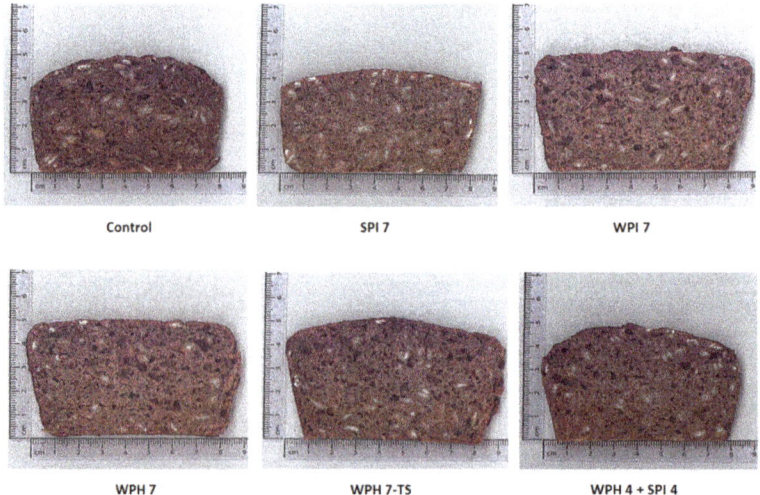

Figure 1. Example photos of cross section of rye bread samples. Labels: numbers indicate the amount of added protein (4 = 4%, and 7 = 7%); TS = texture and taste modified sample; WPH = whey protein hydrolysate; WPI = whey protein isolate; SPI = soy protein isolate.

2.3. Cream Cheese

2.3.1. Recipes of Cream Cheese Prototypes

A total of five cream cheese samples were selected for the descriptive analysis (Table 3). To prepare samples for sensory and consumer evaluation test, ingredients were mixed, put into a 60-mL sample cup and preserved in the refrigerator at 4 °C for more than two hours before being served to assessors. Each sample cup contained 25.0 ± 2.0 g of cream cheese. The total protein content of each prototype (%) and per serving (g) were calculated and are shown in Table 3.

Table 3. Cream cheese recipes (per 100 g).

Sample [1]	Cream Cheese [2] (g)	Protein Fortifier		Texture and Taste Modification [3]	Total Weight (g)	Total Protein Content (%)	Protein Content per Serving [4] (g)
		WPH (g)	WPI (g)	Butter (g)			
Control	100	0	0	0	100	4.5	1.1
WPH 9	91	9	0	0	100	11.9	3.0
WPI 9-TS	81	0	9	10	100	11.6	2.9
WPH 9	91	9	0	0	100	11.9	3.0
WPH 9-TS	81	0	9	10	100	11.6	2.9

[1] Labels of the sample: numbers in the labels indicate the amount of added protein (9 = 9%); TS = texture and taste-modified samples. [2] Arla Buko ® Natural Cream Cheese (Arla Foods, Viby J, Denmark) contains 4.5% protein, 25% fat, and 0.5% salt. [3] Butter was weighed and softened in room temperature for 0.5 h before being mixed with cream cheese, using a hand mixer at slow speed for 1 min. The butter contains 1.0% salt and 0.9% protein. [4] Weight per serving: 25 g.

2.3.2. Descriptive Analysis of Cream Cheese

Panelists

The descriptive analysis of cream cheese was conducted in the sensory evaluation laboratory at the university. In total, nine trained panelists aged 23 to 29 years old participated in the training and assessment sessions. They were recruited from the screened sensory panel at the Department of Food Science. They had experience of at least one year in the sensory evaluation of foods and were familiar with the consumption of cream cheese. Before the test, all panelists signed an informed consent form for the study. Panelists were paid for their participation.

Training

To develop sensory vocabulary of the cream cheese, three 2-h training sessions were conducted. In the first session, panelists tasted samples and generated sensory attributes to describe the cheese. In the second and third sessions, reference standards of each attribute were presented or defined and discussed by the panelists to select the final sensory vocabulary. In the end, the final list of odor, appearance, texture, mouthfeel, flavor, taste, and after-taste attributes of the cream cheese was generated by the panel (Table 4). Trial assessments of cream cheese samples were conducted in the last training session to make sure that panelists had experienced sufficient training to consistently use the attributes to differentiate the products.

Table 4. Sensory attributes and corresponding definitions used in the descriptive analysis of cream cheese.

Category	Attributes	Definitions
Odor	Butter	Odor associated with softened butter
Appearance	Yellow	Degree of color yellowness in the surface of sample
	Glossy	Degree to which the surface of cream cheese is shiny
Texture	Smooth	Absence of any particles or lumps in the sample
	Firmness	Extent of resistance against the palate and tongue during mastication
	Meltdown rate	The amount of "work" required to break down the bolus
	Viscosity	Stickiness between tongue and upper palate

Table 4. *Cont.*

Category	Attributes	Definitions
Mouthfeel	Astringent	The drying and puckering sensation evoked by strong black tea
	Coating	Extent to which the cheese coats the palate and tongue during mastication
Flavor	Creamy	Flavor associated with whipped cream
	Buttermilk	Flavor impression of cultured buttermilk
	Fatty	Flavor associated with butter
	Egg yolk	Flavor associated with cooked egg yolk
	Rancid	Flavor associated with oxidized, rancid cooking oil
	Fresh cheesy	Flavor associated with fresh, mild cheese without mold flavor, e.g., fresh mozzarella or ricotta
Basic taste	Salty	Basic taste elicited by sodium chloride
	Bitter	Basic taste of quinine
	Sour	Basic taste evoked by citric acid
	Sweet	Basic taste evoked by sucrose
	Umami	Basic taste elicited by monosodium glutamate
After-taste	Bitter	Taste sensation of quinine

Assessment

Cream cheese samples were evaluated in triplicate in three assessment sessions conducted at the sensory evaluation laboratory at a temperature of 22 °C. Cream cheese samples were preserved in a refrigerator at 4 °C for more than two hours before serving to the assessors. All samples were labeled with 3-digit codes and served in randomized order. Panelists used the 15-cm linear scale to rate all attributes of each sample. Water and plain crackers were provided for mouth cleansing between samples.

2.4. Consumer Test

The consumer panel consisted of 72 independent older Danish adults (44 females and 28 males; aged 61 to 83 years old) recruited from the external consumer panel of the Department of Food Science. A consumer acceptance test was conducted in individual sensory booths. The test included two sessions for rye bread tasting and cream cheese tasting, respectively. A 15-min break was held between the two sessions.

Based on the results of the descriptive analysis, six rye bread prototypes and all five cream cheese prototypes were selected and included for consumer evaluation. Rye bread samples were preserved and served at room temperature. Cream cheese samples were preserved at refrigerator at 4 °C for more than two hours before serving to the test persons. Samples were labeled with three-digit codes and served in a randomized order. Water, cucumber, and plain white bread cubes were provided for mouth cleansing between samples. Each sample was tasted and then evaluated for overall liking and selected product-evoked emotions, which included satisfied, desire, happy, interested, pleasant, calm, disgusted, unhappy, bored, and disappointed. The 9-point hedonic scale [25] was used to measure overall liking (1 = extreme dislike, 5 = neither like nor dislike, 9 = extreme like). The rate-all-that-apply method (RATA) was applied for emotion evaluation. Consumer participants ticked emotions they felt after tasting and rated the intensity of ticked emotions using a 5-point Likert scale (1 = slightly, 3 = moderately, 5 = extremely) [26]. The emotion attributes which were not checked represented emotions that consumers could not feel and were recorded as "0 points". Consumer demographic characters were also collected, which included age, gender, self-reported health status, living status, education level, and consumption frequency of rye bread and cream cheese. Consumers' perceived healthiness and willingness to trial purchase protein-enriched rye bread and cream cheese were evaluated using a 5-point Likert scale (1 = not at all, 3 = moderately, 5 = extremely). Before the test, all participants signed the informed consent of the study. After the test, each consumer participant received a goodie bag as the reward.

2.5. Data Analysis

The descriptive analysis panel data were analyzed by mixed model analysis of variance (ANOVA) to investigate the significance of each sensory attribute in discriminating products. Products were treated as the fixed factor, and panelists and replications were set as random factors [27]. Principal components analysis (PCA) was performed on average sensory data to relate rye bread and cream cheese products with sensory attributes, respectively. External preference mapping (PREFMAP) was conducted to investigate relationships among consumer acceptance and sensory attributes across rye bread and cream cheese products, respectively. Both PCA and PREFMAP were applied to the significant sensory attributes. Agglomerative hierarchical clustering analysis (AHC) was carried out to investigate the existence of homogeneous clusters of consumers with similar acceptance of rye bread or cream cheese, respectively. One-way ANOVA was conducted on consumer liking data and emotion data with post hoc Fisher's least significant difference (LSD) test. A penalty-lift analysis [28–31] was performed to analyze emotion RATA data in relation to the liking scores. The XLSTAT version 2018.3 (Addinsoft, New York, NY, USA) and SPSS statistics version 24 (IBM, Armonk, NY, USA) software packages were used for data analysis.

3. Results

3.1. Sensory Descriptive Analysis of Rye Bread

Table 2 presents the list of the 29 sensory attributes of rye bread assessed by 10 trained panelists in four replicate sessions. The attributes covered the odor, appearance, mouthfeel, texture, flavor, taste, and the after-taste of crumbs and crust. From an ANOVA analysis of the sensory data, it was found that all attributes, apart from the crumb's beany flavor, grainy flavor, salty taste, and bitter taste, were significantly different ($p < 0.05$) across the rye bread samples tested. This indicated that most of the sensory attributes were useful in characterizing differences across bread samples. Attributes which were not significantly different among rye bread prototypes were not included in further PCA analysis.

The relationship between rye bread samples and significant sensory attributes were visualized by principal component analysis (PCA). Figure 2 presents the PCA bi-plot of sensory attributes for all 15 rye bread samples. The first two principal components (PCs) accounted for 72% of the total variance (46% for PC1, 26% for PC2). PC1 separated the bread samples mainly according to yeasty odor, the crumb's compact appearance, and floury and sticky mouthfeel in the positive direction, and burned odor, the crumb's porous appearance, crumbly texture, and umami taste, and the crust's brown appearance, hard texture, and bitter after-taste in the negative direction. PC2 was positively linked with the sour taste, sour after-taste, and buttermilk flavor located in the positive direction and was negatively associated with the dry texture.

The PCA bi-plot shows that the sample groups spanned the sensory space quite well (Figure 2). WPI-enriched samples (WPI 4, WPI 7, WPI 7-T and WPI 7-TS) were closely linked to dry texture, and negatively related with astringent mouthfeel, sour taste, sour after-taste, and buttermilk flavor. WPH-enriched breads (WPH 4, WPH 7, WPH 7-T, and WPH 7-TS) were characterized by a brown and porous appearance, burned odor, crumbly and elastic texture, umami taste, and bitter after-taste. Moreover, they had a negative correlation with the attributes of yeasty odor, compact appearance, and floury mouthfeel. The three 7% SPI-enriched samples (SPI 7, SPI 7-T and SPI 7-TS) correlated with a yeasty odor, compact appearance, soft texture, and floury and sticky mouthfeel. The 4% SPI-enriched bread (SPI 4) and breads enriched by mixed proteins (WPH 4 + SPI 4 and WPI 4 + SPI 4) were characterized by sour taste, sour after-taste, buttermilk flavor, astringent mouthfeel, and soft texture. Compared with WPI and SPI, WPH-enriched samples were located much closer to the control sample, which demonstrated that WPH enrichment altered the sensory properties of rye bread to a smaller extent. Thus, WPH could be regarded as a more appropriate protein type for enrichment in rye bread in this study.

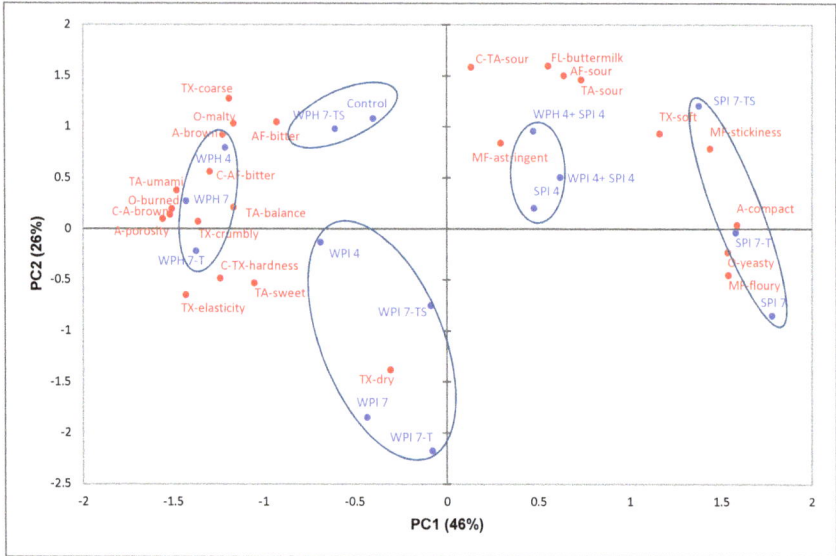

Figure 2. Principal component analysis bi-plot of sensory attributes (red labels) and rye bread samples (blue labels). PC1 = first principal component; PC2 = second principal component. Red labels: sensory attributes; C = attributes for crust; attributes without "C" are attributes for crumbs; O = odor attributes; A = appearance attributes; TA = taste attributes; TX = texture attributes; FL = flavor attributes; MF = mouthfeel attributes; and AF = after taste attributes. Blue labels: rye bread samples; numbers indicate amount of added protein (4 = 4%, and 7 = 7%). T = texture-modified samples; TS = texture and taste-modified samples.

To compare the effects of different protein types on bread sensory characters, it was found that most WPH-enriched samples were located close to burned odor and brown appearance, which could be explained by the enhanced Maillard reactions because of the addition of WPH [32]. Moreover, the three 7% WPI-enriched breads had a less soft and drier texture. The textures of WPH 7 and WPH 7-T were more crumbly, hard, and elastic. Furthermore, compared to the remaining samples, the four WPH -enriched rye breads had higher umami taste and bitter after-taste, which is in line with prior research [32–34]. Crumbs of the three 7% SPI-enriched breads appeared more compact and less porous, and had more floury and sticky mouthfeel and less crumbly texture- (Figure 2).

In terms of influences from taste and texture modification strategies, it was found that compared with WPH 7 and WPH 7-T, sample WPH 7-TS was located much closer to the control sample. This indicated that the taste and texture modification strategies (addition of gluten and sourdough) reached positive effects in counteracting adverse sensory changes caused by the WPH-enrichment. The enrichment of higher percentage of all three kinds of proteins decreased the buttermilk flavor and sour taste, which could be explained by the increased pH value due to protein enrichment. The control sample had pH value of 4.0, while the average pH values of SPI 7, WPI 7, and WPH 7 were 4.6, 4.8, and 4.8 (data not shown), respectively. The addition of dried sourdough adjusted the sour taste in samples SPI 7-TS, WPI 7-TS, and WPH 7-TS so that they had a sour taste intensity closer to that of the control sample.

Moreover, it could be observed that whey protein and soy protein had opposing influences on the texture characters of rye bread. It was found that the addition of 4% SPI to 4% WPI or 4% WPH-enriched rye bread reduced the crumbly texture and increased the soft texture successfully.

Enrichment with the blend of WPI/WPH and SPI not only counteracted each other's effects on bread texture but also resulted in an increase in the total amount of additional protein.

In summary, texture and taste modification strategies had positive effects in counteracting negative sensory changes caused by the protein-enrichment, especially in correcting the crumbly texture, compact appearance, floury mouthfeel, and/or sour taste of breads enriched with the higher percentage of proteins. WPH was found to be the most appropriate ingredient for rye bread enrichment. The 7% WPH-enriched, texture and taste-modified rye bread sample (WPH 7-TS) was the optimal sample, showing little sensory difference with respect to the non-enriched control bread.

3.2. Consumer Liking of Rye Bread

In total, six bread samples (control, WPH 7-TS, WPH 7, WPI 7, SPI 7, WPH 4 + SPI 4) were chosen for consumer evaluation based on the results of sensory descriptive analysis. The sensory space spanned by the 15 rye bread samples (Figure 2) was well-represented by the six bread samples selected for the consumer acceptance test. The average ratings of consumer overall liking of rye breads are shown in Table 5. Consumers who were homogenous in their acceptance towards different rye bread samples were grouped through agglomerative hierarchical clustering (AHC). Figure 3 represents the external preference mapping to demonstrate the correlation between sensory attributes and the overall liking of different consumer clusters, with average sensory data as the explanatory variables (X) and mean liking ratings of three consumer clusters as responses (Y). The mean liking ratings of consumer clusters are also shown in Table 5.

Table 5 showed that the average overall liking ratings of each bread sample ranged from 5.5 to 6.5. Significant differences ($p < 0.05$) of consumer overall liking were found across the sample of six rye breads. WPH 7-TS rye bread (6.0) and WPH 4 + SPI 4 (5.9) were the most accepted protein-enriched samples, amongst which WPH 7-TS showed no significant difference in terms of consumer acceptance compared to the control bread ($p > 0.05$). Moreover, the taste and texture modification of WPH 7-TS increased consumer liking by 0.4 units compared to WPH 7 (5.6). SPI 7 and WPI 7 were the least preferred rye bread samples, with significantly lower liking ratings compared to the other four samples ($p < 0.05$).

Table 5. Mean ratings of consumers' liking for rye bread samples. The size of each cluster is indicated (%).

Sample	Cluster 1 (24%)	Cluster 2 (50%)	Cluster 3 (26%)	Mean (100%)
Control	6.7abA	6.8aA	5.9bA	6.5A
SPI 7	5.8aB	5.9aB	4.4bB	5.5C
WPI 7	5.8aB	4.7bC	6.5aA	5.5C
WPH 7	5.5BC	5.6B	5.7A	5.6BC
WPH 7-TS	4.8bC	6.3aAB	6.6aA	6.0AB
WPH 4+ SPI 4	6.3A	5.7B	6.1A	5.9BC

Different lowercase letters within the same row indicate significant post hoc Fisher's least significant difference (LSD) differences at $p < 0.05$; different capital letters within the same column indicate significant LSD differences at $p < 0.05$.

The external preference mapping plots are presented in Figure 3. AHC identified three consumer clusters representing different patterns of product liking. In cluster 1, 24% of the consumers were located relatively close to the WPH 4 + SPI 4 and control samples, which had significantly higher overall liking ratings (6.3 and 6.7, respectively) as compared to the remaining four samples in cluster 1. The attributes sour taste, soft texture, and sticky mouthfeel which characterized the control and WPH 4 + SPI 4 appeared to influence the consumer liking of cluster 1 positively. WPH 7 and WPH 7-TS, with hard, crumbly, and elastic textures were the least liked in cluster 1. Cluster 2 (50%) liked the control sample (6.8) the most, which was characterized by sour taste, sour after-taste, and a sour-related buttermilk flavor. Cluster 2 showed the least preference towards sample WPI 7 (4.7), which had a dry texture. Consumers of clusters 1 and 2 (74%) could be regarded as 'sour rye bread lovers'. Consumers in cluster 3 (26%) liked sample WPH 7-TS (6.6) the most and sample SPI 7 (4.4) the least.

It appeared that they were attracted by WPH 7-TS with its brown (crust) and porous appearance, burned odor, crumbly and hard (crust) texture, and umami and bitter after-taste, and disliked SPI 7, with its yeasty odor and compact appearance. Thus, it seems that the sourness levels and texture and mouthfeel properties of rye bread might play important roles in influencing the liking of most consumers. Demographic characters were compared across three clusters as well and no significant differences were found. The mean rating of consumers' willingness to trial purchase protein-enriched rye bread was very high (4.0 on the 5-point Likert scale).

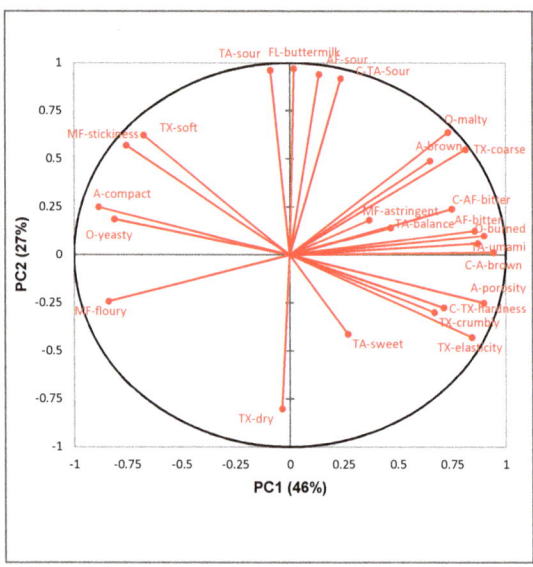

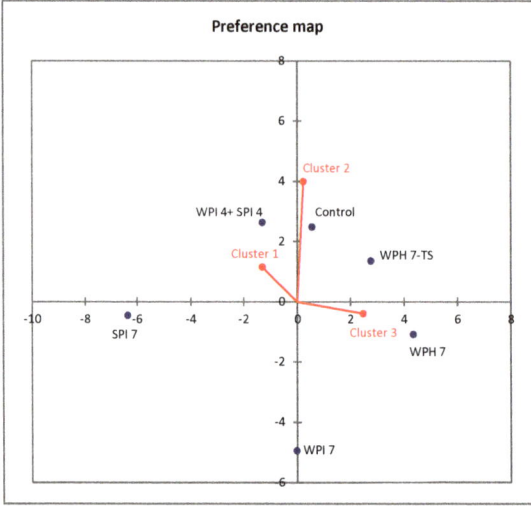

Figure 3. External preference mapping of rye bread. Red labels: O = odor attributes; A = appearance attributes; TA = taste attributes; TX = texture attributes; FL = flavor attributes; MF = mouthfeel attributes; AF = after-taste attributes. Blue labels: numbers indicate amount of added protein (4 = 4%, and 7 = 7%); TS = texture and taste-modified samples.

3.3. Sensory Descriptive Analysis of Cream Cheese

Table 4 shows the list of the descriptive sensory attributes of cream cheese assessed by the nine trained panelists in triplicate. The attributes characterized the odor, appearance, mouthfeel, texture, flavor, taste, and after-taste aspects of cream cheese. The attributes meltdown rate, coating mouthfeel, astringent mouthfeel, egg yolk flavor, and salty, sweet, and umami tastes were not significant in discriminating cheese products ($p > 0.05$), and thus were excluded in further PCA and PREFMAP analyses. Cheese prototypes enriched with SPI were not included in the sensory descriptive analysis due to their poor sensory performance compared with WPI- and WPH-enriched samples.

Figure 4 shows the PCA bi-plot of sensory attributes for five cream cheese samples. The first principal component accounted for 59% of the total variance, while the second principal component explained 32% of the total variance. The first two PCs explained 91% of the total variance. The non-enriched control sample is loaded in the fourth quadrant. It was characterized by buttermilk flavor, sour taste, and firm and viscous texture, and was negatively linked with a yellow and glossy appearance. The 9% WPI-enriched, butter-added sample (WPI 9-TS) is loaded in the first quadrant and was closely correlated with fatty, creamy, and fresh cheesy flavors. WPI 9 was associated with smooth texture, yellow appearance, and glossy appearance in the second quadrant. The two samples enriched by 9% WPH (WPH 9 and WPH 9-TS) are located most closely to the less-desired rancid flavor, bitter taste, and bitter after-taste in the third quadrant. All protein-enriched samples, except WPI 9-TS, are loaded in the left side of the map.

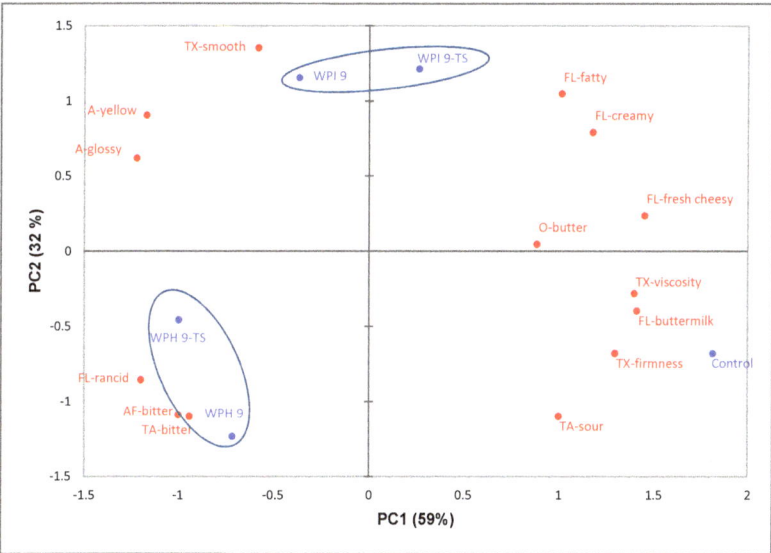

Figure 4. Principal components analysis bi-plot of sensory attributes (red labels) and cream cheese samples (blue labels). Blue labels: numbers indicate amount of added protein (9 = 9%); TS = texture and taste-modified samples. Red labels: O = odor attributes; A = appearance attributes; TA = taste attributes; TX = texture attributes; FL = flavor attributes; AF = aftertaste attributes.

The increased glossiness of cheese samples due to protein enrichment could be explained by the texture changes: increased smoothness and decreased firmness and viscosity. Some panelists used *watery* to describe the surface of protein-enriched cream cheese during the profiling session. The decreased firmness and viscosity might be due to the effects of whey protein on the oil/water emulsion, which led to a decreased extent of partial coalescence and increased extent of fat destabilization [35].

The increased yellowness of protein and/or butter-enriched cheese might be explained by the light-yellow color of dissolved protein powder and/or the higher fat content and larger fat droplets of the cheese [36]. The bitter taste and rancid flavor in WPH-enriched samples could be explained mainly by bitter peptides and some off-flavor compounds in WPH, respectively [37]. Moreover, in contrast to rye bread, the addition of WPH had no significant influence on the umami taste, which could be because the cheesy and creamy flavor masked the umami taste to a large extent. Regarding the taste and texture modification, it appeared that addition of 10% butter in the WPI 9-TS sample helped with the improvement of flavor [36] but not enough to counteract the softening texture effect from protein fortification completely.

In summary, WPI was more adequate for use in cream cheese enrichment when texture and taste treatment was applied, as compared to WPH. The texture and taste modification strategy achieved positive effects in enhancing pleasant flavors in cream cheese.

3.4. Consumer Liking of Cream Cheese

The average ratings of consumer liking are shown in Table 6. For a better understanding of consumer preference, agglomerative hierarchical clustering (AHC) was conducted for a group consumers with a similar acceptance towards different cheese samples. The mean liking ratings per cluster are also shown in Table 6. The external preference mapping plots are presented in Figure 5, which allows a visual representation of the association between cheese samples, sensory attributes, and consumer liking of each cluster.

In Table 6, significant differences ($p < 0.05$) in overall consumer liking were found among the five cheese samples. Acceptance of WPI 9-TS and the control sample was significantly higher than the two WPH-enriched samples ($p < 0.05$). Sample WPI 9-TS was the most liked protein-enriched sample. Besides, acceptance values of WPI 9-TS (6.9) and control sample (6.3) were not significantly different ($p > 0.05$). Compared to cheese enriched with 9% WPI (6.1), the addition of butter in WPI 9-TS successfully enhanced the flavor and increased consumer liking significantly ($p < 0.05$).

Table 6. Mean ratings of consumers' liking towards cream cheese. Size of each cluster was indicated (%).

Sample	Cluster 1 (68%)	Cluster 2 (24%)	Cluster 3 (8%)	Mean (100%)
Control	6.2abB	7.1aA	4.8bAB	6.3AB
WPI 9	6.4aB	5.8abBC	4.5bB	6.1BC
WPI 9-TS	7.2aA	6.8aAB	5.0bAB	6.9A
WPH 9	5.1bC	6.9aA	5.5abAB	5.6C
WPH 9-TS	5.4C	5.5C	6.7A	5.5C

Different lowercase letters within the same row indicate significant LSD differences at $p < 0.05$; different capital letters within the same column indicate significant LSD differences at $p < 0.05$.

The external preference mapping plots of cream cheese are presented in Figure 5. Agglomerative hierarchical clustering identified three consumer clusters. Cluster 1 was the largest group, accounting for 68% of total consumers. This cluster was located in the first quadrant and consumers most liked WPI 9-TS (7.2) characterized by a fatty, creamy and fresh cheesy flavor and butter odor. WPH 9 (5.1), with a rancid flavor and bitter taste, was liked the least by consumer cluster 1. Cluster 2 (24%) expressed the highest liking towards the control sample (7.1) characterized by firmness, viscosity, and a buttermilk flavor, and lowest liking ratings were for WPH 9-TS (5.5), with a bitter taste and rancid flavor, and WPI 9 (5.8), with a yellow and glossy appearance. Cluster 3 (8%) was a small cluster characterized by consumers who liked WPH 9-TS, with a bitter taste, bitter after-taste, and rancid flavor. This might be because a small percentage of older adults may not be sensitive to bitter taste [38]. Demographic data were compared across three clusters, but no significant differences were found. Consumers had moderately high willingness (rated 3.6 on the 5-point scale) towards consumption of protein-enriched cream cheese in general.

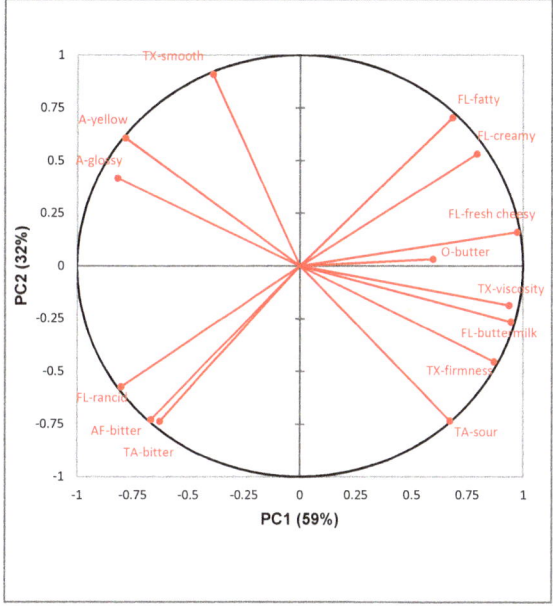
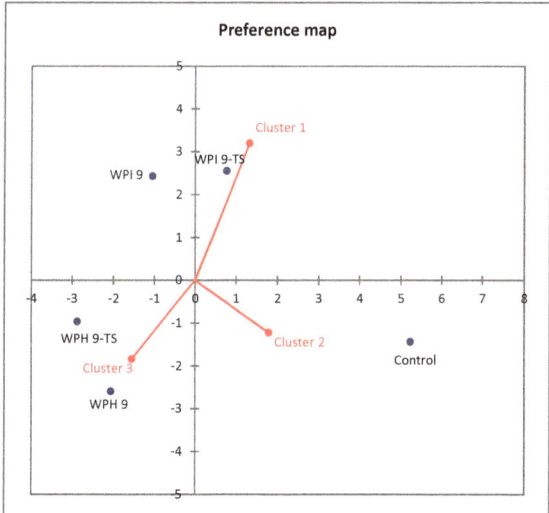

Figure 5. External preference mapping of cream cheese. Red labels: O = odor attributes; A = appearance attributes; TA = taste attributes; TX = texture attributes; FL = flavor attributes; AF = after taste attributes. Blue labels: numbers indicate amount of added protein (9 = 9%), TS = texture and taste-modified samples.

The bitter taste and rancid flavor of WPH restricted its application in cream cheese. WPI-enriched cream cheese with additional butter was regarded as the most promising prototype for its outstanding performance in both sensory and consumer liking evaluations.

3.5. Product-Evoked Emotions

The penalty lift analysis [28–31] was performed to demonstrate the extent that product-evoked emotions affected consumer liking acquisition. All emotion words were applied by more than 20% of consumers; thus, all were included in the analysis [28]. Figure 6 shows the results of penalty-lift analysis of rye bread and cream cheese-evoked emotion data. The elicited positive emotions led to increased consumer liking, and negative emotions indicated reductions of consumer liking, which was in line with former research [31].

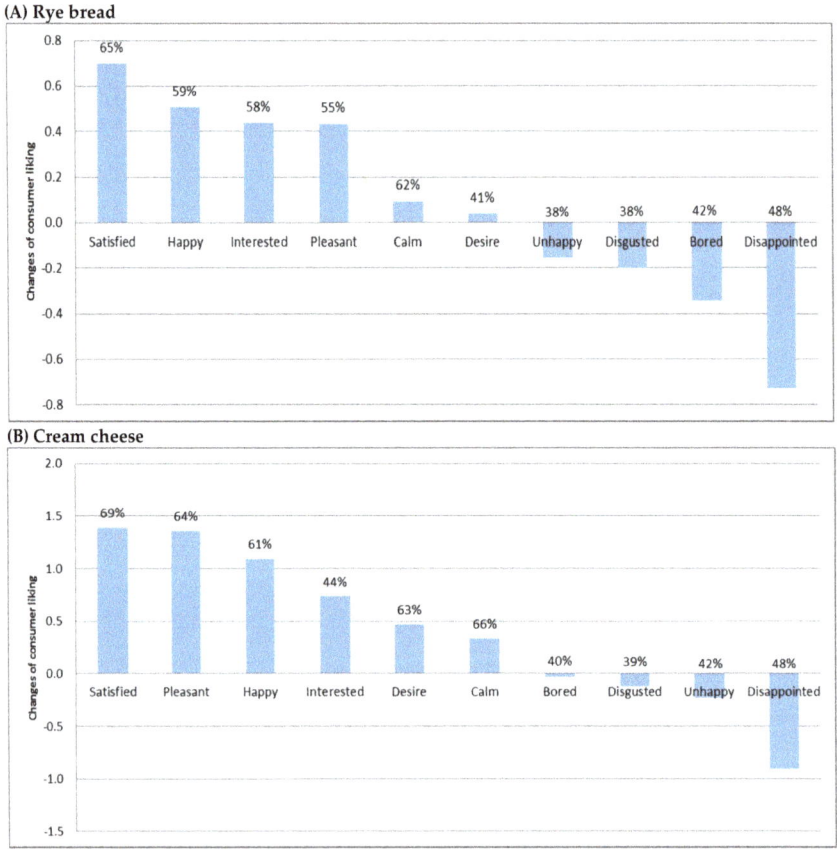

Figure 6. Penalty-lift analysis of emotions' effect on overall liking across (**A**) rye bread samples and (**B**) cheese samples. The frequency (%) of which the emotion descriptors were checked by consumers is also indicated. The values of the vertical axis indicate the unit of change in liking of prototypes for which the respective emotion attribute was checked, compared to liking of prototypes for which the emotion attribute was not checked. The upstand pillars represent the increase in consumer liking and the downward pillars indicate the decrease in consumer liking.

Satisfaction and disappointment represent the gap between consumers' expected liking and experienced liking. The degree of satisfaction indicates the extent that experienced liking goes beyond expectations, while disappointment means the experienced liking does not meet with consumer expectations. Lower expectation and higher experienced liking result in higher satisfaction and lower disappointment. In this study, the liking ratings of satisfied consumers were 0.7 unit and 1.4 units higher than all consumers' average liking ratings of rye bread and cheese, respectively. Disappointment was the most detrimental emotion for liking acquisition of both food matrixes, which reduced the liking ratings for rye bread and cream cheese by 0.7 units and 0.9 units, respectively.

To further investigate the discrimination power of emotions across six rye bread samples and five cream cheese samples, analysis of variance (ANOVA) was also performed on the ratings of emotion descriptors. Results indicated that satisfied, happy, and disappointed performed significantly better in discriminating rye bread samples ($p < 0.05$), whilst satisfied, pleasant, and disappointed went beyond the remaining emotions for discriminating cheese samples ($p < 0.05$).

Moreover, it should be noted that consumers checked desire for cream cheese much more frequently (63%) than rye bread samples (41%). This might be because high-fat foods usually stimulate higher desire to eat and high-fiber and carbohydrate foods often evoke lower consumption desire [39]. The degree of desire often affects the subsequent food intake [20]. To design protein-enriched meals which could stimulate stronger desire and more subsequent food intake, a combination of high-fat foods with high-fiber and carbohydrate foods could be a good option.

In summary, for the two food matrixes, the satisfaction-related emotions satisfied and disappointed were among the most influential emotions on both product liking and discrimination among older consumers. Furthermore, besides experienced liking, desire and satisfaction/disappointment could be useful measurements to indicate prospective food intake, which may guide the design of protein-enriched dishes and meals [24].

4. Discussion

In this study, we explored the sensory and consumer acceptance changes caused by enriching rye bread and cream cheese with whey protein hydrolysate (WPH), whey protein isolate (WPI), and/or soy protein isolate (SPI). Descriptive analysis results showed that different proteins had various influences on the sensory performance of the two food matrixes. Consumers with homogenous acceptance towards rye bread and cream cheese were grouped into their respective clusters. The sensory attributes driving the liking of each consumer cluster were demonstrated.

WPH enrichment led to higher bitter after-taste in rye bread, mainly due to the increased Maillard reaction and content of bitter peptides [30,34]. However, PREFMAP of rye bread showed that bitterness seems had no negative effect on the acceptance of most consumers; a small group of consumers even appeared to be attracted by the bitterness of rye breads. This might be because bitter taste is a typical sensory character in rye bread [40]; even though WPH increased bitter after-taste to some extent, the intensity was not beyond the accepted level among senior consumers. Moreover, the sour taste and sour-related flavor seem to be important in affecting the acceptance among most consumers, which explained the high liking towards WPH 7-TS. It was also noted that WPH increased the umami taste, which might be elicited from the free amino acids released during the hydrolysis of protein [41,42]. This could have advantageous effects in food matrices requiring an umami taste, e.g., a variety of soups and sausages. Regarding the texture changes caused by WPH- and WPI-enrichment, the increased hardness and elasticity could be explained by the heat-induced aggregation of whey protein [43,44]. The foaming property of whey protein may lead to the porous appearance, larger volume, and crumbly texture [45]. The high water-binding capacity of whey protein might be the reason which increases the perceived dryness during mastication [11].

Isolated protein (WPI and SPI)-enriched rye breads had a lower bitter taste compared to WPH. However, the texture and/or mouthfeel of WPI and SPI-enriched breads restricted their application in rye breads. The dry texture among WPI-enriched breads might be the major problem that led to the breads being disliked by at least half of the consumers. SPI enrichment increased the stickiness, floury mouthfeel, and compactness of rye breads, which appeared to decrease the acceptance of more than half the consumers. The sensory changes caused by SPI might be because the soy protein conferred a protective network on partial gluten structure which increased the dense and sticky texture of the dough and bread [15,46]. Enrichment with the blend of WPI/WPH and SPI counteracted each other's effects on rye bread texture and contributed to consumer liking.

In contrast to rye breads, when applying WPH in cream cheese, the increased bitter taste and rancid flavor appeared to reduce consumer acceptance significantly. WPI was regarded as more proper for cream cheese enrichment when additional butter was added for flavor enhancement. The flavor advantage of WPI 9-TS cream cheese might be the major reason explaining its higher liking rating.

The sour taste seems dominate consumer liking in rye breads. More diversity was found in consumer liking towards bread texture/mouthfeel. At least half consumers disliked WPI 7 with dry texture; a quarter of the consumers liked WPH samples characterized by a crumbly texture. The remaining one-quarter of consumers appeared to be attracted by WPH 4 + SPI 4 with sticky mouthfeel and soft texture to some extent. For cream cheese, the liking of most consumers (68%) seems to be mainly affected by the odor and the flavor dimension, which led to the high liking of WPI 9-TS cheese. The liking of the remaining consumers appeared to be dominated by appearance, texture, and flavor aspects, amongst which the viscosity, firmness, and buttermilk flavor which characterized the control sample attracted the most consumers in this group. Compared to cream cheese, the variety in texture preferences towards rye breads could be due to the texture complexity of the products. Moreover, individual differences in the ability or preferred way to manipulate food in their mouth could also contribute to the diversity in texture preference, as shown in a recent study on texture mouth behavior [47].

The palatability of protein-enriched foods largely depends on the protein-carrier 'fitness'. A precise selection of protein type and food carrier which could inhibit or even benefit from the sensory impacts caused by protein enrichment plays a vital role in developing appealing protein-enriched products. From a sensory point of view, in some cases, the mild flavor and taste of WPI made it more proper for protein-enrichment, as compared to WPH [48]. However, from a nutrition point of view, the nutritional value of WPH is relatively higher due to its higher digestibility and absorptivity than WPI [12,13], which makes it worthwhile to put efforts into broadening the use of protein hydrolysate through modifying its production and processing or identifying masking agents in order to improve its sensory quality [34,42,48].

However, the quality of protein ingredients used for enrichment, such as the digestion and absorption rate and amino acid compositions, might be partly affected by the production process of enriched foods. The potential quality changes may further influence the enriched foods' contribution to muscle protein synthesis. Evaluations on the protein quality of enriched foods and clinical trials on the biological utilization of protein-enriched foods might be needed in future studies.

In this study, screened trained panelists aged 23–49 years were used in the sensory descriptive analysis, and provided reliable and clear characterizations of prototypes. The use of older panelists of a similar age to the target consumers as part of the trained panel was considered, however, descriptive analysis with older panels may introduce more noise in characterizing products due to their highly heterogeneous sensitivity [38]. More investigations regarding the proper use of older panels are needed. With increasing age, adults are more receptive to functional foods because of their increased health considerations, especially in the prevention of chronic diseases [49]. In this context, appealing protein-enriched functional products hold a bright future in the market of older consumers. Older consumers had high prospective willingness towards consumption of protein-enriched rye bread and cream cheese in this study. However, besides 'good taste', there are a number of drivers and obstacles for consumption of protein-enriched foods. A better understanding of motivators for consumption of protein-enriched products among target consumers could help the promotion of protein intake.

In the present study, a lab-based consumer acceptance test was conducted to obtain a general perspective on how consumers accept the products. To evaluate consumer acceptance of protein-enriched foods or meals in real life, contextual aspects could be considered and included for exploration in future consumer studies to strengthen the predictive power of the results [50].

The most preferred enriched prototypes of the two food matrices had twice amount of protein as compared to non-enriched controls. Per slice, the WPH 7-TS bread contained 7.0 g protein, which was 4.0 g more than the non-enriched control bread (Table 1). Each serving of WPI 9-TS cream cheese contained 2.9 g protein, 1.8 g more than the control cheese (Table 3). Assuming that older adults could consume two to three slices of bread combined with two to three servings of cream cheese in one meal, the protein intake could increase by 11.6–17.4 g/meal due to protein-enrichment, achieving 19.8–29.7 g/meal in total, which is close to the dietary recommendation for older adults (25–30 g/meal) [8]. However, to evaluate the increase of protein intake through consumption of protein-enriched foods in real life, further studies are needed to investigate the effects of protein-enrichment on food intake and satiety in target older consumers [51].

5. Conclusions

The present study evaluated different kinds of protein-enrichments of rye bread and cream cheese for their sensory acceptability by independent senior citizens. Relationships between sensory properties of the protein fortification in these products were established. Sensory acceptability by senior consumers was different with respect to the sensory properties of appearance, flavor, and texture, indicating that diverse protein fortification strategies should be considered in product development and optimization to be able to satisfy and engage senior consumers in the consumption of such nutritious products.

Author Contributions: All authors contributed to the design of the study. X.S. conducted the tests and wrote the first draft of the manuscript. All authors revised and edited the manuscript.

Acknowledgments: The authors acknowledge support by the University of Copenhagen's excellence program for interdisciplinary research through the project "CALM—Counteracting age-related loss of skeletal muscle mass" (calm.ku.dk). The first author is supported by scholarships from Chinese Scholarship Council and S. C. Van Foundation. We are grateful to Arla Food Ingredients for providing the protein materials. We thank Åse Solvej Hansen and Susanne M. Bølling Laugesen for their help in experiment design.

Conflicts of Interest: All authors declare no conflict of interests.

References

1. World Health Organization. World Report on Ageing and Health 2015. Available online: http://www.who.int/ageing/events/world-report-2015-launch/en/ (accessed on 8 July 2018).
2. Van Staveren, W.A.; de Groot, L.C.P. Evidence-based dietary guidance and the role of dairy products for appropriate nutrition in the elderly. *J. Am. Coll. Nutr.* **2011**, *30*, 429–437. [CrossRef]
3. Brownie, S. Why are elderly individuals at risk of nutritional deficiency? *Int. J. Nurs. Pract.* **2006**, *12*, 110–118. [CrossRef] [PubMed]
4. Doets, E.L.; Kremer, S. The silver sensory experience—A review of senior consumers' food perception, liking and intake. *Food Qual. Prefer.* **2016**, *48*, 316–332. [CrossRef]
5. Lonnie, M.; Hooker, E.; Brunstrom, J.M.; Corfe, B.M.; Green, M.A.; Watson, A.W.; Williams, E.A.; Stevenson, E.J.; Penson, S.; Johnstone, A.M. Protein for life: Review of optimal protein intake, sustainable dietary sources and the effect on appetite in ageing adults. *Nutrients* **2018**, *10*, 360. [CrossRef] [PubMed]
6. Tieland, M.; Borgonjen-Van den Berg, K.J.; Van Loon, L.J.; de Groot, L.C. Dietary protein intake in Dutch elderly people: A focus on protein sources. *Nutrients* **2015**, *7*, 9697–9706. [CrossRef] [PubMed]
7. Von Haehling, S.; Morley, J.E.; Anker, S.D. An overview of sarcopenia: Facts and numbers on prevalence and clinical impact. *J. Cachexia Sarcopenia Muscle* **2010**, *1*, 129–133. [CrossRef] [PubMed]
8. Paddon-Jones, D.; Rasmussen, B.B. Dietary protein recommendations and the prevention of sarcopenia: Protein, amino acid metabolism and therapy. *Curr. Opin. Clin. Nutr. Metab. Care* **2009**, *12*, 86. [CrossRef] [PubMed]
9. Fielding, R.A.; Vellas, B.; Evans, W.J.; Bhasin, S.; Morley, J.E.; Newman, A.B.; Cederholm, T. Sarcopenia: An undiagnosed condition in older adults. Current consensus definition: Prevalence, etiology, and consequences. International working group on sarcopenia. *J. Am. Med. Dir. Assoc.* **2011**, *12*, 249–256. [CrossRef] [PubMed]

10. Robinson, S.; Cooper, C.; Aihie Sayer, A. Nutrition and sarcopenia: A review of the evidence and implications for preventive strategies. *J. Aging Res.* **2012**, *2012*, 510801. [CrossRef] [PubMed]
11. Wendin, K.; Höglund, E.; Andersson, M.; Rothenberg, E. Protein enriched foods and healthy ageing: Effects of protein fortification on muffin characteristics. *Agro Food Ind. Hi-Technol.* **2017**, *28*, 16–18.
12. Phillips, S.M.; Tang, J.E.; Moore, D.R. The role of milk- and soy-based protein in support of muscle protein synthesis and muscle protein accretion in young and elderly persons. *J. Am. Coll. Nutr.* **2009**, *28*, 343–354. [CrossRef] [PubMed]
13. Tang, J.E.; Moore, D.R.; Kujbida, G.W.; Tarnopolsky, M.A.; Phillips, S.M. Ingestion of whey hydrolysate, casein, or soy protein isolate: Effects on mixed muscle protein synthesis at rest and following resistance exercise in young men. *J. Appl. Physiol.* **2009**, *107*, 987–992. [CrossRef] [PubMed]
14. Höglund, E. Protein and energy enriched muffins designed for nutritional needs of older adults. *Nutr. Food Sci. Int. J.* **2017**, *2*. [CrossRef]
15. Tang, X.; Liu, J. A comparative study of partial replacement of wheat flour with whey and soy protein on rheological properties of dough and cookie quality. *J. Food Qual.* **2017**. [CrossRef]
16. Aprodu, I.; Badiu, E.A.; Banu, I. Influence of protein and water addition on gluten-free dough properties and bread quality. *J. Food Eng.* **2016**, *12*, 355–363. [CrossRef]
17. Song, X.; Pérez-Cueto, F.J.A.; Laugesen, S.M.B.; van der Zanden, L.D.T.; Giacalone, D. Older consumers' attitudes towards food carriers for protein-enrichment. *Appetite* **2018**. under review.
18. Van der Zanden, L.D.T.; van Kleef, E.; de Wijk, R.A.; van Trijp, H.C. Examining heterogeneity in elderly consumers' acceptance of carriers for protein-enriched food: A segmentation study. *Food Qual. Prefer.* **2015**, *42*, 130–138. [CrossRef]
19. Ng, M.; Chaya, C.; Hort, J. Beyond liking: Comparing the measurement of emotional response using essense profile and consumer defined check-all-that-apply methodologies. *Food Qual. Prefer.* **2013**, *28*, 193–205. [CrossRef]
20. Kirkmeyer, S.V.; Mattes, R.D. Effects of food attributes on hunger and food intake. *Int. J. Obes.* **2000**, *24*, 1167. [CrossRef]
21. Cardello, A.V. Consumer Expectations and Their Role in Food Acceptance. In *Measurement of Food Preferences*, 1st ed.; MacFie, H.J.H., Thomson, D.M.H., Eds.; Springer: Boston, MA, USA, 1994; pp. 253–259.
22. Den Uijl, L.C.; Jager, G.; de Graaf, C.; Waddell, J.; Kremer, S. It is not just a meal, it is an emotional experience—A segmentation of older persons based on the emotions that they associate with mealtimes. *Appetite* **2014**, *83*, 287–296. [CrossRef] [PubMed]
23. Gutjar, S.; Dalenberg, J.R.; de Graaf, C.; de Wijk, R.A.; Palascha, A.; Renken, R.J.; Jager, G. What reported food-evoked emotions may add: A model to predict consumer food choice. *Food Qual. Prefer.* **2015**, *45*, 140–148. [CrossRef]
24. Köster, E.P.; Mojet, J. From mood to food and from food to mood: A psychological perspective on the measurement of food-related emotions in consumer research. *Food Res. Int.* **2015**, *76*, 180–191. [CrossRef]
25. Peryam, D.R.; Pilgrim, F.J. Hedonic scale method of measuring food preferences. *Food Technol.* **1957**, *11*, 9–14.
26. Ares, G.; Bruzzone, F.; Vidal, L.; Cadena, R.S.; Giménez, A.; Pineau, B.; Hunter, D.C.; Paisley, A.G.; Jaeger, S.R. Evaluation of a rating-based variant of check-all-that-apply questions: Rate-all-that-apply (RATA). *Food Qual. Prefer.* **2014**, *36*, 87–95. [CrossRef]
27. Lawless, H.T.; Heymann, H. *Sensory Evaluation of Food: Principles and Practices*, 2nd ed.; Springer Science & Business Media: New York, NY, USA, 2010; pp. 519–520. ISBN 978-1-4419-6487-8.
28. Plaehn, D. CATA penalty/reward. *Food Qual. Prefer.* **2012**, *24*, 141–152. [CrossRef]
29. Meyners, M.; Castura, J.C.; Carr, B.T. Existing and new approaches for the analysis of CATA data. *Food Qual. Prefer.* **2013**, *30*, 309–319. [CrossRef]
30. Torri, L.; Salini, S. An itinerant sensory approach to investigate consumers' perception and acceptability at a food exhibition. *Food Res. Int.* **2016**, *90*, 91–99. [CrossRef] [PubMed]
31. Waehrens, S.S.; Grønbeck, M.S.; Olsen, K.; Byrne, D.V. Impact of consumer associations, emotions, and appropriateness for use on food acceptability: A CATA and liking evaluation of vegetable and berry beverage. *J. Sens. Stud.* **2018**, e12328. [CrossRef]
32. Ames, J.M. Control of the Maillard reaction in food systems. *Trends Food Sci. Technol.* **1990**, *1*, 150–154. [CrossRef]

33. Cheung, L.K.; Aluko, R.E.; Cliff, M.A.; Li-Chan, E.C. Effects of exopeptidase treatment on antihypertensive activity and taste attributes of enzymatic whey protein hydrolysates. *J. Funct. Foods* **2015**, *13*, 262–275. [CrossRef]
34. Leksrisompong, P.; Gerard, P.; Lopetcharat, K.; Drake, M. Bitter taste inhibiting agents for whey protein hydrolysate and whey protein hydrolysate beverages. *J. Food Sci.* **2012**, *77*, S282–S287. [CrossRef] [PubMed]
35. Daw, E.; Hartel, R.W. Fat destabilization and melt-down of ice creams with increased protein content. *Int. Dairy J.* **2015**, *43*, 33–41. [CrossRef]
36. Wendin, K.; Langton, M.; Caous, L.; Hall, G. Dynamic analyses of sensory and microstructural properties of cream cheese. *Food Chem.* **2000**, *71*, 363–378. [CrossRef]
37. Leksrisompong, P.P.; Miracle, R.E.; Drake, M. Characterization of flavor of whey protein hydrolysates. *J. Agric. Food Chem.* **2010**, *58*, 6318–6327. [CrossRef] [PubMed]
38. Song, X.; Giacalone, D.; Johansen, S.M.B.; Frøst, M.B.; Bredie, W.L.P. Changes in orosensory perception related to aging and strategies for counteracting its influence on food preferences among older adults. *Trends Food Sci. Technol.* **2016**, *53*, 49–59. [CrossRef]
39. Holt, S.H.A.; Delargy, H.J.; Lawton, C.L.; Blundell, J.E. The effects of high-carbohydrate vs high-fat breakfasts on feelings of fullness and alertness, and subsequent food intake. *Int. J. Food Sci. Nutr.* **1999**, *50*, 13–28. [CrossRef] [PubMed]
40. Heiniö, R.L.; Liukkonen, K.H.; Katina, K.; Myllymäki, O.; Poutanen, K. Milling fractionation of rye produces different sensory profiles of both flour and bread. *LWT-Food Sci. Technol.* **2003**, *36*, 577–583. [CrossRef]
41. Rhyu, M.R.; Kim, E.Y. Umami taste characteristics of water extract of Doenjang, a Korean soybean paste: Low-molecular acidic peptides may be a possible clue to the taste. *Food Chem.* **2011**, *127*, 1210–1215. [CrossRef] [PubMed]
42. Fu, Y.; Liu, J.; Hansen, E.T.; Bredie, W.L.P.; Lametsch, R. Structural characteristics of low bitter and high umami protein hydrolysates prepared from bovine muscle and porcine plasma. *Food Chem.* **2018**, *257*, 163–171. [CrossRef] [PubMed]
43. Spiegel, T. Whey protein aggregation under shear conditions–effects of lactose and heating temperature on aggregate size and structure. *Int. J. Food Sci. Technol.* **1999**, *34*, 523–531. [CrossRef]
44. Havea, P.; Singh, H.; Creamer, L.K. Characterization of heat-induced aggregates of β-lactoglobulin, α-lactalbumin and bovine serum albumin in a whey protein concentrate environment. *J. Dairy Res.* **2001**, *68*. [CrossRef]
45. Foegeding, E.A.; Davis, J.P.; Doucet, D.; McGuffey, M.K. Advances in modifying and understanding whey protein functionality. *Trends Food Sci. Technol.* **2002**, *13*, 151–159. [CrossRef]
46. Ziobro, R.; Witczak, T.; Juszczak, L.; Korus, J. Supplementation of gluten-free bread with non-gluten proteins. Effect on dough rheological properties and bread characteristic. *Food Hydrocoll.* **2013**, *32*, 213–220. [CrossRef]
47. Jeltema, M.; Beckley, J.; Vahalik, J. Food texture assessment and preference based on mouth behavior. *Food Qual. Prefer.* **2016**, *52*, 160–171. [CrossRef]
48. Li-Chan, E.C.Y. Bioactive peptides and protein hydrolysates: Research trends and challenges for application as nutraceuticals and functional food ingredients. *Curr. Opin. Food Sci.* **2015**, *1*, 28–37. [CrossRef]
49. Vella, M.N.; Stratton, L.M.; Sheeshka, J.; Duncan, A.M. Exploration of functional food consumption in older adults in relation to food matrices, bioactive ingredients, and health. *J. Nutr. Gerontol. Geriatr.* **2013**, *32*, 122–144. [CrossRef] [PubMed]
50. Meiselman, H.L. The contextual basis for food acceptance, food choice and food intake: The food, the situation and the individual. In *Food Choice, Acceptance and Consumption*, 1st ed.; Meiselman, H.L., MacFie, H.J.H., Eds.; Springer: Boston, MA, USA, 1996; pp. 239–263. ISBN 0-7514-0192-7.
51. Ziylan, C.; Kremer, S.; Eerens, J.; Haveman-Nies, A.; de Groot, L.C. Effect of meal size reduction and protein enrichment on intake and satiety in vital community-dwelling older adults. *Appetite* **2016**, *105*, 242–248. [CrossRef] [PubMed]

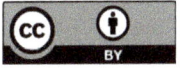

© 2018 by the authors. Licensee MDPI, Basel, Switzerland. This article is an open access article distributed under the terms and conditions of the Creative Commons Attribution (CC BY) license (http://creativecommons.org/licenses/by/4.0/).

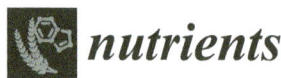

Review

Muscle and Bone Health in Postmenopausal Women: Role of Protein and Vitamin D Supplementation Combined with Exercise Training

Deborah Agostini [1,†], Sabrina Donati Zeppa [1,†], Francesco Lucertini [1], Giosuè Annibalini [1], Marco Gervasi [1], Carlo Ferri Marini [1], Giovanni Piccoli [1], Vilberto Stocchi [1], Elena Barbieri [1,2,*] and Piero Sestili [1]

[1] Department of Biomolecular Sciences, University of Urbino Carlo Bo, 61029 (PU) Urbino, Italy; deborah.agostini@uniurb.it (D.A.); sabrina.zeppa@uniurb.it (S.D.Z.); francesco.lucertini@uniurb.it (F.L.); giosue.annibalini@uniurb.it (G.A.); marco.gervasi@uniurb.it (M.G.); carlo.ferrimarini@uniurb.it (C.F.M.); giovanni.piccoli@uniurb.it (G.P.); vilberto.stocchi@uniurb.it (V.S.); piero.sestili@uniurb.it (P.S.)
[2] Interuniversity Institute of Myology (IIM), University of Urbino Carlo Bo, 61029 (PU) Urbino, Italy
* Correspondence: elena.barbieri@uniurb.it; Tel.: +39-0722-303-417; Fax: +39-0722-303-401
† These Authors contributed equally to this review.

Received: 17 July 2018; Accepted: 13 August 2018; Published: 16 August 2018

Abstract: Menopause is an age-dependent physiological condition associated with a natural decline in oestrogen levels, which causes a progressive decrease of muscle mass and strength and bone density. Sarcopenia and osteoporosis often coexist in elderly people, with a prevalence of the latter in elderly women. The profound interaction between muscle and bone induces a negative resonance between the two tissues affected by these disorders worsening the quality of life in the postmenopausal period. It has been estimated that at least 1 in 3 women over age 50 will experience osteoporotic fractures, often requiring hospitalisation and long-term care, causing a large financial burden to health insurance systems. Hormonal replacement therapy is effective in osteoporosis prevention, but concerns have been raised with regard to its safety. On the whole, the increase in life expectancy for postmenopausal women along with the need to improve their quality of life makes it necessary to develop specific and safe therapeutic strategies, alternative to hormonal replacement therapy, targeting both sarcopenia and osteoporosis progression. This review will examine the rationale and the effects of dietary protein, vitamin D and calcium supplementation combined with a specifically-designed exercise training prescription as a strategy to counteract these postmenopausal-associated disorders.

Keywords: postmenopausal women; sarcopenia; osteoporosis; exercise; dietary protein; vitamin D

1. Introduction

Sarcopenia was firstly described at the end of the twentieth century by Rosenberg as a degenerative depletion in muscle mass [1] associated with age. It also involves the loss of muscle functionality leading to mobility restriction, functional impairment and physical disability [2] and finally loss of independence and reduced quality of life.

Even though there is still heterogeneity in diagnostic criteria and modalities to detect sarcopenia, the most used is the definition adopted by the European Working Group on Sarcopenia in Older People (EWGSOP) [3]. The group recommended, for the diagnosis of sarcopenia, that low muscle mass should be associated with low muscle function (defined as strength and performance) and proposed an algorithm for case finding in older individuals based on measurements of gait speed, grip strength and muscle mass. They also described measurement tools and specific age/gender cut off points to distinguish between presarcopenia, sarcopenia and severe sarcopenia [3]. Afterwards, an International Working Group on Sarcopenia (IWGS) incorporated sex-specific threshold values for muscle mass [4] while the Foundation of NIH (FNIH) Sarcopenia Project proposed a different definition for sarcopenia [5].

Although it is challenging to distinguish among sarcopenia, frailty and cachexia, they do represent different conditions: frailty has been defined by Morley et al. as "a medical syndrome with multiple causes and contributors that is characterized by diminished strength, endurance and reduced physiologic function that increases an individual's vulnerability for developing increased dependency and/or death," of which sarcopenia can be an aspect [6]; cachexia, characterized by weight and muscle mass loss, can be a cause of sarcopenia having a great inflammatory component [7].

The loss of muscle mass begins substantially at the age of 50 and continues afterwards [8] with similar gender-independent changes, such as increased inflammation and satellite cell senescence, reduced myocyte regeneration and protein synthesis [9] and several other gender-dependent alterations caused by the age-associated decrease of sex hormones [10]. Due to the decrease of testosterone in men and oestrogens in women, people of both genders experience sarcopenia. Although in general, men show a greater decay in muscle mass, women frequently present sarcopenia, since their muscle mass level in young age is physiologically much lower [11,12]. In a recent meta-analysis, Shafiee et al. examined the overall prevalence of sarcopenia in both women and men aged >60 years using the EWGSOP, IWGS and Asian Working Group for Sarcopenia criteria: they reported a prevalence of about 10% in adults, without global gender differences [13]. Hormonal replacement therapy (HRT) aimed at preventing the modifications and chronic somatic diseases caused by age-related oestrogen decrease, results in greater muscle strength in 50–65 years women, while in older women studies are not conclusive [14,15].

Several studies highlighted an association between sarcopenia and osteoporosis, another age-related disease involving low bone mineral density (BMD), bone tissue frailty and risk of fractures [16]. Osteoporosis is diagnosed by BMD criteria or occurrence of fragility factors [17]. Osteoporosis is more prevalent among older individuals with a far higher prevalence in women, where the onset often coincides with menopause. Indeed, it is estimated that the overall effect of menopause is an annual bone loss of about 2% during the first six years and 0.5–1% thereafter [18]. In western countries, the risk of osteoporotic fractures during the lifetime is about 40–50% in women and 13–22% in men [19]. Osteoporotic fractures often require hospitalisation and long-term care; thus, osteoporosis represents a significant health challenge worldwide. The Women's Health Initiative is a long-term health study focused on strategies for preventing disease in postmenopausal women, aimed to analyse and suggest strategies to manage postmenopausal related problems effectively. During the project, eleven clinically risk factors have been identified, providing new insights into the epidemiology of osteoporosis [20].

Muscle-bone physiological interaction is increasingly reputed to be essential to prevent disease and disability in the elderly: in particular, Sjöblom et al. reported that women suffering from sarcopenia have more than a double higher risk of fracture and falls compared to those without the disease [21]. Among multiple factors, the musculoskeletal decline is also linked to protein, calcium and vitamin D availability and decrease in physical activity level. Deterioration in muscle and bone health is majorly caused by an inadequate protein intake associated with a significant demand due to an aging-related increase of protein anabolic resistance, chronic inflammation and oxidative processes [22]. The lack of physical activity, often affecting elderly people, accelerates muscle catabolism and is another major risk factor. Collectively, these problems may lead to a vicious cycle of muscle loss, injury and inefficient repair, causing elderly people to become progressively sedentary over time. Thus, therapeutic and/or nutritional strategies improving muscle mass and regeneration in the aged are nowadays required. Importantly, these strategies could also allow to maintain the capacity of sustaining and practicing physical exercise. Indeed, exercise is known to mitigate several deleterious effects of aging, such as insulin resistance, mitochondrial dysfunction and inflammation in muscle [23] and represent one of the best strategies to counteract sarcopenia. Resistance exercise is a trigger for muscle protein synthesis and can work in synergy with adequate protein intake [24].

In the elderly vitamin D deficiency often occurs and it is associated with sarcopenia, bone loss and disability. Vitamin D is highly interconnected with phosphate and calcium metabolism, as first demonstrated by Harrison and Harrison in 1961 [25]. The 1,25-dihydroxyvitamin D, D (1,25(OH)2D) the active metabolite of vitamin D, also known as calcitriol, increases intestinal phosphate absorption enhancing the expression of type 2b sodium–phosphate co-transporter [26,27]. Moreover, a deficiency of phosphate stimulates 1α-hydroxylase to convert vitamin D to calcitriol, which in turn stimulates phosphate absorption in the small intestine. Furthermore, calcitriol can also induce the secretion of Fibroblast-like growth factor-23 by osteocytes in bone, which lead to phosphate excretion in the kidney [28], as well as feedback on vitamin D metabolism. Since vitamin D is responsible for adequate intestinal absorption of calcium and phosphate, it maintains appropriate circulating concentrations of these minerals, which enable normal mineralization of the bone contributing to muscle health. Thus, adequate intake of calcium and vitamin D, associated with a correct lifestyle, is suggested during aging [29].

On the whole, the increase in life expectancy for postmenopausal women along with the need to improve their quality of life makes it necessary to develop specific therapeutic strategies, in association with HRT or as an alternative to it. Here we discuss the effect of protein intake, vitamin D supplementation, physical activity and of their synergistic administration in maintaining musculoskeletal health in postmenopausal women.

2. Mechanisms Involved in Muscle and Bone Loss in Postmenopausal Women

One of the most responsive pathways involved in musculoskeletal health is the Mammalian target of rapamycin (mTOR), involved in several anabolic processes in skeletal muscle [30]. mTOR is an evolutionarily conserved serine/threonine kinase known to play critical roles in protein synthesis. A better understanding of mTOR signalling in the maintenance of skeletal muscle mass might favour the development of mTOR-targeted treatments to prevent muscle wasting with particular attention at the healthy muscle in postmenopausal women conditions [31]. A well-known upstream stimulator of mTOR in skeletal muscle is insulin-like growth factor 1 (IGF-1), recognized as indispensable for muscle growth and regeneration [32–34] IGF-1 binds to the IGF-1 receptor (IGF1-R), a receptor tyrosine-kinase and subsequently recruits insulin receptor substrate-1. The specific role of each IGF-1 isoform and their post-translational modifications [35] must be taken into consideration for their effect in the proper tissue or microenvironment context. Furthermore, IGF-1 is directly involved in mitogenesis and neoplastic transformation, suggesting that this signalling pathway plays an important role in cancer promotion. IGF-1-therapeutic strategies must be viewed in the appropriate tissue context and in function of the IGF-1 circulating level and depending on IGFBP availability.

In women, the age-related decline of skeletal muscle mass and strength accelerates with the beginning of menopause. Oestrogen signalling of muscle satellite cell activation and proliferation is mediated via oestrogen receptor-alpha (ERα) placed on skeletal muscle and activates several signalling pathways including IGF-1 signalling, nitric oxide signalling or activation of the phosphor-inositide-3 kinase/protein kinase B (Akt) pathway which then act to positively influence muscle satellite cells and promote protein synthesis [31]. Recent investigations demonstrated that IGF-1 and its receptor IGF1-R were not necessary for the induction of hypertrophy and the activation of Akt/mTOR in mechanical loading [36]. The expression of dominant negative (DN)-IGF-1 receptor specifically in skeletal muscle promoted muscle hypertrophy using an increased functional overload model induced by synergistic ablation [36]. Of notice, DN-IGF-I receptor-expressing muscle showed a comparable level of Akt and p70S6K1 activation. This data does not exclude an alternative upstream mediator for IGF1-R that could regulate Akt/mTOR signalling in skeletal muscle hypertrophy. In women, recent studies showed that the expression of IGF1-R in skeletal muscle cells increased in postmenopausal period after oestrogen replacement [37]. Moreover, it is known that oestrogen has an anabolic influence on muscle stimulating IGF-1R [38]. ERs are also expressed in human muscles [39]. In this regard, Wiik et al. have described the form of ERα and ERβ in both myonuclei and capillaries [40]. Their expression and distribution in muscle fibres appear greater in men, women and children, compared to postmenopausal women [40]. Notably, ERs can be also activated through IGF-1 that acts in stimulating their transcriptional activity [41]. Indeed, ERs could take part in muscle strength increase through the effect of both oestrogen and IGF-1. Despite that, both oestrogen and IGF-1 reduced at menopause, probably affecting muscle mass and strength.

Accordingly, estradiol plays an important role in the morphological muscle status increasing translocation of the glucose transporter, GLUT-4 to the plasma membrane through Akt pathway. Indeed, it causes an increase of myogenin and myosin heavy chain levels, which are important in skeletal muscles remodelling [42,43]. Estradiol also induces the Akt phosphorylation in myoblasts and its administration in postmenopausal women up-regulates the expression of mTOR genes [44]. As known, muscle wasting occurs when catabolic states overcome anabolic states. Sex hormones (i.e., androgens and oestrogen) play different roles in muscle mass maintenance and their decrease during aging negatively affects musculoskeletal health. Testosterone promotes an anabolic state activating protein synthesis and muscular regeneration through the androgen receptor, expressed in mesenchymal stem cells, satellite cells and fibroblasts [45]. Furthermore, it acts increasing circulating and intramuscular IGF-1 [46]. The catabolic state is promoted by the ubiquitin-proteasome system (UPS), autophagy-lysosomal system and apoptosis. Myostatin and inflammatory cytokines promote Forkhead box O (FOXO) protein activation that induces UPS and autophagy-lysosomal systems. Oestrogen is likely to promote an anti-inflammatory and anti-catabolic influence on muscle, especially after exercise, even though a complete characterization of mechanisms is lacking [10].

Several studies demonstrated an association between sarcopenia and osteoporosis, another age-related disease characterized by low BMD leading to bone tissue frailty and risk of fractures [16], with a higher prevalence in women. Biomechanical and biochemical interactions in the musculoskeletal unit are of great importance in the regulation and maintenance of tissue function. As functional units, muscles and long bones adapt to respond to metabolic and mechanical demand in health and they deteriorate together with ageing because of the same biomechanical and biochemical link between these two tissues [47]. The 'mechanostat' theory of Frost states that bone adjusts itself to sustain strain in a physiological window [48]: bone formation occurs if a greater strain is requested (i.e., physical activity), while lower strains (i.e., inactivity) will promote bone resorption. Accordingly, there will be an increase or a decrease, respectively, in muscle mass. Alongside biomechanical coupling in the musculoskeletal unit, also biochemical communication should be considered in muscle-bone crosstalk since both muscle and bone act as endocrine organs secreting respectively "myokines" and "osteokines" [49]. Skeletal muscle releases several hundred proteins and peptides capable of influencing bone health. The myokine [50] and osteokine [51] irisin, for example, is increased by exercise and has anabolic effects on muscle [50] and on osteoblast lineage by enhancing differentiation and activity of bone-forming cells [52]. Also, myostatin—that is, a negative regulator of muscle growth and interleukin-6 (IL-6)—is reported to have effects on bone [53]. Furthermore, skeletal muscle expresses high levels of several microRNAs that can be delivered by exosomes [54]. Information regarding the endocrine and paracrine effects of muscle-derived exosomes is limited but they are likely to play a role also in bone [53].

Also, tendons, ligaments, cartilage and connective tissue can affect muscle bone cross-talk [49]; periosteum, that separates muscle and bone, is semi-permeable and molecules such as IGF-1, IL-5 and prostaglandin E2 could permeate this membrane [55]. Taking into account the tight connection between muscle and bone, maintaining healthy skeletal muscles (i.e., through adequate exercise and nutrition) can help in counteracting osteoporosis in postmenopausal women.

Oestrogen-based HRT has an important role in maintaining and enhancing muscle mass and strength and also in protecting against muscle damage. The benefits of oestrogen for the skeletal muscle coupled with their additional positive actions on bone and metabolic health in older females provide further incentives for HRT use to enhance overall health in postmenopausal women. HRT is associated with an improved contractile function and power in 50–65-year-old women [15], while research is not conclusive in older, postmenopausal women. Analysing coronary heart disease and mortality, HRT showed many benefits in early observational data for use in younger healthy women (50–60 years) but age stratification revealed no benefit and increased harm in >60 year women, together with an increased breast cancer risk [56]. Recently the US Preventive Services Task Force recommended against the prevention of chronic condition in menopause using a combined oestrogen and progestin therapy and against oestrogen alone in postmenopausal women after hysterectomy [57], due to well documented harmful effects. Marjoribanks et al., in a systematic review on long-term HRT for perimenopausal and postmenopausal women, concluded that even though HRT is effective in osteoporosis prevention, it should be recommended as an option only when the risk of disease is very high and no other strategy is available [58]. They suggest that the adoption of HRT, if necessary, should be short-termed, provided that there is no increased risk of cardiovascular and thromboembolic disease and of several types of cancer [58]. The disadvantages related to the menopause, however, are not always manifested all at the same time and in all women; in some it seems not to be completely, in others there are only some disturbances, in others, finally, these disadvantages occur together and can also be very evident and frustrating.

The risks associated with taking a pharmacological substitution therapy is much debated, but, in light of the most recent scientific acquisitions, menopause can be tackled by acquiring healthy habits that prevent the related disorders. Thanks to the better understanding of the causes, the ease of access to the diagnosis and the possibility of treatment before fractures occurrence today, a real prevention of both sarcopenia and osteoporosis and associated complications is possible. First of all, the fact is that muscle and bone health is a process that must develop throughout life in both males and females. Building a strong and healthy muscle-skeletal structure in childhood and adolescence can be the best defence. The further key steps that should be pursued at all ages for a successful prevention should consider: monitor a balanced diet rich in protein sources, calcium, magnesium and vitamin D that could interfere with anabolic mediators for both muscle and bone; practice exercise to enhance muscle strength, power output, neuromuscular activity and muscle mass; follow healthy lifestyles (avoiding alcohol, smoke and drugs) and, when appropriate, perform tests to define bone mineral density and possibly undergo appropriate treatment.

3. Exercise

Given the strict association between loss of muscle (namely, sarcopenia) and bone mass (namely, osteoporosis) that accompany aging, physical activity and exercise represent effective preventive and therapeutic strategies able to slow down sarcopenia progression and prevent/delay the onset of and treat, osteoporosis. Indeed, exercise has beneficial effects on muscle mass, muscle strength and physical performance [59–61], which counteract the reduced ability to perform activities of daily living and the increased risk of musculoskeletal injuries related to sarcopenia [62,63]. Exercise has also been shown to delay the onset of osteoporosis [64–66] and to improve balance [67] and muscular fitness [64–66,68] thus it is generally regarded as the primary non-pharmacological treatment for the prevention of osteoporosis and fall-related fractures. Since menopause occurs approximately with the onset of sarcopenia, aging non-physically active postmenopausal women should switch as soon as possible to an active lifestyle to prevent osteoporosis, while those already osteoporotic should exercise regularly to improve bone health and reduce the risk of fractures. It is well known that exercise, particularly progressive resistance exercise training (RET), is effective in increasing muscle mass, strength and endurance. Specific recommendations and guidance to prescribe exercise to treat sarcopenia, which update and extend those of the American College of Sports Medicine (ACSM) to promote muscle hypertrophy, strength and power [69], have recently appeared in literature [70]. Exercise that enhances muscle strength and mass also increases bone mass (i.e., bone mineral density and content) and bone strength of the specific bones stressed and may serve as a valuable measure to prevent, slow, or reverse the loss of bone mass in individuals with osteoporosis. Although further studies are still needed to determine optimal exercise prescription parameters for preventing osteoporosis and fractures [64–66] a recent consensus on physical activity and exercise recommendations for adults with osteoporosis [71] has stated the appropriateness of the current physical activity guidelines [68,72] for those without spine fractures and has proposed safer exercise guidance and strategies for those with a history of vertebral fractures. The ACSM's framework for exercise prescription employs the so-called FITT-VP principle [73], which reflects the frequency (F), intensity (I), time (T) and type (T) of exercise and its volume (V) and progression (P) over time, in an individualized exercise training program. A detailed description of the FITT-VP principle for each type of exercise i.e., aerobic, resistance, flexibility and balance- adapted to postmenopausal ageing women according to the abovementioned studies, is provided in the following tables (Tables 1–4).

Literature put a strong emphasis on resistance training for all individuals with osteoporosis [71] and recommend moderate to high intensity RET to treat sarcopenia [70]. Therefore, since preventing the loss of -or increasing- muscle strength and endurance is a cross-cutting goal for both sarcopenic and osteoporotic postmenopausal women, emphasis on progressive RET has been proposed. As a consequence of this approach, in this population there is the need to account for daily protein intake and, even, timing of protein supplementation [74].

Table 1. Aerobic (cardiorespiratory endurance) exercise recommendations for ageing postmenopausal women.

Intensity—I	Frequency—F	Time—T (Duration)	Type—T (Mode) [Examples]	Volume—V (Quantity)	Progression—P (Rate of)	Specific Notes
Moderate: 40–59% of VO$_2$R or HRR; 64–75% HR$_{max}$; 4–5 RPE	At least 5 day·week^{-1}	30 to 60 min each session (i.e., at least 150 min·week^{-1})	Weight-bearing activity [walking, jogging, dancing, or other activities where full body weight is supported by limbs]	≥500–1000 MET·min·week^{-1}	Increase gradually any of the FITT components (as tolerated). Initiate increasing exercise duration: an example is adding 5–10 min every 1–2 week over the first 4–6 week and adjusting upward over the next 4–8 months to meet the recommended FITT components	If tolerated, moderate to vigorous intensity and 3–5 day·week^{-1} frequency is recommended but lower intensities and frequencies are still beneficial when the current physical activity level is low. For individuals with a history of vertebral fracture vigorous intensity may not be appropriate because it might increase the risk of falls or fractures: in those patients, moderate intensity is recommended
Vigorous: 60–89% of VO$_2$R or HRR; 76–95% HR$_{max}$; 6–8 RPE	At least 3 day·week^{-1}	20 to 60 min each session (i.e., at least 75 min·week^{-1})				

Modified from [69,70,72]. MET·min: metabolic equivalents (MET) of energy expenditure for a physical activity performed for a given number of minutes (min), calculated as MET × min; VO$_2$R: oxygen uptake reserve, calculated as the difference between maximal oxygen uptake and resting oxygen uptake; HRR: heart rate reserve, calculated as the difference between maximal heart rate and resting heart rate; HR$_{max}$: maximal heart rate; RPE: rate of perceived exertion, on the 0–10 scale.

Table 2. Resistance (strength) exercise recommendations for ageing postmenopausal women.

Intensity—I	Frequency—F	Time—T (Duration)	Type—T (Mode) [Examples]	Volume—V (Quantity)	Progression—P (Rate of)	Specific Notes
Novice exercisers: ~8 to 12 repetitions performed near task failure (i.e., ~10 to 14-RM or 5–8 on the 0–10 RPE scale)	1–2 day·week^{-1}	Depends on exercise volume (number of sets, repetitions for each set and rest intervals in-between) and is not associated with effectiveness	Any form of movement designed to improve muscular fitness by exercising a muscle or a muscle group against external resistance: exercise and breathing techniques are of paramount importance [free weights, resistance machines, weight-bearing functional tasks, etc.]	1 set of 8–12 repetitions (no more than 8–10 exercises per session)	Progress with small increments possible [e.g., 2–10% 1-RM, depending on muscular size and involvement, is recommended]. If a break is taken, lower the level of resistance by 2 weeks' worth of no exercise	Avoid making absolute restrictions about amount of weight allowed, instead place emphasis on safe movement recommendations; avoid rapid, repetitive, weighted, or end-range flexion or rotation of the spine; avoid lifting from or lowering to the floor; avoid exercises to improve strength/endurance in "core" or "abdominal" muscles involving repeated flexion or rotation of the spine (isometric exercises, or holds are preferable. In individuals with a history of vertebral fracture a consultation with an exercise specialist/therapist with training in exercise prescription for osteoporosis is highly recommended (in the absence of such consultation, it may be advisable to limit resistance exercises to those that use body weight, the floor, or the wall to provide resistance)
Intermediate to experienced exercisers: ~8 to 12 repetitions performed to task failure (i.e., ~8 to 12-RM or >8 on the 0–10 RPE scale)	2–3 day·week^{-1}			2 sets of 8–12 repetitions (no more than 8–10 exercises per session)		

Modified from [69,70,72]. RPE: rate of perceived exertion, on the 0–10 scale; 1-RM: one repetition maximum, that is, the load that can be lifted one time only; multiple RM: the load that can be lifted no more than the specified times.

Table 3. Flexibility (stretching) exercise recommendations for ageing postmenopausal women.

Intensity—I	Frequency—F	Time—T (Duration)	Type—T (Mode) [Examples]	Volume—V (Quantity)	Progression—P (Rate of)	Specific Notes
Stretch to the point of feeling tightness or slight discomfort	≥2–3 day·week^{-1} (stretching on a daily basis is most effective)	Hold a static stretch for at least 10–30 s (30–60 s may confer greater benefit). Accumulate a total of 60 s of stretching for each flexibility exercise by adjusting time/duration and repetitions (see volume) according to individual needs	Stretching exercise that increase the ability to move a joint through its complete ROM (provided individual specific conditions are accounted for) (static active flexibility; static passive flexibility; dynamic flexibility; ballistic flexibility; proprioceptive neuromuscular facilitation; etc.)	Repeat each exercise 2–4 times in order to attain the goal of 60 s stretch time [e.g.: two 30-s stretches or four 15-s stretches]. A stretching routine can be completed approximately in ≤10 min	Optimal progression is still unknown	Focus on joints with low ROM. Flexibility exercises are most effective when the muscles are warm

Modified from [69,70,72]. ROM: range of motion.

Table 4. Balance exercise recommendations for ageing postmenopausal women.

Intensity—I	Frequency—F	Time—T (Duration)	Type—T (Mode) [Examples]	Volume—V (Quantity)	Progression—P (Rate of)	Specific Notes
Not applicable	Daily	≥15–20 min	Exercises include those that reduce the base of support in static stance [e.g., semi-tandem, tandem, or one-legged stand], a dynamic or three-dimensional balance challenge [e.g., Tai Chi, tandem walk, walking on heels or toes], or other strategies to challenge balance systems [e.g., weight shifting, reduced contact with support objects, dual-tasking, close eyes during static balance challenges, etc.]	Cumulative time: 2 h per week	Progress from "standing still" to "dynamic" exercises. Progression of the balance challenge should occur over time [e.g., moving to a more difficult exercise, removing vision or contact with support object, or dual-tasking, etc.]	Balance can be exercised during daily walks or activities, while standing still reduce the base of support, semi-tandem stance, one-leg stand; shift weight between heels and toes or during dynamic movements [e.g., Tai Chi; tandem walk, dancing, etc.]

Modified from [69,70,72].

4. Dietary Protein

Aged skeletal muscle possesses a reduced ability to respond to amino acid and insulin levels, leading to the concept of anabolic resistance, influenced by dietary protein digestion and amino acid absorption, plasma availability and hormonal response [75]. Moreau et al. reported differences in splanchnic protein metabolism during aging, with a maintained muscle protein synthesis (MPS), in a condition of an adequate rate of plasma levels of essential amino acids [76]. Alongside a reduced ability to use protein, a greater demand and a reduced intake are often present [22]. Chronic low-grade inflammation, that is often linked to oestrogen decrease and to visceral adipose tissue, favours proteolysis over synthesis and leads to an increased MPS demand [77]. Recommendations for dietary protein intake in general population with a moderate physical activity is 0.8 g of protein per kilogram of body weight per day [78]; however, due to increased protein demand in healthy older people, the European Society for Clinical Nutrition and Metabolism has proposed a daily recommended amount of 1.0–1.2 g/kg body weight/day as optimal for a healthy older individual [79,80]. Physical activity and exercise require a higher protein intake than sedentary condition [81].

Data from the National Health and Nutrition Examination Survey (NHANES) showed that, despite recommendations, daily protein intake decreases in the elderly and at least 8% of women consume an insufficient amount of protein [82]. 35% of institutionalized elderly people do not reach the recommended daily allowance (RDA) [83]. Gregorio et al. analysed the association of dietary protein amount with physical performance in postmenopausal women [84]. A sample of 387 healthy women has been studied, revealing an average consumption of 1.1 g/kg body weight/day and a percentage of 25% of subjects resulted below the RDA: they reported that subjects within the low protein group possess an impaired upper and lower extremity functionality than those in higher consumption group and that subjects with higher BMI and fat/lean ratio often consume protein below the RDA [84]. It should be remembered that higher fat mass is associated with impaired muscle metabolism [85] and insulin resistance, which is recognised as precursor of frailty [86].

Increased availability of amino acids has positive effects on muscle anabolism [87] improving lean body mass [88]. Protein intake also increases IGF-1 plasma concentration [89], together with muscle mass and strength [90]. In addition to the bone anabolic effect of IGF-1, increased protein intake has also been shown to reduce bone resorption [91]; furthermore, protein can act modifying calcitriol and intestinal calcium absorption, increasing bone health [92]. As explained, protein intake above RDA may be of benefits in postmenopausal women and Antonio et al. demonstrated the safety and effectiveness of three-fold higher dose in increasing lean mass, in both genders in association with resistance exercise [93]. In young women, the author also excluded a dangerous effect of high protein intake (more than 2.2 g/kg body weight/day for six months) on bone mineral content [94].

The best daily frequency for consuming protein, that is, single versus fractionated intakes, is still under debate. Indeed, some studies reported that daily protein should be consumed in a single meal, since a protein pulse feeding was more efficient than protein spread feeding in improving protein retention [95] and increasing plasma postprandial amino acid concentrations [96]. However, Kim et al. [97] found no differences comparing the effect of protein distribution pattern on functional outcome and protein kinetics; other studies reported that within-day protein distribution was more efficient in improving protein synthesis [98] and was negatively correlated with frailty [99]. Finally, a more frequent consumption of meals containing 30–45 g of protein [100] or protein supplementation at breakfast and lunch [101] have been recently associated with better lean mass preservation in older people.

Several factors can influence postprandial MPS: in particular, muscle disuse as a consequence of sarcopenia or immobilization causes a decrease in basal metabolic rate and muscle strength [102] and dietary protein consumption fails to act in this pathological condition [103]. On the contrary essential amino acid induces an enhanced effect on MPS if ingested following a resistance training session [104]. The mechanism involved in exercise-improvement of dietary protein effect depends on an increased amino acid delivery to the muscle through blood flow [105] and on mTOR pathway activation (after resistance exercise), that lead to muscle mass enhancement if an adequate amino acid pool is present: notably, this process seems to be delayed in elderly [106].

Alongside total protein amount and within-day protein distribution, quality of protein and their sources should be considered [107] in terms of essential amino acids and leucine content and of digestion/absorption kinetics. Pennings et al. [108] demonstrated that whey stimulates postprandial muscle protein accretion more effectively than casein and casein hydrolysate in older men, and attributed this effect to whey's faster digestion and absorption kinetics and to higher leucine content.

More recently, Zhu et al. demonstrated that in older postmenopausal well-nourished healthy women (70–80 years old) 30 g/day of extra protein did not improve the maintenance of muscle mass or physical function despite muscle deterioration in the upper limb. The authors attributed the lack of effects to the high habitual protein intake of women involved in this study, suggesting that protein intervention could be more effective in not well-nourished population. Furthermore, the intervention was not carried out in combination with resistance exercise, which has been demonstrated to improve protein effect [109]. Daly et al. reported that a protein-enriched diet equivalent to 1.3 g/kg body weight/day achieved through lean red meat consumption is safe and useful for enhancing the effects of resistance training on lean body mass and muscle strength and reducing circulating IL-6 concentrations in elderly women [110]. In this study, women were in a broader age range (60–90) and more than 40% had a history of HRT: these differences, in combination with training, could explain the discrepancies in muscle response.

Figueiredo Braggion et al. compared the effects of diets rich in vegetable protein versus animal protein in ovariectomized old female rats (a condition that may only mimic human menopause) in association or not with resistance training. They demonstrated that animal protein diet combined with training promoted muscle remodelling (reduction in type I and IIA fibres with an increase in type IIB fibres in medial gastrocnemius muscle, with increased collagen volume density) more efficiently compared to other conditions applied [111]. More importantly, a very recent human study showed that animal derived protein consumption, combined with physical activity, is positively associated with muscle mass and strength across ages in men and women [112].

Milk is a high-quality protein source, able of increasing muscle synthesis to a similar extent that whey [113] and beef [114]. However, the proposed protein amount of protein/meal of 30 g would require the consumption of one litre of milk [115]; for this reason, Orsatti et al. have recently proposed the addition of soy protein to milk to enhance the effect of resistance training in postmenopausal women muscle [116]. Soy represents a good alternative to animal products, even though it is less effective in promoting muscle protein synthesis than animal sources [117], due to the high amount of isoflavones. Isoflavones are, in turn, often used as a natural alternative to hormone therapies and have been demonstrated to reduce the loss of bone mass and inflammation [118] that occur in menopause. Orsatti et al. observed that the addition of soy protein to milk, in association to resistance exercise, improves muscle strength but not muscle mass and attributed the latter to leucine content, that is lower with respect to the values suggested for maximizing protein synthesis [116].

Besides the effect of global amino acid availability, specific amino acids such as leucine, glutamine and arginine can play an important muscle health effect. Leucine (an essential amino acid) supplementation has been proposed as a strategy to counteract anabolic resistance in older muscle since it acts as a signalling molecule able to activate mTOR and thus protein synthesis [119]. Also, Xia et al. suggested an increase of leucine consumption in the diet, together with concurrent training, to counteract sarcopenia associated with chronic low-grade inflammation, often present during menopause [77]. Glutamine and arginine can also differentially regulate mTOR [120,121]. The nonessential amino acid glycine has anti-inflammatory and antioxidant properties and seems to promote the preservation of muscle mass. In a mice model of inflammation, glycine has been demonstrated to counteract anabolic resistance, since the improvement in leucine-stimulated protein synthesis was accompanied by higher phosphorylation status of mTOR, ribosomal protein S6 kinase and eukaryotic translation initiation factor 4E binding protein 1 compared with L-alanine-treated controls [122].

Taken together, the above evidence suggests that postmenopausal women need an adequate protein intake, in association with exercise (according to the modalities described in Tables 1–4) to counteract sarcopenia and related bone loss.

5. Vitamin D

Vitamin D is known to significantly contribute to the regulation of calcium and phosphorus homeostasis and skeletal mineralization through endocrine effects on bone, intestine, parathyroid glands and kidney [123]. Vitamin D has both skeletal and extra-skeletal beneficial effects. There is growing evidence that vitamin D regulates many other cell functions and its potential effect on skeletal muscle mass and strength is receiving greater attention. The biological actions of vitamin D on muscle cell differentiation, metabolism and function may be multiple, acting through direct and indirect, genomic and non-genomic pathways.

Vitamin D can be cutaneous synthesized from 7-dehydrocholesterol (7-DHC) (80–90%), a precursor of cholesterol, after exposure to ultraviolet B light. This endogenous synthesis mainly depends on the intensity of solar radiation. Very limited number of foods contains vitamin D such as fatty fish (like salmon and mackerel) or mushrooms, whereas milk products and eggs contain only small amounts of vitamin D. Calcitriol can be produced both by dietary sources and endogenous vitamin D through two hydroxylation reactions. The diet provides about 10–20% of the daily requirement of vitamin D. 25-hydroxyvitamin D (25(OH)D), the precursor of calcitriol, is the major circulating form of vitamin D and is considered the best biomarker to assess the vitamin D status; it circulates bound to a specific plasma carrier protein, vitamin D binding protein, that also transports the calcitriol.

The Institute of Medicine defines plasma concentration of 25(OH)D as adequate (25(OH)D concentrations > 50 nmol/L or > 20 ng/mL), insufficient (25(OH)D concentration between 30–50 nmol/L or 12–20 ng/mL), or as deficient (25(OH)D levels < 30 nmol/L or < 12 ng/mL). The committee stated that 50 nmol/L is the serum 25(OH)D level that covers the need of 97.5% of the population. Serum concentrations >125 nmol/L or > 50 ng/mL are associated with potential adverse effects [124].

Serum 25(OH)D levels < 50 nmol/L are associated with increased bone turnover, bone loss and possibly mineralization defects and poorer outcomes for frailty, hip fracture and all-cause mortality [29]; furthermore, it may exacerbate osteoporosis in elderly or postmenopausal women by increasing the rate of bone turnover. Aging decreases the capacity of human skin to produce vitamin D, in particular, 7-DHC concentration, the precursor of vitamin D, declines in the elderly [125]. During aging, the combined effect of a decline in intestinal calcium absorption, in the ability of the kidney to synthesize calcitriol and an increase in its catabolism contributes to age-related bone loss [123]. In addition, with aging there is a defect in 1 α hydroxylation [123].

High levels of dietary calcium intake and/or calcium supplements can significantly improve bone mineral content and density in postmenopausal women, however, some studies suggest that calcium supplements alone may not be sufficient to reduce fracture risk and that additional vitamin D supplementation is required; calcium, in combination with vitamin D supplementation, reduces the risk of fragility fractures and increases the survival in the elderly [126,127].

Furthermore, an increased level of calcium intake during the period of childhood and adolescence can lead to a reduction in the risk of osteoporosis during old age and post menopause [128].

Vitamin D has a pivotal role in the regulation and uptake of calcium in muscle cells, promoting protein synthesis and calcium and phosphate transport in muscle, which is important for muscle strength and contractile activity. Vitamin D appears to optimize the effect of dietary protein on skeletal muscle anabolism [29]. Both direct and indirect effects of vitamin D seem to play a role in muscle functionality, although most of them are attributed to the concomitant hypocalcaemia and hypophosphatemia [128]. Vitamin D plays a key role in regulating calcium-dependent functions of muscle, such as contraction, mitochondrial function and insulin sensitivity [128]. Loss of muscle mass is related to vitamin D deficiency [129,130]. The mechanisms by which vitamin D affects muscle strength and function have not yet fully clarified but are likely mediated by the vitamin D receptor (VDR); VDR and 1-alpha hydroxylase are both expressed in muscle tissue [131].

The presence of nuclear VDRs in muscle tissue suggests that vitamin D acts on muscle via a genomic transcriptional effect. Mechanistically, it has been suggested that 1,25-dihydroxyvitamin D binds to the nuclear VDR in muscle resulting in de novo protein synthesis [132]. Salles et al. have reported an anabolic effect of vitamin D in murine C2C12 myotubes through an increased insulin receptor and VDR mRNA expression [133]. Both the transcriptional induction of these genes and the enhancement of the insulin and leucine action on the related protein is one of the cardinal processes of vitamin D effect on skeletal muscle anabolism [133].

Furthermore, vitamin D signalling via VDR regulates gene transcription and activates further intracellular signalling pathways involved in calcium metabolism and it has been suggested to be involved in myoblast proliferation and differentiation [134]. Proximal myopathy (proximal weakness), characterizes patients with VDR-dependent rickets, an evidence arisen from studies in either older or younger populations [128]. Additionally, VDR-knockout mice are characterized by abnormal muscle morphology/physical function, while VDR polymorphisms have been associated with differences in muscle strength [135]. Muscle and bone VDR and 1-alpha hydroxylase expression decrease with aging [131,136,137] and it might be involved in intramuscular inflammation, since it has been associated with an increase of IL-6 and TNF-alpha levels in human skeletal muscle [138]. This process leads to the inhibition of muscle protein synthesis, to skeletal muscle apoptosis [139] and increased differentiation of myogenic precursor cells into adipocytes [140]. Recently, several authors have demonstrated that vitamin D supplementation can modulate VDR expression [131]. From a pathogenic point of view, reversible atrophy of type II muscle fibres and fatty infiltration of skeletal muscles have been reported in patients with vitamin D deficiency [131,141]. In younger adults, serum 25(OH)D concentration is inversely related to muscle fat infiltration, independently from body mass index and physical activity [142]. Such changes in muscle lipid content may have important implications for musculoskeletal function. Hence, since low vitamin D status is common in many elderly populations [143], attention should be paid to the potential therapeutic benefits of its supplementation. To this regard, European guidance for the diagnosis and management of osteoporosis in postmenopausal women recommends a daily intake of at least 1000 mg/day for calcium, 800 IU/day for vitamin D and 1 g/kg body weight of protein for all women aged over 50 years [29]. On the whole, vitamin D deficiency is associated with a loss of muscle mass and strength in elderly people and with a decline in physical performance. A nutritional intervention of vitamin D and amino acid supplementation could be a strategy to support muscle protein availability and synthesis in sarcopenia condition.

6. Conclusions

Osteoporosis and sarcopenia are two disorders affecting elderly people; their increasing incidence, due to the longer life expectancy in most western countries, might become an uncontrolled clinical and financial burden in the next few years. Early diagnosis, prevention and treatment of these disorders represent a very current but actually unmet, social and medical need. The evidence of profound interactions between bone and muscle causes a sort of negative resonance between the two tissues when they are simultaneously affected by osteoporosis and sarcopenia, respectively. Indeed, the coexistence of this twin condition in ageing leads to an accelerated worsening of the quality of life, poor clinical perspectives and high utilization of health resources. Due to the age- and/or gender-associated prevalence of sarcopenia and osteoporosis, postmenopausal women are potentially more prone to such a joint clinical situation. Nutritional and lifestyle factors may positively affect muscle and bone mass and function and have the advantage to be cheap and safe. To this regard, protein, vitamin D and calcium supplementation combined with a specifically-designed training protocol, emphasizing progressive RET, are capable of directly targeting some of the major physio-pathological causes of the twin condition progression and could simultaneously and coherently delay or revert the vicious cycle leading to the reciprocally-induced deterioration and wasting of osteoporotic bone and sarcopenic muscle (Figure 1).

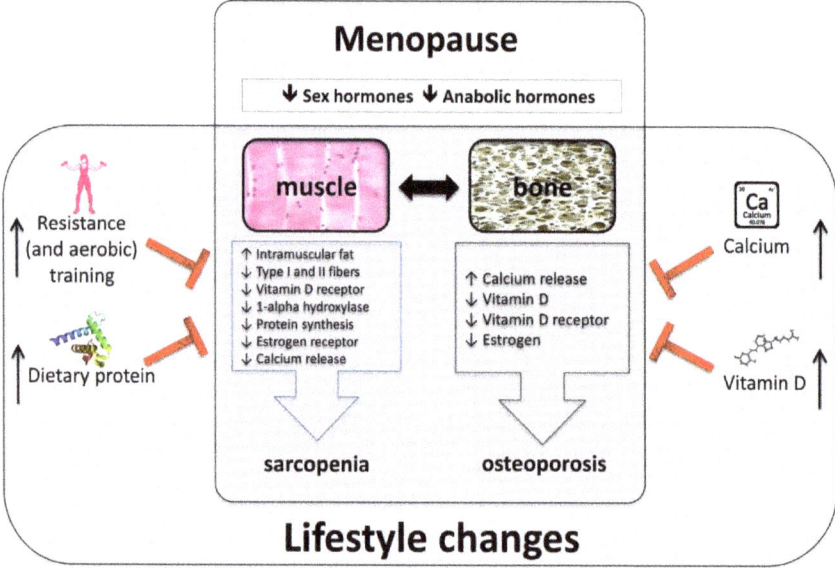

Figure 1. Menopause-related factors affecting muscle and bone and their possible prevention through a rationale strategy based on protein and vitamin D supplementation regimens in combination with specifically-designed training protocols.

The medical and social relevance of strategies alternative to HRT targeting both sarcopenia and osteoporosis progression based on a female-specific rationale would be invaluable. To this regard, the development of controlled and selected protein and vitamin D supplementation regimens in combination with specifically-designed exercise training protocols may represent a cheaper and safer alternative to oestrogen replacement therapies.

Author Contributions: Conceptualization, D.A., S.D.Z., E.B., P.S.; Methodology, F.L., C.F.M.; Software, G.A. and M.G.; Resources, G.P.; Supervision, V.S., P.S.; Writing-Review & Editing, D.A., S.D.Z, F.L., E.B., P.S.

Funding: This research was funded by "Progetti di Valorizzazione 2017", granted by the Department of Biomolecular Sciences, University of Urbino Carlo Bo, Italy.

Conflicts of Interest: The authors declare no conflict of interest.

References

1. Rosemberg, I. Epidemiologic and methodologic problems in determining nutritional status of older persons. Proceedings of a conference. Albuquerque, New Mexico, October 19–21, 1988. *Am. J. Clin. Nutr.* **1989**, *50*, 1121–1235.
2. Janssen, I.; Heymsfield, S.B.; Ross, R. Low relative skeletal muscle mass (sarcopenia) in older persons is associated with functional impairment and physical disability. *J. Am. Geriatr. Soc.* **2002**, *50*, 889–896. [CrossRef] [PubMed]
3. Cruz-Jentoft, A.J.; Baeyens, J.P.; Bauer, J.M.; Boirie, Y.; Cederholm, T.; Landi, F.; Martin, F.C.; Michel, J.P.; Rolland, Y.; Schneider, S.M.; et al. Sarcopenia: European consensus on definition and diagnosis: Report

4. Fielding, R.A.; Vellas, B.; Evans, W.J.; Bhasin, S.; Morley, J.E.; Newman, A.B.; Abellan van Kan, G.; Andrieu, S.; Bauer, J.; Breuille, D.; et al. Sarcopenia: An undiagnosed condition in older adults. Current consensus definition: Prevalence, etiology and consequences. International working group on sarcopenia. *J. Am. Med. Dir. Assoc.* **2011**, *12*, 249–256. [CrossRef] [PubMed]
5. Studenski, S.A.; Peters, K.W.; Alley, D.E.; Cawthon, P.M.; McLean, R.R.; Harris, T.B.; Ferrucci, L.; Guralnik, J.M.; Fragala, M.S.; Kenny, A.M.; et al. The FNIH sarcopenia project: Rationale, study description, conference recommendations and final estimates. *J. Gerontol.* **2014**, *69*, 547–558. [CrossRef] [PubMed]
6. Morley, J.E.; Vellas, B.; van Kan, G.A.; Anker, S.D.; Bauer, J.M.; Bernabei, R.; Cesari, M.; Chumlea, W.C.; Doehner, W.; Evans, J.; et al. Frailty consensus: A call to action. *J. Am. Med. Dir. Assoc.* **2013**, *14*, 392–397. [CrossRef] [PubMed]
7. Rolland, Y.; Abellan van Kan, G.; Gillette-Guyonnet, S.; Vellas, B. Cachexia versus sarcopenia. *Curr. Opin. Clin. Nutr. Metab. Care* **2011**, *14*, 15–21. [CrossRef] [PubMed]
8. Dennison, E.M.; Sayer, A.A.; Cooper, C. Epidemiology of sarcopenia and insight into possible therapeutic targets. *Nat. Rev. Rheumatol.* **2017**, *13*, 340–347. [CrossRef] [PubMed]
9. Bentzinger, C.F.; Rudnicki, M.A. Rejuvenating aged muscle stem cells. *Nat. Med.* **2014**, *20*, 234–235. [CrossRef] [PubMed]
10. Anderson, L.J.; Liu, H.; Garcia, J.M. Sex Differences in Muscle Wasting. *Adv. Exp. Med. Biol.* **2017**, *1043*, 153–197. [PubMed]
11. Churchward-Venne, T.A.; Breen, L.; Phillips, S.M. Alterations in human muscle protein metabolism with aging: Protein and exercise as countermeasures to offset sarcopenia. *Biofactors* **2014**, *40*, 199–205. [CrossRef] [PubMed]
12. Janssen, I.; Heymsfield, S.B.; Wang, Z.M.; Ross, R. Skeletal muscle mass and distribution in 468 men and women aged 18-88 yr. *J. Appl. Physiol.* **2000**, *89*, 81–88. [CrossRef] [PubMed]
13. Shafiee, G.; Keshtkar, A.; Soltani, A.; Ahadi, Z.; Larijani, B.; Heshmat, R. Prevalence of sarcopenia in the world: A systematic review and meta-analysis of general population studies. *J. Diabetes Metab. Disord.* **2017**, *16*, 21. [CrossRef] [PubMed]
14. Hansen, M. Female hormones: Do they influence muscle and tendon protein metabolism? *Proc. Nutr. Soc.* **2018**, *77*, 32–41. [CrossRef] [PubMed]
15. Qaisar, R.; Renaud, G.; Hedstrom, Y.; Pollanen, E.; Ronkainen, P.; Kaprio, J.; Alen, M.; Sipila, S.; Artemenko, K.; Bergquist, J.; et al. Hormone replacement therapy improves contractile function and myonuclear organization of single muscle fibres from postmenopausal monozygotic female twin pairs. *J. Physiol.* **2013**, *591*, 2333–2344. [CrossRef] [PubMed]
16. Stevenson, J.C. A woman's journey through the reproductive, transitional and postmenopausal periods of life: Impact on cardiovascular and musculo-skeletal risk and the role of estrogen replacement. *Maturitas* **2011**, *70*, 197–205. [CrossRef] [PubMed]
17. Kanis, J.A. Assessment of fracture risk and its application to screening for postmenopausal osteoporosis: Synopsis of a WHO report. WHO Study Group. *Osteoporos. Int.* **1994**, *4*, 368–381. [CrossRef] [PubMed]
18. Dobbs, M.B.; Buckwalter, J.; Saltzman, C. Osteoporosis: The increasing role of the orthopaedist. *Iowa Orthop. J.* **1999**, *19*, 43–52. [PubMed]
19. Johnell, O.; Kanis, J. Epidemiology of osteoporotic fractures. *Osteoporos. Int.* **2005**, *16* (Suppl. 2), S3–S7. [CrossRef]
20. Jackson, R.D.; Mysiw, W.J. Insights into the epidemiology of postmenopausal osteoporosis: The Women's Health Initiative. *Semin. Reprod. Med.* **2014**, *32*, 454–462. [PubMed]
21. Sjoblom, S.; Suuronen, J.; Rikkonen, T.; Honkanen, R.; Kroger, H.; Sirola, J. Relationship between postmenopausal osteoporosis and the components of clinical sarcopenia. *Maturitas* **2013**, *75*, 175–180. [CrossRef] [PubMed]
22. Bauer, J.; Biolo, G.; Cederholm, T.; Cesari, M.; Cruz-Jentoft, A.J.; Morley, J.E.; Phillips, S.; Sieber, C.; Stehle, P.; Teta, D.; et al. Evidence-based recommendations for optimal dietary protein intake in older people: A position paper from the PROT-AGE Study Group. *J. Am. Med. Dir. Assoc.* **2013**, *14*, 542–559. [CrossRef] [PubMed]

23. Cartee, G.D.; Hepple, R.T.; Bamman, M.M.; Zierath, J.R. Exercise Promotes Healthy Aging of Skeletal Muscle. *Cell Metab.* **2016**, *23*, 1034–1047. [CrossRef] [PubMed]
24. Moore, D.R.; Tang, J.E.; Burd, N.A.; Rerecich, T.; Tarnopolsky, M.A.; Phillips, S.M. Differential stimulation of myofibrillar and sarcoplasmic protein synthesis with protein ingestion at rest and after resistance exercise. *J. Physiol.* **2009**, *587*, 897–904. [CrossRef] [PubMed]
25. Harrison, H.E.; Harrison, H.C. Intestinal transport of phosphate: Action of vitamin D, calcium and potassium. *Am. J. Physiol.* **1961**, *201*, 1007–1012. [CrossRef] [PubMed]
26. Kido, S.; Kaneko, I.; Tatsumi, S.; Segawa, H.; Miyamoto, K. Vitamin D and type II sodium-dependent phosphate cotransporters. *Contrib. Nephrol.* **2013**, *180*, 86–97. [PubMed]
27. Xu, H.; Bai, L.; Collins, J.F.; Ghishan, F.K. Age-dependent regulation of rat intestinal type IIb sodium-phosphate cotransporter by 1,25-(OH)(2) vitamin D(3). *Am. J. Physiol. Cell. Physiol.* **2002**, *282*, C487–C493. [CrossRef] [PubMed]
28. Liu, N.; Nguyen, L.; Chun, R.F.; Lagishetty, V.; Ren, S.; Wu, S.; Hollis, B.; DeLuca, H.F.; Adams, J.S.; Hewison, M. Altered endocrine and autocrine metabolism of vitamin D in a mouse model of gastrointestinal inflammation. *Endocrinology* **2008**, *149*, 4799–4808. [CrossRef] [PubMed]
29. Rizzoli, R.; Stevenson, J.C.; Bauer, J.M.; van Loon, L.J.; Walrand, S.; Kanis, J.A.; Cooper, C.; Brandi, M.L.; Diez-Perez, A.; Reginster, J.Y.; et al. The role of dietary protein and vitamin D in maintaining musculoskeletal health in postmenopausal women: A consensus statement from the European Society for Clinical and Economic Aspects of Osteoporosis and Osteoarthritis (ESCEO). *Maturitas* **2014**, *79*, 122–132. [CrossRef] [PubMed]
30. Yoon, M.S. mTOR as a Key Regulator in Maintaining Skeletal Muscle Mass. *Front. Physiol.* **2017**, *8*, 788. [CrossRef] [PubMed]
31. Maltais, M.L.; Desroches, J.; Dionne, I.J. Changes in muscle mass and strength after menopause. *J. Musculoskelet. Neuronal. Interact.* **2009**, *9*, 186–197. [PubMed]
32. Musaro, A.; McCullagh, K.; Paul, A.; Houghton, L.; Dobrowolny, G.; Molinaro, M.; Barton, E.R.; Sweeney, H.L.; Rosenthal, N. Localized Igf-1 transgene expression sustains hypertrophy and regeneration in senescent skeletal muscle. *Nat. Genet.* **2001**, *27*, 195–200. [CrossRef] [PubMed]
33. Pelosi, L.; Giacinti, C.; Nardis, C.; Borsellino, G.; Rizzuto, E.; Nicoletti, C.; Wannenes, F.; Battistini, L.; Rosenthal, N.; Molinaro, M.; et al. Local expression of IGF-1 accelerates muscle regeneration by rapidly modulating inflammatory cytokines and chemokines. *FASEB. J.* **2007**, *21*, 1393–1402. [CrossRef] [PubMed]
34. Rabinovsky, E.D.; Gelir, E.; Gelir, S.; Lui, H.; Kattash, M.; DeMayo, F.J.; Shenaq, S.M.; Schwartz, R.J. Targeted expression of IGF-1 transgene to skeletal muscle accelerates muscle and motor neuron regeneration. *FASEB. J.* **2003**, *17*, 53–55. [CrossRef] [PubMed]
35. Annibalini, G.; Contarelli, S.; De Santi, M.; Saltarelli, R.; Di Patria, L.; Guescini, M.; Villarini, A.; Brandi, G.; Stocchi, V.; Barbieri, E. The intrinsically disordered E-domains regulate the IGF-1 prohormones stability, subcellular localisation and secretion. *Sci. Rep.* **2018**, *8*, 8919. [CrossRef] [PubMed]
36. Spangenburg, E.E.; Le Roith, D.; Ward, C.W.; Bodine, S.C. A functional insulin-like growth factor receptor is not necessary for load-induced skeletal muscle hypertrophy. *J. Physiol.* **2008**, *586*, 283–291. [CrossRef] [PubMed]
37. Olivieri, F.; Ahtiainen, M.; Lazzarini, R.; Pollanen, E.; Capri, M.; Lorenzi, M.; Fulgenzi, G.; Albertini, M.C.; Salvioli, S.; Alen, M.J.; et al. Hormone replacement therapy enhances IGF-1 signaling in skeletal muscle by diminishing miR-182 and miR-223 expressions: A study on postmenopausal monozygotic twin pairs. *Aging. Cell* **2014**, *13*, 850–861. [CrossRef] [PubMed]
38. Sitnick, M.; Foley, A.M.; Brown, M.; Spangenburg, E.E. Ovariectomy prevents the recovery of atrophied gastrocnemius skeletal muscle mass. *J. Appl. Physiol.* **2006**, *100*, 286–293. [CrossRef] [PubMed]
39. Lemoine, S.; Granier, P.; Tiffoche, C.; Rannou-Bekono, F.; Thieulant, M.L.; Delamarche, P. Estrogen receptor alpha mRNA in human skeletal muscles. *Med. Sci. Sports Exerc.* **2003**, *35*, 439–443. [CrossRef] [PubMed]
40. Wiik, A.; Ekman, M.; Johansson, O.; Jansson, E.; Esbjornsson, M. Expression of both oestrogen receptor alpha and beta in human skeletal muscle tissue. *Histochem. Cell Biol.* **2009**, *131*, 181–189. [CrossRef] [PubMed]
41. Ciana, P.; Raviscioni, M.; Mussi, P.; Vegeto, E.; Que, I.; Parker, M.G.; Lowik, C.; Maggi, A. In vivo imaging of transcriptionally active estrogen receptors. *Nat. Med.* **2003**, *9*, 82–86. [CrossRef] [PubMed]

42. Galluzzo, P.; Rastelli, C.; Bulzomi, P.; Acconcia, F.; Pallottini, V.; Marino, M. 17beta-Estradiol regulates the first steps of skeletal muscle cell differentiation via ER-alpha-mediated signals. *Am. J. Physiol. Cell Physiol.* **2009**, *297*, C1249–C1262. [CrossRef] [PubMed]
43. Lluis, F.; Perdiguero, E.; Nebreda, A.R.; Munoz-Canoves, P. Regulation of skeletal muscle gene expression by p38 MAP kinases. *Trends. Cell biol.* **2006**, *16*, 36–44. [CrossRef] [PubMed]
44. Pollanen, E.; Ronkainen, P.H.; Horttanainen, M.; Takala, T.; Puolakka, J.; Suominen, H.; Sipila, S.; Kovanen, V. Effects of combined hormone replacement therapy or its effective agents on the IGF-1 pathway in skeletal muscle. *Growth Horm. IGF Res.* **2010**, *20*, 372–379. [CrossRef] [PubMed]
45. Dubois, V.; Laurent, M.; Boonen, S.; Vanderschueren, D.; Claessens, F. Androgens and skeletal muscle: Cellular and molecular action mechanisms underlying the anabolic actions. *Cell. Mol. Life Sci.* **2012**, *69*, 1651–1667. [CrossRef] [PubMed]
46. Carson, J.A.; Manolagas, S.C. Effects of sex steroids on bones and muscles: Similarities, parallels and putative interactions in health and disease. *Bone* **2015**, *80*, 67–78. [CrossRef] [PubMed]
47. Reginster, J.Y.; Beaudart, C.; Buckinx, F.; Bruyere, O. Osteoporosis and sarcopenia: Two diseases or one? *Curr. Opin. Clin. Nutr. Metab. Care* **2016**, *19*, 31–36. [CrossRef] [PubMed]
48. Frost, H.M. Bone's mechanostat: A 2003 update. *Anat. Rec. A Discov. Mol. Cell. Evol. Biol.* **2003**, *275*, 1081–1101. [CrossRef] [PubMed]
49. Maurel, D.B.; Jahn, K.; Lara-Castillo, N. Muscle-Bone Crosstalk: Emerging Opportunities for Novel Therapeutic Approaches to Treat Musculoskeletal Pathologies. *Biomedicines* **2017**, *5*. [CrossRef] [PubMed]
50. Mahgoub, M.O.; D'Souza, C.; Al Darmaki, R.; Baniyas, M.; Adeghate, E. An update on the role of irisin in the regulation of endocrine and metabolic functions. *Peptides* **2018**, *104*, 15–23. [CrossRef] [PubMed]
51. Colaianni, G.; Cuscito, C.; Mongelli, T.; Oranger, A.; Mori, G.; Brunetti, G.; Colucci, S.; Cinti, S.; Grano, M. Irisin enhances osteoblast differentiation in vitro. *Int. J. Endocrinol.* **2014**, *2014*, 902186. [CrossRef] [PubMed]
52. Colaianni, G.; Grano, M. Role of Irisin on the bone-muscle functional unit. *Bonekey Rep.* **2015**, *4*, 765. [CrossRef] [PubMed]
53. Cardozo, C.P.; Graham, Z.A. Muscle-bone interactions: Movement in the field of mechano-humoral coupling of muscle and bone. *Ann. N. Y. Acad. Sci.* **2017**, *1402*, 10–17. [CrossRef] [PubMed]
54. Guescini, M.; Canonico, B.; Lucertini, F.; Maggio, S.; Annibalini, G.; Barbieri, E.; Luchetti, F.; Papa, S.; Stocchi, V. Muscle Releases Alpha-Sarcoglycan Positive Extracellular Vesicles Carrying miRNAs in the Bloodstream. *PLoS ONE* **2015**, *10*, e0125094. [CrossRef] [PubMed]
55. Lai, X.; Price, C.; Lu, X.L.; Wang, L. Imaging and quantifying solute transport across periosteum: Implications for muscle-bone crosstalk. *Bone* **2014**, *66*, 82–89. [CrossRef] [PubMed]
56. Lobo, R.A. Hormone-replacement therapy: Current thinking. *Nat. Rev. Endocrinol.* **2017**, *13*, 220–231. [CrossRef] [PubMed]
57. U. S. Preventive Services Task Force; Grossman, D.C.; Curry, S.J.; Owens, D.K.; Barry, M.J.; Davidson, K.W.; Doubeni, C.A.; Epling, J.W., Jr.; Kemper, A.R.; Krist, A.H.; et al. Hormone Therapy for the Primary Prevention of Chronic Conditions in Postmenopausal Women: US Preventive Services Task Force Recommendation Statement. *JAMA* **2017**, *318*, 2224–2233. [PubMed]
58. Marjoribanks, J.; Farquhar, C.; Roberts, H.; Lethaby, A.; Lee, J. Long-term hormone therapy for perimenopausal and postmenopausal women. *Cochrane Database Syst. Rev.* **2017**, *1*, CD004143. [CrossRef] [PubMed]
59. Landi, F.; Marzetti, E.; Martone, A.M.; Bernabei, R.; Onder, G. Exercise as a remedy for sarcopenia. *Curr. Opin. Clin. Nutr. Metab. Care* **2014**, *17*, 25–31. [CrossRef] [PubMed]
60. Gervasi, M.; Sisti, D.; Amatori, S.; Andreazza, M.; Benelli, P.; Sestili, P.; Rocchi, M.B.L.; Calavalle, A.R. Muscular viscoelastic characteristics of athletes participating in the European Master Indoor Athletics Championship. *Eur. J. Appl. Physiol.* **2017**, *117*, 1739–1746. [CrossRef] [PubMed]
61. Annibalini, G.; Lucertini, F.; Agostini, D.; Vallorani, L.; Gioacchini, A.; Barbieri, E.; Guescini, M.; Casadei, L.; Passalia, A.; Del Sal, M.; et al. Concurrent Aerobic and Resistance Training Has Anti-Inflammatory Effects and Increases Both Plasma and Leukocyte Levels of IGF-1 in Late Middle-Aged Type 2 Diabetic Patients. *Oxid. Med. Cell. Longev.* **2017**, *2017*, 3937842. [CrossRef] [PubMed]
62. Freiberger, E.; Sieber, C.; Pfeifer, K. Physical activity, exercise and sarcopenia -future challenges. *Wien. Med. Wochenschr.* **2011**, *161*, 416–425. [CrossRef] [PubMed]

63. Montero-Fernandez, N.; Serra-Rexach, J.A. Role of exercise on sarcopenia in the elderly. *Eur. J. Phys. Rehabil. Med.* **2013**, *49*, 131–143. [PubMed]
64. Bolam, K.A.; van Uffelen, J.G.; Taaffe, D.R. The effect of physical exercise on bone density in middle-aged and older men: A systematic review. *Osteoporos. Int.* **2013**, *24*, 2749–2762. [CrossRef] [PubMed]
65. Kemmler, W.; Haberle, L.; von Stengel, S. Effects of exercise on fracture reduction in older adults A systematic review and meta-analysis. *Osteoporosis Int.* **2013**, *24*, 1937–1950. [CrossRef] [PubMed]
66. Polidoulis, I.; Beyene, J.; Cheung, A.M. The effect of exercise on pQCT parameters of bone structure and strength in postmenopausal women—A systematic review and meta-analysis of randomized controlled trials. *Osteoporos. Int.* **2012**, *23*, 39–51. [CrossRef] [PubMed]
67. Cadore, E.L.; Rodriguez-Manas, L.; Sinclair, A.; Izquierdo, M. Effects of Different Exercise Interventions on Risk of Falls, Gait Ability and Balance in Physically Frail Older Adults: A Systematic Review. *Rejuvenation Res.* **2013**, *16*, 105–114. [CrossRef] [PubMed]
68. American College of Sports Medicine; Chodzko-Zajko, W.J.; Proctor, D.N.; Fiatarone Singh, M.A.; Minson, C.T.; Nigg, C.R.; Salem, G.J.; Skinner, J.S. American College of Sports Medicine position stand. Exercise and physical activity for older adults. *Med. Sci. Sports Exerc.* **2009**, *41*, 1510–1530. [CrossRef] [PubMed]
69. American College of Sports Medicine. American College of Sports Medicine position stand. Progression models in resistance training for healthy adults. *Med. Sci. Sports Exerc.* **2009**, *41*, 687–708. [CrossRef] [PubMed]
70. Law, T.D.; Clark, L.A.; Clark, B.C. Resistance Exercise to Prevent and Manage Sarcopenia and Dynapenia. *Annu. Rev. Gerontol. Geriatr.* **2016**, *36*, 205–228. [CrossRef] [PubMed]
71. Giangregorio, L.M.; McGill, S.; Wark, J.D.; Laprade, J.; Heinonen, A.; Ashe, M.C.; MacIntyre, N.J.; Cheung, A.M.; Shipp, K.; Keller, H.; et al. Too Fit To Fracture: Outcomes of a Delphi consensus process on physical activity and exercise recommendations for adults with osteoporosis with or without vertebral fractures. *Osteoporos. Int.* **2015**, *26*, 891–910. [CrossRef] [PubMed]
72. American College of Sports Medicine. American College of Sports Medicine position stand. Osteoporosis and exercise. *Med. Sci. Sports Exerc.* **1995**, *27*, i–vii. [CrossRef]
73. American College of Sports Medicine; Riebe, D.; Ehrman, J.K.; Liguori, G.; Magal, M. *ACSM's Guidelines for Exercise Testing and Prescription*, 10th ed.; Wolters Kluwer Health: Philadelphia, PA, USA, 2018; p. 472.
74. Phu, S.; Boersma, D.; Duque, G. Exercise and Sarcopenia. *J. Clin. Densitom.* **2015**, *18*, 488–492. [CrossRef] [PubMed]
75. Burd, N.A.; Gorissen, S.H.; van Loon, L.J. Anabolic resistance of muscle protein synthesis with aging. *Exerc. Sport Sci. Rev.* **2013**, *41*, 169–173. [CrossRef] [PubMed]
76. Moreau, K.; Walrand, S.; Boirie, Y. Protein redistribution from skeletal muscle to splanchnic tissue on fasting and refeeding in young and older healthy individuals. *J. Am. Med. Dir. Assoc.* **2013**, *14*, 696–704. [CrossRef] [PubMed]
77. Xia, Z.; Cholewa, J.; Zhao, Y.; Shang, H.Y.; Yang, Y.Q.; Araujo Pessoa, K.; Su, Q.S.; Lima-Soares, F.; Zanchi, N.E. Targeting Inflammation and Downstream Protein Metabolism in Sarcopenia: A Brief Up-Dated Description of Concurrent Exercise and Leucine-Based Multimodal Intervention. *Front. Physiol.* **2017**, *8*, 434. [CrossRef] [PubMed]
78. Joint WHO/FAO/UNU Expert Consultation. Protein and amino acid requirements in human nutrition. *World Health Organ. Tech. Rep. Ser.* **2007**, 1–265.
79. Deutz, N.E.; Bauer, J.M.; Barazzoni, R.; Biolo, G.; Boirie, Y.; Bosy-Westphal, A.; Cederholm, T.; Cruz-Jentoft, A.; Krznaric, Z.; Nair, K.S.; et al. Protein intake and exercise for optimal muscle function with aging: Recommendations from the ESPEN Expert Group. *Clin. Nutr.* **2014**, *33*, 929–936. [CrossRef] [PubMed]
80. Volpi, E.; Campbell, W.W.; Dwyer, J.T.; Johnson, M.A.; Jensen, G.L.; Morley, J.E.; Wolfe, R.R. Is the Optimal Level of Protein Intake for Older Adults Greater Than the Recommended Dietary Allowance? *J. Gerontol. A Biol. Sci. Med. Sci.* **2013**, *68*, 677–681. [CrossRef] [PubMed]
81. Wu, G. Dietary protein intake and human health. *Food Funct.* **2016**, *7*, 1251–1265. [CrossRef] [PubMed]
82. Fulgoni, V.L., 3rd. Current protein intake in America: Analysis of the National Health and Nutrition Examination Survey, 2003–2004. *Am. J. Clin. Nutr.* **2008**, *87*, 1554S–1557S. [CrossRef] [PubMed]

83. Tieland, M.; Borgonjen-Van den Berg, K.J.; van Loon, L.J.; de Groot, L.C. Dietary protein intake in community-dwelling, frail and institutionalized elderly people: Scope for improvement. *Eur. J. Nutr.* **2012**, *51*, 173–179. [CrossRef] [PubMed]
84. Gregorio, L.; Brindisi, J.; Kleppinger, A.; Sullivan, R.; Mangano, K.M.; Bihuniak, J.D.; Kenny, A.M.; Kerstetter, J.E.; Insogna, K.L. Adequate dietary protein is associated with better physical performance among post-menopausal women 60-90 years. *J. Nutr. Health Aging* **2014**, *18*, 155–160. [CrossRef] [PubMed]
85. Beals, J.W.; Sukiennik, R.A.; Nallabelli, J.; Emmons, R.S.; van Vliet, S.; Young, J.R.; Ulanov, A.V.; Li, Z.; Paluska, S.A.; De Lisio, M.; et al. Anabolic sensitivity of postprandial muscle protein synthesis to the ingestion of a protein-dense food is reduced in overweight and obese young adults. *Am. J. Clin. Nutr.* **2016**, *104*, 1014–1022. [CrossRef] [PubMed]
86. Barzilay, J.I.; Blaum, C.; Moore, T.; Xue, Q.L.; Hirsch, C.H.; Walston, J.D.; Fried, L.P. Insulin resistance and inflammation as precursors of frailty: The Cardiovascular Health Study. *Arch. Intern. Med.* **2007**, *167*, 635–641. [CrossRef] [PubMed]
87. Volpi, E.; Ferrando, A.A.; Yeckel, C.W.; Tipton, K.D.; Wolfe, R.R. Exogenous amino acids stimulate net muscle protein synthesis in the elderly. *J. Clin. Investig.* **1998**, *101*, 2000–2007. [CrossRef] [PubMed]
88. Dillon, E.L.; Sheffield-Moore, M.; Paddon-Jones, D.; Gilkison, C.; Sanford, A.P.; Casperson, S.L.; Jiang, J.; Chinkes, D.L.; Urban, R.J. Amino acid supplementation increases lean body mass, basal muscle protein synthesis and insulin-like growth factor-I expression in older women. *J. Clin. Endocrinol. Metab.* **2009**, *94*, 1630–1637. [CrossRef] [PubMed]
89. Castaneda, C.; Gordon, P.L.; Fielding, R.A.; Evans, W.J.; Crim, M.C. Marginal protein intake results in reduced plasma IGF-I levels and skeletal muscle fiber atrophy in elderly women. *J. Nutr. Health Aging* **2000**, *4*, 85–90. [PubMed]
90. Bonjour, J.P.; Kraenzlin, M.; Levasseur, R.; Warren, M.; Whiting, S. Dairy in adulthood: From foods to nutrient interactions on bone and skeletal muscle health. *J. Am. Coll. Nutr.* **2013**, *32*, 251–263. [CrossRef] [PubMed]
91. Dawson-Hughes, B.; Harris, S.S.; Rasmussen, H.; Song, L.; Dallal, G.E. Effect of dietary protein supplements on calcium excretion in healthy older men and women. *J. Clin. Endocrinol. Metab.* **2004**, *89*, 1169–1173. [CrossRef] [PubMed]
92. Kerstetter, J.E.; Kenny, A.M.; Insogna, K.L. Dietary protein and skeletal health: A review of recent human research. *Curr. Opin. Lipidol.* **2011**, *22*, 16–20. [CrossRef] [PubMed]
93. Antonio, J.; Ellerbroek, A.; Silver, T.; Orris, S.; Scheiner, M.; Gonzalez, A.; Peacock, C.A. A high protein diet (3.4 g/kg/d) combined with a heavy resistance training program improves body composition in healthy trained men and women–a follow-up investigation. *J. Int. Soc. Sports Nutr.* **2015**, *12*, 39. [CrossRef] [PubMed]
94. Antonio, J.; Ellerbroek, A.; Evans, C.; Silver, T.; Peacock, C.A. High protein consumption in trained women: Bad to the bone? *J. Int. Soc. Sports Nutr.* **2018**, *15*, 6. [CrossRef] [PubMed]
95. Arnal, M.A.; Mosoni, L.; Boirie, Y.; Houlier, M.L.; Morin, L.; Verdier, E.; Ritz, P.; Antoine, J.M.; Prugnaud, J.; Beaufrere, B.; et al. Protein pulse feeding improves protein retention in elderly women. *Am. J. Clin. Nutr.* **1999**, *69*, 1202–1208. [CrossRef] [PubMed]
96. Bouillanne, O.; Neveux, N.; Nicolis, I.; Curis, E.; Cynober, L.; Aussel, C. Long-lasting improved amino acid bioavailability associated with protein pulse feeding in hospitalized elderly patients: A randomized controlled trial. *Nutrition* **2014**, *30*, 544–550. [CrossRef] [PubMed]
97. Kim, I.Y.; Schutzler, S.; Schrader, A.M.; Spencer, H.J.; Azhar, G.; Wolfe, R.R.; Ferrando, A.A. Protein intake distribution pattern does not affect anabolic response, lean body mass, muscle strength or function over 8 weeks in older adults: A randomized-controlled trial. *Clin. Nutr.* **2018**, *37*, 488–493. [CrossRef] [PubMed]
98. Mamerow, M.M.; Mettler, J.A.; English, K.L.; Casperson, S.L.; Arentson-Lantz, E.; Sheffield-Moore, M.; Layman, D.K.; Paddon-Jones, D. Dietary protein distribution positively influences 24-h muscle protein synthesis in healthy adults. *J. Nutr.* **2014**, *144*, 876–880. [CrossRef] [PubMed]
99. Bollwein, J.; Diekmann, R.; Kaiser, M.J.; Bauer, J.M.; Uter, W.; Sieber, C.C.; Volkert, D. Distribution but not amount of protein intake is associated with frailty: A cross-sectional investigation in the region of Nurnberg. *Nutr. J.* **2013**, *12*, 109. [CrossRef] [PubMed]
100. Loenneke, J.P.; Loprinzi, P.D.; Murphy, C.H.; Phillips, S.M. Per meal dose and frequency of protein consumption is associated with lean mass and muscle performance. *Clin. Nutr.* **2016**, *35*, 1506–1511. [CrossRef] [PubMed]

101. Norton, C.; Toomey, C.; McCormack, W.G.; Francis, P.; Saunders, J.; Kerin, E.; Jakeman, P. Protein Supplementation at Breakfast and Lunch for 24 Weeks beyond Habitual Intakes Increases Whole-Body Lean Tissue Mass in Healthy Older Adults. *J. Nutr.* **2016**, *146*, 65–69. [CrossRef] [PubMed]
102. Kim, T.N.; Choi, K.M. Sarcopenia: Definition, epidemiology and pathophysiology. *J. Bone Metab.* **2013**, *20*, 1–10. [CrossRef] [PubMed]
103. Phillips, S.M.; Glover, E.I.; Rennie, M.J. Alterations of protein turnover underlying disuse atrophy in human skeletal muscle. *J. Appl. Physiol.* **2009**, *107*, 645–654. [CrossRef] [PubMed]
104. Atherton, P.J.; Smith, K. Muscle protein synthesis in response to nutrition and exercise. *J. Physiol.* **2012**, *590*, 1049–1057. [CrossRef] [PubMed]
105. Biolo, G.; Tipton, K.D.; Klein, S.; Wolfe, R.R. An abundant supply of amino acids enhances the metabolic effect of exercise on muscle protein. *Am. J. Physiol. Endocrinol. Metab.* **1997**, *273*, E122–E129. [CrossRef] [PubMed]
106. Drummond, M.J.; Dreyer, H.C.; Pennings, B.; Fry, C.S.; Dhanani, S.; Dillon, E.L.; Sheffield-Moore, M.; Volpi, E.; Rasmussen, B.B. Skeletal muscle protein anabolic response to resistance exercise and essential amino acids is delayed with aging. *J. Appl. Physiol.* **2008**, *104*, 1452–1461. [CrossRef] [PubMed]
107. Guimaraes-Ferreira, L.; Cholewa, J.M.; Naimo, M.A.; Zhi, X.I.; Magagnin, D.; de Sa, R.B.; Streck, E.L.; Teixeira Tda, S.; Zanchi, N.E. Synergistic effects of resistance training and protein intake: Practical aspects. *Nutrition* **2014**, *30*, 1097–1103. [CrossRef] [PubMed]
108. Pennings, B.; Boirie, Y.; Senden, J.M.; Gijsen, A.P.; Kuipers, H.; van Loon, L.J. Whey protein stimulates postprandial muscle protein accretion more effectively than do casein and casein hydrolysate in older men. *Am. J. Clin. Nutr.* **2011**, *93*, 997–1005. [CrossRef] [PubMed]
109. Zhu, K.; Kerr, D.A.; Meng, X.; Devine, A.; Solah, V.; Binns, C.W.; Prince, R.L. Two-Year Whey Protein Supplementation Did Not Enhance Muscle Mass and Physical Function in Well-Nourished Healthy Older Postmenopausal Women. *J. Nutr.* **2015**, *145*, 2520–2526. [CrossRef] [PubMed]
110. Daly, R.M.; O'Connell, S.L.; Mundell, N.L.; Grimes, C.A.; Dunstan, D.W.; Nowson, C.A. Protein-enriched diet, with the use of lean red meat, combined with progressive resistance training enhances lean tissue mass and muscle strength and reduces circulating IL-6 concentrations in elderly women: A cluster randomized controlled trial. *Am. J. Clin. Nutr.* **2014**, *99*, 899–910. [CrossRef] [PubMed]
111. Figueiredo Braggion, G.; Ornelas, E.; Carmona Sattin Cury, J.; Edviges Alves Lima, N.; Aquino, R.C.; Affonso Fonseca, F.L.; Maifrino, L.B. Morphological and Biochemical Effects on the Skeletal Muscle of Ovariectomized Old Female Rats Submitted to the Intake of Diets with Vegetable or Animal Protein and Resistance Training. *Oxid. Med. Cell. Longev.* **2016**, *2016*, 9251064. [CrossRef] [PubMed]
112. Landi, F.; Calvani, R.; Tosato, M.; Martone, A.M.; Picca, A.; Ortolani, E.; Savera, G.; Salini, S.; Ramaschi, M.; Bernabei, R.; et al. Animal-Derived Protein Consumption Is Associated with Muscle Mass and Strength in Community-Dwellers: Results from the Milan EXPO Survey. *J. Nutr. Health Aging* **2017**, *21*, 1050–1056. [CrossRef] [PubMed]
113. Mitchell, C.J.; McGregor, R.A.; D'Souza, R.F.; Thorstensen, E.B.; Markworth, J.F.; Fanning, A.C.; Poppitt, S.D.; Cameron-Smith, D. Consumption of Milk Protein or Whey Protein Results in a Similar Increase in Muscle Protein Synthesis in Middle Aged Men. *Nutrients* **2015**, *7*, 8685–8699. [CrossRef] [PubMed]
114. Burd, N.A.; Gorissen, S.H.; van Vliet, S.; Snijders, T.; van Loon, L.J.C. Differences in postprandial protein handling after beef compared with milk ingestion during postexercise recovery: A randomized controlled trial. *Am. J. Clin. Nutr.* **2015**, *102*, 828–836. [CrossRef] [PubMed]
115. van Vliet, S.; Burd, N.A.; van Loon, L.J. The Skeletal Muscle Anabolic Response to Plant- versus Animal-Based Protein Consumption. *J. Nutr.* **2015**, *145*, 1981–1991. [CrossRef] [PubMed]
116. Orsatti, F.L.; Maesta, N.; de Oliveira, E.P.; Nahas Neto, J.; Burini, R.C.; Nunes, P.R.P.; Souza, A.P.; Martins, F.M.; Nahas, E.P. Adding Soy Protein to Milk Enhances the Effect of Resistance Training on Muscle Strength in Postmenopausal Women. *J. Diet. Suppl.* **2018**, *15*, 140–152. [CrossRef] [PubMed]
117. Phillips, S.M. Nutrient-rich meat proteins in offsetting age-related muscle loss. *Meat. Sci.* **2012**, *92*, 174–178. [CrossRef] [PubMed]
118. Chilibeck, P.D.; Cornish, S.M. Effect of estrogenic compounds (estrogen or phytoestrogens) combined with exercise on bone and muscle mass in older individuals. *Appl. Physiol. Nutr. Metab.* **2008**, *33*, 200–212. [CrossRef] [PubMed]

119. De Bandt, J.P. Leucine and Mammalian Target of Rapamycin-Dependent Activation of Muscle Protein Synthesis in Aging. *J. Nutr.* **2016**, *146*, 2616S–2624S. [CrossRef] [PubMed]
120. Chantranupong, L.; Scaria, S.M.; Saxton, R.A.; Gygi, M.P.; Shen, K.; Wyant, G.A.; Wang, T.; Harper, J.W.; Gygi, S.P.; Sabatini, D.M. The CASTOR Proteins Are Arginine Sensors for the mTORC1 Pathway. *Cell* **2016**, *165*, 153–164. [CrossRef] [PubMed]
121. Jewell, J.L.; Kim, Y.C.; Russell, R.C.; Yu, F.X.; Park, H.W.; Plouffe, S.W.; Tagliabracci, V.S.; Guan, K.L. Metabolism. Differential regulation of mTORC1 by leucine and glutamine. *Science* **2015**, *347*, 194–198. [CrossRef] [PubMed]
122. Ham, D.J.; Caldow, M.K.; Chhen, V.; Chee, A.; Wang, X.; Proud, C.G.; Lynch, G.S.; Koopman, R. Glycine restores the anabolic response to leucine in a mouse model of acute inflammation. *Am. J. Physiol. Endocrinol. Metab.* **2016**, *310*, E970–E981. [CrossRef] [PubMed]
123. Veldurthy, V.; Wei, R.; Oz, L.; Dhawan, P.; Jeon, Y.H.; Christakos, S. Vitamin D, calcium homeostasis and aging. *Bone Res.* **2016**, *4*, 16041. [CrossRef] [PubMed]
124. Ross, A.C.; Manson, J.E.; Abrams, S.A.; Aloia, J.F.; Brannon, P.M.; Clinton, S.K.; Durazo-Arvizu, R.A.; Gallagher, J.C.; Gallo, R.L.; Jones, G.; et al. The 2011 report on dietary reference intakes for calcium and vitamin D from the Institute of Medicine: What clinicians need to know. *J. Clin. Endocrinol. Metab.* **2011**, *96*, 53–58. [CrossRef] [PubMed]
125. MacLaughlin, J.; Holick, M.F. Aging decreases the capacity of human skin to produce vitamin D3. *J. Clin. Investig.* **1985**, *76*, 1536–1538. [CrossRef] [PubMed]
126. Chapuy, M.C.; Pamphile, R.; Paris, E.; Kempf, C.; Schlichting, M.; Arnaud, S.; Garnero, P.; Meunier, P.J. Combined calcium and vitamin D3 supplementation in elderly women: Confirmation of reversal of secondary hyperparathyroidism and hip fracture risk: The Decalyos II study. *Osteoporos. Int.* **2002**, *13*, 257–264. [CrossRef] [PubMed]
127. Saini, A.K.; Dawe, E.J.C.; Thompson, S.M.; Rosson, J.W. Vitamin D and Calcium Supplementation in Elderly Patients Suffering Fragility Fractures; The Road not Taken. *Open Orthop. J.* **2017**, *11*, 1230–1235. [CrossRef] [PubMed]
128. Broe, K.E.; Chen, T.C.; Weinberg, J.; Bischoff-Ferrari, H.A.; Holick, M.F.; Kiel, D.P. A higher dose of vitamin d reduces the risk of falls in nursing home residents: A randomized, multiple-dose study. *J. Am. Geriatr. Soc.* **2007**, *55*, 234–239. [CrossRef] [PubMed]
129. O'Donnell, S.; Moher, D.; Thomas, K.; Hanley, D.A.; Cranney, A. Systematic review of the benefits and harms of calcitriol and alfacalcidol for fractures and falls. *J. Bone Miner. Metab.* **2008**, *26*, 531–542. [CrossRef] [PubMed]
130. Richy, F.; Dukas, L.; Schacht, E. Differential effects of D-hormone analogs and native vitamin D on the risk of falls: A comparative meta-analysis. *Calcif. Tissue Int.* **2008**, *82*, 102–107. [CrossRef] [PubMed]
131. Robinson, S.M.; Reginster, J.Y.; Rizzoli, R.; Shaw, S.C.; Kanis, J.A.; Bautmans, I.; Bischoff-Ferrari, H.; Bruyere, O.; Cesari, M.; Dawson-Hughes, B.; et al. Does nutrition play a role in the prevention and management of sarcopenia? *Clin. Nutr.* **2018**, *37*, 1121–1132. [CrossRef] [PubMed]
132. Bischoff-Ferrari, H.A. Relevance of vitamin D in muscle health. *Rev. Endocr. Metab. Disord.* **2012**, *13*, 71–77. [CrossRef] [PubMed]
133. Salles, J.; Chanet, A.; Giraudet, C.; Patrac, V.; Pierre, P.; Jourdan, M.; Luiking, Y.C.; Verlaan, S.; Migne, C.; Boirie, Y.; et al. 1,25(OH)2-vitamin D3 enhances the stimulating effect of leucine and insulin on protein synthesis rate through Akt/PKB and mTOR mediated pathways in murine C2C12 skeletal myotubes. *Mol. Nutr. Food Res.* **2013**, *57*, 2137–2146. [CrossRef] [PubMed]
134. Garcia, L.A.; King, K.K.; Ferrini, M.G.; Norris, K.C.; Artaza, J.N. 1,25(OH)2vitamin D3 stimulates myogenic differentiation by inhibiting cell proliferation and modulating the expression of promyogenic growth factors and myostatin in C2C12 skeletal muscle cells. *Endocrinology* **2011**, *152*, 2976–2986. [CrossRef] [PubMed]
135. Grundberg, E.; Brandstrom, H.; Ribom, E.L.; Ljunggren, O.; Mallmin, H.; Kindmark, A. Genetic variation in the human vitamin D receptor is associated with muscle strength, fat mass and body weight in Swedish women. *Eur. J. Endocrinol.* **2004**, *150*, 323–328. [CrossRef] [PubMed]
136. Al-Said, Y.A.; Al-Rached, H.S.; Al-Qahtani, H.A.; Jan, M.M. Severe proximal myopathy with remarkable recovery after vitamin D treatment. *Can. J. Neurol. Sci.* **2009**, *36*, 336–339. [CrossRef] [PubMed]

137. Wicherts, I.S.; van Schoor, N.M.; Boeke, A.J.; Visser, M.; Deeg, D.J.; Smit, J.; Knol, D.L.; Lips, P. Vitamin D status predicts physical performance and its decline in older persons. *J. Clin. Endocrinol. Metab.* **2007**, *92*, 2058–2065. [CrossRef] [PubMed]
138. Stockton, K.A.; Mengersen, K.; Paratz, J.D.; Kandiah, D.; Bennell, K.L. Effect of vitamin D supplementation on muscle strength: A systematic review and meta-analysis. *Osteoporos. Int.* **2011**, *22*, 859–871. [CrossRef] [PubMed]
139. Ryan, K.J.; Daniel, Z.C.; Craggs, L.J.; Parr, T.; Brameld, J.M. Dose-dependent effects of vitamin D on transdifferentiation of skeletal muscle cells to adipose cells. *J. Endocrinol.* **2013**, *217*, 45–58. [CrossRef] [PubMed]
140. Peake, J.; Della Gatta, P.; Cameron-Smith, D. Aging and its effects on inflammation in skeletal muscle at rest and following exercise-induced muscle injury. *Am. J. Physiol. Regul. Integr. Comp. Physiol.* **2010**, *298*, R1485–R1495. [CrossRef] [PubMed]
141. Somjen, D.; Weisman, Y.; Kohen, F.; Gayer, B.; Limor, R.; Sharon, O.; Jaccard, N.; Knoll, E.; Stern, N. 25-hydroxyvitamin D3-1alpha-hydroxylase is expressed in human vascular smooth muscle cells and is upregulated by parathyroid hormone and estrogenic compounds. *Circulation* **2005**, *111*, 1666–1671. [CrossRef] [PubMed]
142. Gilsanz, V.; Kremer, A.; Mo, A.O.; Wren, T.A.; Kremer, R. Vitamin D status and its relation to muscle mass and muscle fat in young women. *J. Clin. Endocrinol. Metab.* **2010**, *95*, 1595–1601. [CrossRef] [PubMed]
143. Ter Borg, S.; Verlaan, S.; Hemsworth, J.; Mijnarends, D.M.; Schols, J.M.; Luiking, Y.C.; de Groot, L.C. Micronutrient intakes and potential inadequacies of community-dwelling older adults: A systematic review. *Br. J. Nutr.* **2015**, *113*, 1195–1206. [CrossRef] [PubMed]

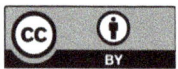

© 2018 by the authors. Licensee MDPI, Basel, Switzerland. This article is an open access article distributed under the terms and conditions of the Creative Commons Attribution (CC BY) license (http://creativecommons.org/licenses/by/4.0/).

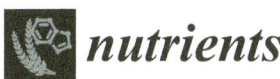

Article

Impact of Meeting Different Guidelines for Protein Intake on Muscle Mass and Physical Function in Physically Active Older Women

Andreas Nilsson *, Diego Montiel Rojas and Fawzi Kadi

School of Health Sciences, Örebro University, 702 81 Örebro, Sweden; diego.montiel@oru.se (D.M.R.); fawzi.kadi@oru.se (F.K.)
* Correspondence: andreas.nilsson@oru.se; Tel.: +46-19-303553

Received: 2 July 2018; Accepted: 21 August 2018; Published: 24 August 2018

Abstract: The role of dietary protein intake on muscle mass and physical function in older adults is important for the prevention of age-related physical limitations. The aim of the present study was to elucidate links between dietary protein intake and muscle mass and physical function in older women meeting current guidelines of objectively assessed physical activity. In 106 women (65 to 70 years old), protein intake was assessed using a 6-day food record and participants were classified into high and low protein intake groups using two Recommended Dietary Allowance (RDA) thresholds (0.8 g·kg^{-1} bodyweight (BW) and 1.1 g·kg^{-1} BW). Body composition, aerobic fitness, and quadriceps strength were determined using standardized procedures, and self-reported physical function was assessed using the SF-12 Health Survey. Physical activity was assessed by accelerometry and self-report. Women below the 0.8 g·kg^{-1} BW threshold had a lower muscle mass ($p < 0.05$) with no differences in physical function variables. When based on the higher RDA threshold (1.1 g·kg^{-1} BW), in addition to significant differences in muscle mass, women below the higher threshold had a significantly ($p < 0.05$) higher likelihood of having physical limitations. In conclusion, the present study supports the RDA threshold of 0.8 g·kg^{-1} BW of proteins to prevent the loss of muscle mass and emphasizes the importance of the higher RDA threshold of at least 1.1 g·kg^{-1} BW to infer additional benefits on constructs of physical function. Our study also supports the role of protein intake for healthy ageing, even in older adults meeting guidelines for physical activity.

Keywords: elderly; muscle strength; nutrition; physical activity; physical functioning; Recommended Dietary Allowance (RDA); sarcopenia

1. Introduction

A large body of research has highlighted the role of dietary proteins as primary anabolic stimuli responsible for the maintenance of muscle mass. At an adult population level, a protein intake of 0.8 g·kg^{-1} of bodyweight (BW) represents a recommended daily allowance (RDA) of protein needed for preservation of muscle mass and strength [1–3]. However, given the reduced anabolic response to protein ingestion that seems to occur in older adults, an increased protein allowance in the range of 1.0–1.2 g·kg^{-1} BW has been proposed [4]. Indeed, accelerated decline in muscle mass and strength occurs in old adults and is related to impaired physical function, disability, and reduced quality of life [5]. Interestingly, inter-individual variability in the rate of muscle mass wasting and functional decline suggests that lifestyle behaviors, including diet and physical activity, may be key factors for the promotion of health ageing [6]. Therefore, the study of the influence of dietary protein intake on muscle mass and physical function in older adults has received growing attention. It has been shown that a higher protein intake can be associated with preservation of muscle mass [7,8]. For example, a lower protein intake at baseline was associated with a greater loss of lean mass over a

3-year follow-up period in older adults [7]. In contrast, a higher body mass including both fat and lean mass was reported in older women with a protein intake below 0.8 g·kg^{-1} BW [9]. Besides muscle mass, whether protein intake may confer positive effects on functional capacity is important to clarify given the age-related impairment in physical function. Interestingly, higher protein intake has been associated with reduced risk of frailty in older women [10–13]. Beneficial effects of higher protein intake on physical function, including handgrip strength [8,14,15], the short physical performance battery (SPPB) scores [9], and self-reported physical function [8,15–17] have also been reported. However, results from others do not support a significant impact of total protein intake on muscle strength, SPPB scores, and walking speed [18–21]. These conflicting results may be explained by several factors obscuring the link between dietary protein intake, muscle mass, and physical function. For example, different methods to assess dietary protein intake, including the use of RDA thresholds for classification of high and low intakes, will affect study outcomes. Likewise, which dimension of the physical function and whether objective or self-report assessment methods are used are other relevant factors. In addition, variations in health status among the elderly population must be taken into consideration when evaluating the impact of protein intake on muscle mass and physical function. Differences in study samples regarding the prevalence of diseases and physical impairment likely limit comparability between studies. Noteworthy, as physical function is partly determined by body composition, variations in muscle mass must be considered in order to determine the true impact of protein intake on measures of physical function. Furthermore, physical activity (PA) is a lifestyle behavior with the potential to have a substantial impact on physical function. Indeed, PA has been recognized as an important anabolic stimulus for the regulation of muscle mass [22]. Therefore, when investigating links between protein intake, body composition, and physical function, the influence of PA level should be taken into consideration. However, most previous studies rely on self-reported PA, which is prone to recall bias and less accurate than objective methods [23]. Alongside total weekly amount of PA, accounting for strengthening activities according to PA guidelines for healthy ageing could further clarify the true impact of protein on physical function.

Therefore, the aim of the present study was to elucidate links between dietary protein intake, muscle mass, and objective and self-reported measures of physical function in older community-dwelling women meeting current guidelines of objectively assessed PA.

2. Materials and Methods

2.1. Subjects

One hundred and twenty-two women aged between 65 and 70 years old were recruited through local advertisement and were subsequently screened for inclusion in the study. To be included in the study, participants had to meet the current guidelines of 150 min per week of moderate-to-vigorous physical activity and be free of diagnosed coronary heart disease, diabetes mellitus, have no disability with respect to mobility, and be non-smokers. A total of 106 women fulfilled inclusion criteria. All procedures were conducted according to standards set by the Declaration of Helsinki. Written informed consent was obtained from all participants and the study was approved by the regional ethics committee of Uppsala (2011/033).

2.2. Anthropometry and Body Composition

Body weight (kg) and height (cm) were measured using a digital scale and a portable stadiometer to the nearest 0.1 kg and 0.5 cm, respectively. Subjects having a body mass index (BMI) ≥ 25 kg·m^{-2} were classified as overweight. Skeletal muscle mass index (SMI) was assessed using bioelectrical impedance analysis (BIA) and derived using the equation by Janssen et al. [24].

2.3. Assessment of Physical Function

A standardized submaximal exercise on a cycle ergometer (model 874 E; Monark, Varberg, Sweden) was performed during 6 min at a constant workload to assess aerobic fitness [25]. Maximal isometric quadriceps strength was measured using a force sensor (K. TOYO 333A, Toyo-Korea, Seoul, Korea) as previously described [26]. Self-reported physical function limitation was assessed by the 12-item Short Form Health Survey (SF-12) [27]. Participants answered two questions related to the ability to accomplish various daily activities questions on a three-item response scale (limited a lot; limited a little; not limited at all). Participants who reported "limited a little" or "limited a lot" on at least one of the two questions were classified as having a physical limitation, and all other participants were subsequently classified as not having any physical limitation.

2.4. Assessment of Adherence to Physical Activity Guidelines

Accelerometer-based assessment of PA during a week was performed using the Actigraph GT3x activity monitor (Actigraph, Pensacola, FL, USA) as previously described [28]. A cut-point of >1324 counts per minute, specifically developed for women over 60 years of age [29], was used to define time spent in moderate-to-vigorous PA (MVPA). Engagement in strengthening activities during the past 12 months was assessed using the EPAQ2 questionnaire [30]. From a list of strengthening activities, such as resistance exercise, participants reported the frequency and average time spent per session. Subsequently, we classified participants in two groups based on whether they engaged in strengthening activities at least twice a week or not.

2.5. Dietary Protein Intake

Dietary intake was monitored using a food record over a period of 6 days. Participants were instructed by a nutritionist on how to register their daily food intake with the assistance of a portion size guide developed by the Swedish National Food Agency. Total energy intake and relative macronutrient intakes (E%) were derived using Dietist XP software (Kost och Näringsdata, Bromma, Sweden). Daily protein intake was normalized to bodyweight and expressed as g·kg-1 bodyweight. In accordance with guidelines for protein intake (0.8 g·kg^{-1} BW or 1.1 g·kg^{-1} BW) [1–4], participants were classified into higher or lower protein intakes.

2.6. Statistics

Data are presented as mean ± standard deviation. All variables were checked for normality and transformed when necessary. Between-group differences in continuous variables were first assessed by using independent samples t-test. Since variations in body composition were related to physical function, adjustment for SMI was performed using analysis of covariance. Binary logistic regression was used to examine the likelihood of having physical limitations in the two protein intake groups based on different RDA thresholds. The model was further adjusted for SMI. A priori statistical power calculations showed that moderate effect sizes were detectable with a power of ≥80% when based on our sample size. Statistical significance was set at $p < 0.05$ and all procedures were performed using SPSS software version 24 (IBM Corporation, New York, NY, USA).

3. Results

3.1. Characteristics of the Study Population

The mean age, weight, and BMI of the study sample was 67.5 ± 1.8 years, 67.9 ± 11.6 kg, and 25.1 ± 4.0 kg·m^{-2}, respectively. The average time spent in MVPA was 67 ± 25 min·day^{-1}. Aerobic fitness and isometric quadriceps strength averaged 28.7 ± 7.2 mL O^2·min^{-1}·kg^{-1} BW and 2.7 ± 0.7 N·kg^{-1} BW, respectively. A total of 31.4% reported physical limitations. Compared to women without physical limitations, those reporting limitations had a higher BMI (24.2 ± 3.7 vs. 27.1 ± 3.9;

$p < 0.05$), lower SMI (31.4 ± 4.1 vs. 29.2 ± 3.1; $p < 0.05$), lower aerobic fitness (30.1 ± 7.4 vs. 25.2 ± 6.1; $p < 0.05$), and lower isometric quadriceps strength (2.8 ± 0.7 vs. 2.5 ± 0.6; $p < 0.05$). A total of 34% of women reported engagement in strengthening activities at least twice a week and there were no significant differences in body composition variables nor physical function measures between those involved and not involved in this type of activities.

The average energy intake of the study population was 1705 ± 380 kcal·day^{-1}, with 46% ± 6%, 34% ± 5%, and 17% ± 2% of the energy derived from carbohydrates, fat, and protein, respectively. There were no significant differences in energy distribution of macronutrients (E%) between groups of protein intakes regardless of whether based on the lower (0.8 g·kg^{-1} BW) or the higher (1.1 g·kg^{-1} BW) protein intake guideline. There were no significant differences in total energy intake or energy distribution of macronutrients (E%) between physically limited and not limited older women.

3.2. Influence of Protein Intake on Muscle Mass and Physical Function

The average daily protein intake of the entire sample was 1.03 ± 0.26 g·kg^{-1} BW. When categorizing participants in high and low protein intake based on the lower RDA threshold of 0.8 g·kg^{-1} BW, women in the low protein intake group had a higher BMI and a lower SMI (Table 1) regardless of total energy intake. Similar differences in body composition variables were observed between protein groups based on the higher RDA threshold (1.1 g·kg^{-1} BW). In addition, SMI was significantly lower in those with an intake of <0.8 g·kg^{-1} BW compared to those having an intake of ≥1.1 g·kg^{-1} BW (28.5 ± 3.3 vs. 32.4 ± 3.9, $p < 0.05$).

Table 1. Participant characteristics by groups of protein intake.

	Protein Intake [c]			
	<0.8	≥0.8	<1.1	≥1.1
N	22	84	67	39
Protein intake, g·day^{-1}	54.0 ± 9.6	72.4 ± 13.6 *	61.9 ± 10.8	80.2 ± 13.7 *
Relative protein intake, g·kg^{-1} BW·day^{-1}	0.71 ± 0.09	1.12 ± 0.23 *	0.87 ± 0.14	1.31 ± 0.18 *
Total energy intake, Kcal·day^{-1}	1304 ± 306	1810 ± 324 *	1551 ± 316	1968 ± 336 *
Carbohydrate, % of energy	45.4 ± 6.4	46.2 ± 6.2	46.6 ± 6.1	45.2 ± 6.3
Fat, % of energy	34.0 ± 5.2	34.5 ± 5.3	33.8 ± 5.1	35.3 ± 5.3
Protein, % of energy	17.3 ± 3.5	16.4 ± 2.0	16.5 ± 2.5	16.7 ± 2.1
Body composition Weight, kg Height, cm BMI, kg·m^{-2} SMI, % BW	76.1 ± 12.6 164 ± 5 28.1 ± 4.2 28.5 ± 3.3	65.7 ± 10.3 * 164 ± 6 24.3 ± 3.6 * 31.4 ± 3.9 *	71.7 ± 11.5 165 ± 5 26.4 ± 4.0 29.9 ± 3.8	61.4 ± 8.4 * 164 ± 6 22.9 ± 3.1 * 32.4 ± 3.9 *
Objective Physical Performance VO$_2$ max, mlO$_2$·kg^{-1} BW·min^{-1} [a] Isometric Quadriceps Strength, N·kg^{-1} BW	27.5 ± 7.9 2.5 ± 0.7	29.0 ± 7.1 2.8 ± 0.7	28.0 ± 6.7 2.6 ± 0.7	29.8 ± 7.9 3.0 ± 0.7 *
Self-Reported Physical Limitation, % yes [b]	55.0	25.6 *	42.9	12.8 *

BW, Body Weight; BMI, Body Mass Index; SMI, Skeletal Muscle Index. [a] Based on n = 94. [b] Based on n = 102. [c] g·kg^{-1} of BW per day. Data expressed as mean ± standard deviation, unless indicated. * $p < 0.05$.

When comparing objective measures of physical function between protein intake groups, the significant difference in isometric quadriceps strength observed when based on the 1.1 g·kg^{-1} BW threshold (Table 1) became attenuated (p = 0.081) after SMI adjustment. No corresponding differences were observed when based on the lower protein intake threshold (0.8 g·kg^{-1} BW).

When based on the lower RDA threshold (0.8 g·kg^{-1} BW), women in the low protein intake group had a higher likelihood of having physical limitations. However, adjustment for SMI attenuated the observed effect (Table 2). Interestingly, when further comparing those below 0.8 g·kg^{-1} BW to those with an intake of ≥ 1.1 g·kg^{-1} BW exclusively, a significantly higher likelihood of having physical limitations was found in the former group (Odds ratio: 5.48, 95% Confidence interval: 1.34–22.43) even after SMI adjustment. When based on the protein intake threshold of 1.1 g·kg^{-1} BW, those with lower intakes showed a higher likelihood of having physical limitations compared to those meeting this threshold even after SMI adjustment (Table 2).

Finally, we reanalyzed all data adjusted for overweight status (BMI ≥ 25 kg·m^{-2}) instead of SMI, which left the results unchanged.

Table 2. Odds ratios (OR, 95% CI) of having a physical limitation for women below the RDA thresholds with those above set as reference.

	Model 1			Model 2		
	OR	95% CI	p	OR	95% CI	p
Protein intake						
<0.8 g·kg^{-1} BW	3.55	(1.29–9.76)	0.014	2.56	(0.88–7.42)	0.083
<1.1 g·kg^{-1} BW	5.10	(1.76–14.77)	0.003	3.94	(1.31–11.83)	0.015

CI, Coefficient Interval; BW, Body Weight; RDA, Recommended Dietary Allowance. Model 1: unadjusted. Model 2: adjusted for SMI.

4. Discussion

This study highlights the detrimental effects of not meeting the lowest RDA guideline of protein intake on both muscle mass and physical function in elderly women. Importantly, while beneficial effects on muscle mass are obtained by meeting the lower RDA level, meeting the higher RDA intake seems necessary to infer an additional impact on physical function. As all women were physically active, our findings support the role of protein intake for healthy ageing even in older adults meeting guidelines for PA.

Estimation of the daily protein intake necessary to infer beneficial effects on body composition and physical function in the ageing population is a debated question, since the RDA threshold for proteins of 0.8 g·kg^{-1} BW is based on the single endpoint of nitrogen balance [31]. Our findings support the assumption that meeting the RDA intake of 0.8 g·kg^{-1} BW per day is a key factor to prevent the decline in muscle mass in older adults. This is in line with recent data suggesting that reaching this threshold was associated with higher percentage of fat free mass among older men and women [32]. Additionally, a 6-month randomized controlled trial in functionally limited older men indicated that adherence to the RDA of 0.8 g·kg^{-1} BW for protein was sufficient to maintain lean body mass, whereas an intake above 1.3 g·kg^{-1} BW did not infer additional effects on muscle mass or enhance the testosterone-induced anabolic response [33]. While an RDA of 0.8 g·kg^{-1} BW seems to be a protein amount sufficient to prevent sarcopenic loss of muscle mass, our findings indicate that this threshold is insufficient to preserve physical function. Indeed, not meeting an intake of 1.1 g·kg^{-1} BW was associated with a higher likelihood of having physical limitations and lower muscle strength. Conflicting results exist regarding the role and amount of dietary proteins in the maintenance of physical function in older adults. For instance, while ten Haaf et al. failed to demonstrate a relationship between total protein intake, SPPB scores, and handgrip strength in a sample of older community dwelling adults [20], Gregorio et al. reported a significant impact of higher protein intakes on SPPB but not on the physical component of the quality of life questionnaire or handgrip strength [9]. In contrast, lower decreases in handgrip strength were reported in older men and women with higher protein intakes during a 6-year follow-up [14]. In our study, physical function was assessed using both objective measures and self-reported constructs, and women reporting physical limitations had poorer aerobic fitness and strength. Meeting the RDA for proteins was not related to aerobic fitness in our sample of older women, which underlines that protein intake may not be a main factor determining cardiovascular health. Together with data from previous studies, it is suggested that associations between protein intake and physical function are partly dependent on the selected aspect of physical capability.

It is important to note that variations in muscle mass are likely to exert a considerable influence on physical function [34] and it may thus confound the link between protein intake and function. Indeed, associations between protein intake and physical function have been shown to become attenuated following adjustment for body composition [35]. In our study, the association between leg strength and protein intake was attenuated after accounting for variations in muscle mass, which indicates that protein intake may indirectly influence muscle strength through its impact on muscle mass. Importantly, by considering a construct covering a broad range of physical capabilities rather than a single aspect of physical function, our data show that those meeting the higher RDA threshold were less likely to have physical limitations compared to the lower intake group regardless of variation in body composition.

A novel approach used in this study was to exclusively include older women meeting current PA guidelines for good health in order to attenuate the well documented effects of PA on muscle mass and physical function. To further consider the potential influence of PA, we additionally assessed regular engagement in strengthening activities. Based on this approach, our findings support the assumption that protein intake plays an important role in the maintenance of muscle mass and preservation of physical function even in older individuals adhering to health-related PA behaviors.

Although the dietary record method is a widely accepted standard method for assessing energy intakes, under-reporting is likely to have occurred, which may underestimate true means of total energy intake. Notably, average levels of total energy intake and macronutrient distribution presented in our study were within the range of reference data reported for corresponding age and gender groups [36]. Furthermore, because our sample exclusively comprised apparently healthy and physically active women, our conclusions do not cover groups with more sedentary lifestyles or with overt disease. Of note, skeletal muscle mass was assessed using bioelectrical impedance analysis. In this respect, despite the higher accuracy of other body composition methods including computed tomography or magnetic resonance imaging, bioelectrical impedance analysis is widely used in the diagnosis of sarcopenia. When performed under standardized conditions and using age-specific cross-validated equations, bioelectrical impedance analysis is currently considered to be an accurate measurement of functioning muscle mass in clinical settings and epidemiological studies. Another aspect worth highlighting is that previous studies either did not consider the role of PA or typically relied on crude measures of self-reported PA. In our study, PA levels were objectively assessed and information on specific types of activities relevant for the study outcomes was additionally collected by self-report. Finally, the cross-sectional design of the study prevents us from making inference on causality. Therefore, study outcomes suggesting causal relationships should be interpreted with caution and experimental settings are warranted to determine the true nature of such relationships.

In conclusion, the present study supports the RDA of $0.8 \text{ g} \cdot \text{kg}^{-1}$ BW of proteins to prevent the loss of muscle mass and physical function in the elderly. Our findings also emphasize that a higher intake of at least $1.1 \text{ g} \cdot \text{kg}^{-1}$ BW is required to infer additional benefits on constructs of physical function preventing the occurrence of physical limitations in the elderly. Finally, our findings were evident in women who met guidelines for PA, supporting the role of dietary habits in general and protein intake in particular in the promotion of healthy ageing.

Author Contributions: Conceptualization: A.N., D.M.R., and F.K.; Methodology: A.N., D.M.R., and F.K.; Validation: A.N., D.M.R., and F.K.; Formal Analysis: A.N., D.M.R., and F.K.; Investigation: A.N., D.M.R., and F.K.; Writing—Original Draft Preparation: A.N., D.M.R., and F.K.; Visualization: A.N., D.M.R., and F.K.; Supervision: A.N. and F.K.; Project Administration: A.N. and F.K.; Funding Acquisition: F.K.

Funding: This research was funded by the Swedish National Centre for Research in Sports, grant numbers [P2012-102, P2014-117, and P2015-120].

Conflicts of Interest: The authors declare no conflict of interest. The funders had no role in the design of the study; in the collection, analyses, or interpretation of data; in the writing of the manuscript, and in the decision to publish the results.

References

1. Wolfe, R.R. The role of dietary protein in optimizing muscle mass, function and health outcomes in older individuals. *Br. J. Nutr.* **2012**, *108*, 88–93. [CrossRef] [PubMed]
2. Baum, J.I.; Kim, I.Y.; Wolfe, R.R. Protein consumption and the elderly: What is the optimal level of intake? *Nutrients* **2016**, *8*, 359. [CrossRef] [PubMed]
3. Wolfe, R.R.; Miller, S.L.; Miller, K.B. Optimal protein intake in the elderly. *Clin. Nutr.* **2008**, *27*, 675–684. [CrossRef] [PubMed]
4. Bauer, J.; Biolo, G.; Cederholm, T.; Cesari, M.; Cruz-Jentoft, A.J.; Morley, J.E.; Phillips, S.; Sieber, C.; Stehle, P.; Teta, D.; et al. Evidence-Based Recommendations for Optimal Dietary Protein Intake in Older People: A Position Paper From the PROT-AGE Study Group. *J. Am. Med. Dir. Assoc.* **2013**, *14*, 542–559. [CrossRef] [PubMed]
5. Dodds, R.M.; Roberts, H.C.; Cooper, C.; Sayer, A.A. The Epidemiology of Sarcopenia. *J. Clin. Densitom.* **2015**, *18*, 461–466. [CrossRef] [PubMed]
6. Nowson, C.; O'Connell, S. Protein Requirements and Recommendations for Older People: A Review. *Nutrients* **2015**, *7*, 6874–6899. [CrossRef] [PubMed]
7. Houston, D.K.; Nicklas, B.J.; Ding, J.; Harris, T.B.; Tylavsky, F.A.; Newman, A.B.; Lee, J.S.; Sahyoun, N.R.; Visser, M.; Kritchevsky, S.B. Dietary protein intake is associated with lean mass change in older, community-dwelling adults: The Health, Aging, and Body Composition (Health ABC) Study. *Am. J. Clin. Nutr.* **2008**, *87*, 150–155. [CrossRef] [PubMed]
8. Beasley, J.M.; Wertheim, B.C.; LaCroix, A.Z.; Prentice, R.L.; Neuhouser, M.L.; Tinker, L.F.; Kritchevsky, S.; Shikany, J.M.; Eaton, C.; Chen, Z.; et al. Biomarker-Calibrated Protein Intake and Physical Function in the Women's Health Initiative. *J. Am. Geriatr. Soc.* **2013**, *61*, 1863–1871. [CrossRef] [PubMed]
9. Gregorio, L.; Brindisi, J.; Kleppinger, A.; Sullivan, R.; Mangano, K.M.; Bihuniak, J.D.; Kenny, A.M.; Kerstetter, J.E.; Insogna, K.L. Adequate dietary protein is associated with better physical performance among post-menopasual women 60–90 years. *J. Nutr. Health Aging* **2014**, *18*, 155–160. [CrossRef] [PubMed]
10. Kobayashi, S.; Suga, H.; Sasaki, S. Diet with a combination of high protein and high total antioxidant capacity is strongly associated with low prevalence of frailty among old Japanese women: A multicenter cross-sectional study. *Nutr. J.* **2017**, *16*, 1–12. [CrossRef] [PubMed]
11. Nanri, H.; Yamada, Y.; Yoshida, T.; Okabe, Y.; Nozawa, Y.; Itoi, A.; Yoshimura, E.; Watanabe, Y.; Yamaguchi, M.; Yokoyama, K.; et al. Sex Difference in the Association Between Protein Intake and Frailty: Assessed Using the Kihon Checklist Indexes Among Older Adults. *J. Am. Med. Dir. Assoc.* **2018**, 30174–30179. [CrossRef] [PubMed]
12. Lorenzo-López, L.; Maseda, A.; De Labra, C.; Regueiro-Folgueira, L.; Rodríguez-Villamil, J.L.; Millán-Calenti, J.C. Nutritional determinants of frailty in older adults: A systematic review. *BMC Geriatr.* **2017**, *17*, 1–13. [CrossRef] [PubMed]
13. Beasley, J.M.; Lacroix, A.Z.; Neuhouser, M.L.; Huang, Y.; Tinker, L.; Woods, N.; Michael, Y.; Curb, J.D.; Prentice, R.L. Protein Intake and Incident Frailty in the Women's Health Initiative Observational Study. *J. Am. Geriatr. Soc.* **2010**, *58*, 1063–1071. [CrossRef] [PubMed]
14. McLean, R.R.; Mangano, K.M.; Hannan, M.T.; Kiel, D.P.; Sahni, S. Dietary Protein Intake Is Protective Against Loss of Grip Strength Among Older Adults in the Framingham Offspring Cohort. *J. Gerontol. Ser. A Biol. Sci. Med. Sci.* **2016**, *71*, 356–361. [CrossRef] [PubMed]
15. Granic, A.; Mendonça, N.; Sayer, A.A.; Hill, T.R.; Davies, K.; Adamson, A.; Siervo, M.; Mathers, J.C.; Jagger, C. Low protein intake, muscle strength and physical performance in the very old: The Newcastle 85+ Study. *Clin. Nutr.* **2017**, *44*, 1–11. [CrossRef] [PubMed]
16. Houston, D.K.; Tooze, J.A.; Garcia, K.; Visser, M.; Rubin, S.; Harris, T.B.; Newman, A.B.; Kritchevsky, S.B. Protein Intake and Mobility Limitation in Community-Dwelling Older Adults: The Health ABC Study. *J. Am. Geriatr. Soc.* **2017**, *65*, 1705–1711. [CrossRef] [PubMed]
17. Rondanelli, M.; Klersy, C.; Terracol, G.; Talluri, J.; Maugeri, R.; Guido, D.; Faliva, M.A.; Solerte, B.S.; Fioravanti, M.; Lukaski, H.; et al. Whey protein, amino acids, and vitamin D supplementation with physical activity increases fat-free mass and strength, functionality, and quality of life and decreases inflammation in sarcopenic elderly. *Am. J. Clin. Nutr.* **2016**, *103*, 830–840. [CrossRef] [PubMed]

18. Sahni, S.; Mangano, K.M.; Hannan, M.T.; Kiel, D.P.; McLean, R.R. Higher Protein Intake Is Associated with Higher Lean Mass and Quadriceps Muscle Strength in Adult Men and Women. *J. Nutr.* **2015**, *145*, 1569–1575. [CrossRef] [PubMed]
19. Scott, D.; Blizzard, L.; Fell, J.; Giles, G.; Jones, G. Associations Between Dietary Nutrient Intake and Muscle Mass and Strength in Community-Dwelling Older Adults: The Tasmanian Older Adult Cohort Study. *J. Am. Geriatr. Soc.* **2010**, *58*, 2129–2134. [CrossRef] [PubMed]
20. Ten Haaf, D.; van Dongen, E.; Nuijten, M.; Eijsvogels, T.; de Groot, L.; Hopman, M. Protein Intake and Distribution in Relation to Physical Functioning and Quality of Life in Community-Dwelling Elderly People: Acknowledging the Role of Physical Activity. *Nutrients* **2018**, *10*, 506. [CrossRef] [PubMed]
21. Chan, R.; Leung, J.; Woo, J.; Kwok, T. Associations of dietary protein intake on subsequent decline in muscle mass and physical functions over four years in ambulant older Chinese people. *J. Nutr. Health Aging* **2014**, *18*, 171–177. [CrossRef] [PubMed]
22. Robinson, S.M.M.; Reginster, J.Y.Y.; Rizzoli, R.; Shaw, S.C.C.; Kanis, J.A.A.; Bautmans, I.; Bischoff-Ferrari, H.; Bruyère, O.; Cesari, M.; Dawson-Hughes, B.; et al. Does nutrition play a role in the prevention and management of sarcopenia? *Clin. Nutr.* **2018**, *37*, 1121–1132. [CrossRef] [PubMed]
23. Shad, B.J.; Wallis, G.; van Loon, L.J.C.; Thompson, J.L. Exercise prescription for the older population: The interactions between physical activity, sedentary time, and adequate nutrition in maintaining musculoskeletal health. *Maturitas* **2016**, *93*, 78–82. [CrossRef] [PubMed]
24. Janssen, I.; Heymsfield, S.B.; Baumgartner, R.N.; Ross, R. Estimation of skeletal muscle mass by bioelectrical impedance analysis. *J. Appl. Physiol.* **2000**, *89*, 465–471. [CrossRef] [PubMed]
25. Åstrand, I. Aerobic work capacity in men and women with special reference to age. *Acta Physiol. Scand. Suppl.* **1960**, *49*, 1–92. [PubMed]
26. Edholm, P.; Strandberg, E.; Kadi, F. Lower limb explosive strength capacity in elderly women: Effects of resistance training and healthy diet. *J. Appl. Physiol.* **2017**, *123*, 190–196. [CrossRef] [PubMed]
27. Gandek, B.; Ware, J.E.; Aaronson, N.K.; Apolone, G.; Bjorner, J.B.; Brazier, J.E.; Bullinger, M.; Kaasa, S.; Leplege, A.; Prieto, L.; et al. Cross-Validation of Item Selection and Scoring for the SF-12 Health Survey in Nine Countries. *J. Clin. Epidemiol.* **1998**, *51*, 1171–1178. [CrossRef]
28. Nilsson, A.; Wåhlin-Larsson, B.; Kadi, F.; Britta, W.; Kadi, F. Physical activity and not sedentary time per se influences on clustered metabolic risk in elderly community-dwelling women. *PLoS ONE* **2017**, *12*, e0175496. [CrossRef] [PubMed]
29. Evenson, K.R.; Wen, F.; Herring, A.H.; Di, C.; LaMonte, M.J.; Tinker, L.F.; Lee, I.-M.; Rillamas-Sun, E.; LaCroix, A.Z.; Buchner, D.M. Calibrating physical activity intensity for hip-worn accelerometry in women age 60 to 91 years: The Women's Health Initiative OPACH Calibration Study. *Prev. Med. Rep.* **2015**, *2*, 750–756. [CrossRef] [PubMed]
30. Wareham, N.J.; Jakes, R.W.; Rennie, K.L.; Mitchell, J.; Hennings, S.; Day, N.E. Validity and repeatability of the EPIC-Norfolk Physical Activity Questionnaire. *Int. J. Epidemiol.* **2002**, *31*, 168–174. [CrossRef] [PubMed]
31. Rand, W.M.; Pellett, P.L.; Young, V.R. Meta-analysis of nitrogen balance studies for estimating protein requirements in healthy adults. *Am. J. Clin. Nutr.* **2003**, *77*, 109–127. [CrossRef] [PubMed]
32. Beasley, J.M.; Deierlein, A.L.; Morland, K.B.; Granieri, E.C.; Spark, A. Is meeting the recommended dietary allowance (RDA) for protein related to body composition among older adults? Results from the Cardiovascular Health of Seniors and Built Environment Study. *J. Nutr. Health Aging* **2016**, *20*, 790–796. [CrossRef] [PubMed]
33. Bhasin, S.; Apovian, C.M.; Travison, T.G.; Pencina, K.; Moore, L.L.; Huang, G.; Campbell, W.W.; Li, Z.; Howland, A.S.; Chen, R.; et al. Effect of Protein Intake on Lean Body Mass in Functionally Limited Older Men. *JAMA Intern. Med.* **2018**, *178*, 530–541. [CrossRef] [PubMed]
34. Bea, J.W.; Going, S.B.; Wertheim, B.C.; Bassford, T.L.; LaCroix, A.Z.; Wright, N.C.; Nicholas, J.S.; Heymsfield, S.B.; Chen, Z. Body composition and physical function in the Women's Health Initiative Observational Study. *Prev. Med. Rep.* **2018**, *11*, 15–22. [CrossRef] [PubMed]

35. Isanejad, M.; Mursu, J.; Sirola, J.; Kröger, H.; Rikkonen, T.; Tuppurainen, M.; Erkkilä, A.T. Dietary protein intake is associated with better physical function and muscle strength among elderly women. *Br. J. Nutr.* **2016**, *115*, 1281–1291. [CrossRef] [PubMed]
36. Livsmedelsverket. *Riksmaten—Vuxna 2010–2011 Livsmedels-Och Näringsintag Bland Vuxna i Sverige*; Livsmedelsverket: Uppsala, Sweden, 2012; ISBN 978 91 7714 216 4.

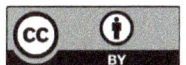

© 2018 by the authors. Licensee MDPI, Basel, Switzerland. This article is an open access article distributed under the terms and conditions of the Creative Commons Attribution (CC BY) license (http://creativecommons.org/licenses/by/4.0/).

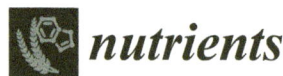

Review

Relative Protein Intake and Physical Function in Older Adults: A Systematic Review and Meta-Analysis of Observational Studies

Hélio José Coelho-Júnior [1,2,*], Luiz Milano-Teixeira [1], Bruno Rodrigues [1], Reury Bacurau [3], Emanuele Marzetti [2] and Marco Uchida [1]

1. Applied Kinesiology Laboratory–AKL, School of Physical Education, University of Campinas, Av. Érico Veríssimo, 701, Cidade Universitária "Zeferino Vaz", Barão Geraldo, Campinas-SP 13.083-851, Brazil; teixeira.luisfelipe@gmail.com (L.M.-T.); prof.brodrigues@gmail.com (B.R.); uchida@g.unicamp.br (M.U.)
2. Department of Geriatrics, Neurosciences and Orthopedics, Teaching Hospital "Agostino Gemelli", Catholic University of the Sacred Heart, 00168 Rome, Italy; emarzetti@live.com
3. School of Arts, Sciences and Humanities, University of São Paulo, Rua Arlindo Béttio, 1000-Ermelino Matarazzo, São Paulo-SP 03828-000, Brazil; reurybacurau@usp.br
* Correspondence: coelhojunior@hotmail.com.br; Tel.: +55-119-493-98302

Received: 22 July 2018; Accepted: 13 September 2018; Published: 19 September 2018

Abstract: (1) Background: The present work aims to conduct a systematic review and meta-analysis of observational studies, in order to investigate the association of relative protein intake and physical function in older adults; (2) Methods: Observational studies, that investigated the association between protein intake and physical function in older adults, were retrieved from MEDLINE, SCOPUS, CINAHL, AgeLine, EMBASE, and Cochrane-CENTRAL. Two independent researchers conducted study selection and data extraction; (3) Results: Very high protein intake ($\geq$1.2 g/kg/day) and high protein intake ($\geq$1.0 g/kg/day) groups showed better lower limb physical functioning and walking speed (WS) performance, respectively, in comparison to individuals who present relative low protein (<0.80 g/kg/day) intake. On the other hand, relative high protein intake does not seem to propitiate a better performance on isometric handgrip (IHG) and chair rise in comparison to relative low protein intake. In addition, there were no significant differences in the physical functioning of high and middle protein intake groups; (4) Conclusions: In conclusion, findings of the present study indicate that a very high ($\geq$1.2 g/kg/day) and high protein intake ($\geq$1.0 g/kg/day) are associated with better lower-limb physical performance, when compared to low protein (<0.80 g/kg/day) intake, in community-dwelling older adults. These findings act as additional evidence regarding the potential need to increase protein guidelines to above the current recommendations. However, large randomized clinical trials are needed to confirm the addictive effects of high-protein diets ($\geq$1.0 g/kg/day) in comparison to the current recommendations on physical functioning. All data are available in the Open ScienceFramework.

Keywords: sarcopenia; protein intake; physical function

1. Introduction

Sarcopenia is a geriatric condition characterized by progressive muscle atrophy accompanied by loss of muscle strength and/or function [1]. The incidence of sarcopenia rises with aging and its prevalence is markedly increased in older subjects [2]. In the absence of targeted interventions, the clinical course of sarcopenia is marked by higher odds of mobility disability, loss of independence, and mortality [3–6]. In this sense, adequate protein intake and physical exercise have been suggested as the two main strategies to counteract sarcopenia, and prevent its deleterious effects [7,8].

Although protein supplementation may be advisable in the management of sarcopenia, the optimal protein requirement for older adults is presently unclear. Indeed, the established guidelines recommended for a number of agencies, such as the Dietary Allowance (RDA), RDI (recommended daily intake) [9], and the RNI (reference nutrient intake) [10] have been questioned, and researchers have discussed if the recommended protein intake is enough to maintain the functional status or even prevent its decline and muscle atrophy in older adults [11,12]. Most critical are regarding the RDA, so that the main concern is that the amount of protein recommended is based on nitrogen balance studies, which may be associated with a methodological bias [11,13].

Opinion articles and consensus statements have argued that older people should be encouraged to consume greater quantities of protein than the RDA (1.0–1.5 g/kg) [11–14]. Findings from observational studies are in line with these inferences, since higher protein consumption is associated with lower risk of frailty, loss of lean body mass, slow walking speed, dynapenia, and poor balance [15–18]. Nevertheless, there is a lack of direct evidence testing the proposed cut-off points for protein consumption. The few available studies have reported incongruent results regarding the association of protein intake and physical function [17,19–21]. However, to the best of our knowledge, meta-analyses have not been performed to determine the pool of results.

Therefore, the present work aimed at conducting a systematic review and meta-analysis of observational studies to investigate the association of relative protein intake and physical function in older adults.

2. Materials and Methods

We conducted a systematic review and meta-analysis of observational studies to assess the association between relative protein intake and physical function in older adults. The study was fully performed by investigators and no librarians were part of the team. This study complies with the criteria proposed by the Primary Reporting Items for Systematic Reviews and Meta-analyses (PRISMA) Statement [22], and the Meta-analysis of Observational Studies in Epidemiology (MOOSE) guidelines [23]. All data are available in the Open Science Framework at https://doi.org/10.17605/OSF.IO/JP5SB.

2.1. Eligibility Criteria

The inclusion criteria consisted of: (a) Observational studies, including cross-sectional and case-control studies, which investigated as primary or secondary outcome the association of relative protein intake and physical function in older adults. Longitudinal cohort studies were also included if crude baseline data were available; (b) participant age of 60 years or older; (c) direct assessment of at least one physical function domain (studies provided self-reported physical function were excluded); (d) provided the comparison of at least two groups with different relative protein intakes; (e) mean values and a measure of dispersion (standard deviation or confidence interval) were provided; (f) published studies (English language). We excluded randomized-clinical trials (RCTs), quasi-experimental, cross-over studies and any kind of investigation that examined the effects of a nutritional intervention associated or not with other interventions (e.g., physical exercise) on physical function. Studies that enrolled institutionalized participants or non-institutionalized participants with cognitive impairment and/or disorder, gastrointestinal and/or renal diseases, anorexia, cancer or any kind of condition that may directly impair protein metabolism (e.g., maple syrup urine disease, tyrosinemia) were also excluded. Sarcopenic and frailty older people were included.

2.2. Search Strategy and Selection Criteria

Studies published on or before August 2018 were retrieved from the following three electronic databases by one investigator (H.J.C.J): (1) MEDLINE (PubMed interface); (2) the Cochrane Library (Wiley interface); (3) SCOPUS (Elsevier interface); (4) CINAHL (EBSCO interface); (5) AgeLine (EBSCO interface); and (6) EMBASE (EBSCO interface). Reference lists for reviews and retrieved articles for additional studies were checked and citation searches on key articles were performed in Google Scholar and ResearchGate for additional reports. Initially, a search strategy was designed using keywords, MeSH terms, and free text words, such as *protein consumption, physical function, older adults*. Additionally, keywords and subject headings were exhaustively combined using Boolean operators. The complete search strategy used for the PubMed is shown in List S1. Only eligible full texts in English language were considered for review. Authors were contacted if necessary.

2.3. Data Extraction and Quality Assessment

Titles and abstracts of retrieved articles were screened for eligibility by two researchers (H.J.C.-J. and B.R.). If an abstract did not provide enough information for evaluation, the full-text was retrieved. Disagreements were solved by a third reviewer (M.U.). Reviewers were not blinded to authors, institutions, or manuscript journals. Studies that provided data for more than two groups—for example, low, middle, high, and very high relative protein intake were also added—since the volunteers were not shared among the groups. Data extraction were independently performed by two reviewers (H.J.C.-J. and L.M.-T) using a standardized coding form. Disagreements were solved by a third reviewer (M.U.). Coded variables included methodological quality and the characteristics of the studies, including: Year, authors, country, study design, setting, sample size (n), age, prevalence of female, body mass index (BMI), lean mass, appendicular muscle mass, dietary intake assessment method, total protein intake, relative protein intake.

Afterwards, studies were allocated into four different groups (*low* (<0.8 g/kg/day), *middle* (0.8–0.99 g/kg/day), *high* ($\geq$1.0 g/kg/day), and *very high* ($\geq$1.2 g/kg/day) protein intake). These cutoffs were selected according to previous research. Indeed, longitudinal [24,25] and review [11–14] studies have arguing that older adults should consume at least 1.0 g/kg/day of protein (i.e., *high*) to maintain muscle mass and optimal physical functioning, so that values below the RDA (<0.8 g/kg/day) may be considered *low*, while values higher than the RDA, but lower than the recommended for these aforementioned studies may be considered *middle*. In addition, some evidence has proposed that a minimum of 1.2 g/kg/day of protein should be consumed by older adults in attempt to avoid poor health-related outcomes and maintain functional performance, regardless the presence of chronic diseases [26,27]. In this sense, investigations that showed a mean protein intake of at least 1.2 g/kg/day were allocated in the *very high* group.

The quality of reporting for each study was performed by two researchers (H.J.C.-J. and L.M.-T) using the Strengthening the Reporting of Observational Studies in Epidemiology (STROBE) instrument [28]. The agreement rate between reviewers was κ = 0.96 for quality assessment.

2.4. Statistical Analysis

Meta-analyses were conducted using Revman V.5. Effect size (ES) were measured using standard mean difference (SMD) and mean difference and are reported with 95% confidence intervals (95% CI). SMD was used in the comparisons between *High protein intake* and *Very high protein intake* versus *Low protein intake* in relation to *Mobility* and *Lower limb physical functioning*, respectively, since the investigations assessed the same outcome, but using different tools. However, the mean difference was used in the remaining comparisons, since all the other studies used the same outcome. If the required outcome metric was not reported in the study, values were calculated using available data. Due to the different characteristics of the included studies, a random-effect model was used to calculate the pooled ES. Heterogeneity across studies was tested using Q-statistics and I^2 index was used to assess inconsistency [29]. The I^2 index was classified as not important (0–40%), moderate (30–60%), substantial (50–90%), and considerable (75–100%).

3. Results

3.1. Characteristics and Quality of Included Studies

Table 1 provides a general description of the included studies. Of the 4392 registers recovered from electronic databases and hand search, 4253 records were excluded based on duplicate data, title or abstract. One hundred thirty-nine studies were fully reviewed and assessed for eligibility. Finally, seven studies met the inclusion criteria (Figure 1).

Included studies were published between 2014 and 2018, the majority had a prospective longitudinal cohort design [17,30–32], while two had a cross-sectional design [20,33] and one study was a case-control [21]. Overall, a total of 8754 community-dwelling older adults from six different countries were included. Volunteers were characterized as healthy in three studies [17,31,34], post-menopausal in two studies [20,31], sarcopenic in one study [21], and diabetic in one study [32]. Mean age of the subjects ranged from 67.8 to 83.0 years, and the percentage of women among total subject population of various study groups varied from 10% to 100%. Mean BMI ranged from 23.7 kg/m^2 to 29.5 kg/m^2, so that one study investigated volunteers with normal BMI [34], while the other six studies investigated overweight individuals [17,20,21,31–33]. Limited information was available regarding the clinical characteristics of study participants. Nevertheless, osteoporosis, diabetes, hypertension, depression, rheumatoid arthritis, and heart diseases were diagnosed among the included individuals. Lean mass and appendicular skeletal muscle represented 55.8% and 24.4%, respectively, of the total weight. Twenty-nine percent of the volunteers reported an episode of fall in the 12 months before the investigations. Physical and functional evaluations included isometric handgrip strength (IHG), knee extensor strength, one-leg stance, usual walking speed (WS), chair rise, tandem walk speed, narrow walk speed, short physical performance battery (SPPB), and timed 8-foot walk. However, only IHG, WS, knee extensor strength, SPPB, and chair rise were included in the final analysis, due to availability of data. According to protein intake per kg of body weight, volunteers could be divided into four major groups: *Low* (<0.8 g/kg/day), *middle* (0.8–0.99 g/kg/day), *high* (≥1.0 g/kg/day), and *very high* (≥1.2 g/kg/day). Methods to evaluate dietary intake included 24-h dietary recall (28.5%), 3-day dietary intake record (28.5%), 4-day dietary intake record (14.3%), food frequency questionnaire (14.3%), and the Semi Quantitative-Food Frequency Questionnaire (SQFFQ) (14.3%).

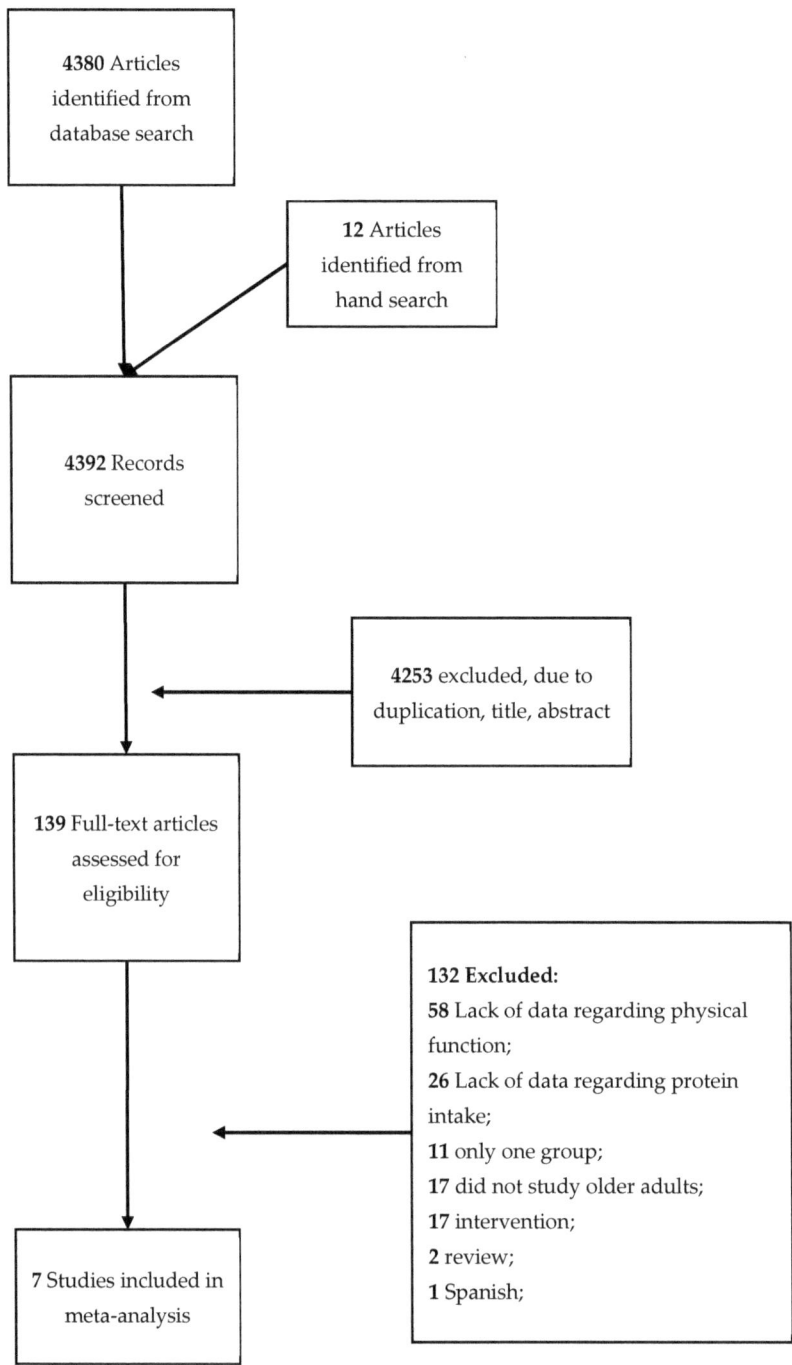

Figure 1. Flowchart of the present study.

Table 1. General description of the included studies.

Year	Authors	Country	Study Design	Population	Setting	Sample Size	Age	Female (%)	BMI	Lean Mass	Appendicular Muscle Mass	Dietary Intake Assessment Method	Total Protein Intake (g/Day)	STROBE Score
2018	ten Haaf et al.	Netherland	Cross-sectional	Healthy	Community-dwelling	HP: 80; LP: 60	83.0	10	26.1	—	—	24-h dietary recall	HP: 89.5; LP: 64.7	19
2016	Isanejad et al.	Finland	Longitudinal	Healthy	Community-dwelling	HP = 112; MP = 269; LP = 171	67.8	100	26.6	HP: 41.3, 16.4, 6.5; MP:40.1, 15.9, 6.7; LP: 39.1, 15.6, 6.6	—	3-day dietary intake record	HP: 83.4; MP:65.0; LP: 51.4	20
2016	Rahi et al.	Canada	Longitudinal	Diabetic	Community-dwelling	HP: 73; LP: 99	75.0	62	29.5	—	—	24-h dietary recall	HP: 91; LP: 64.3	20
2015	Larocque et al.	United States	Longitudinal	Post-menopausal women	Community-dwelling	LP = 1756; HP = 2889	80.1	100	26.8	—	—	Food frequency questionnaire	LP = 42.6; HP = 71.6	17
2015	Verlaan et al.	United Kingdom	Case-control	Sarcopenic and non-sarcopenic	Community-dwelling	Sarcopenic: 66; Non-sarcopenic: 66	71.1	39	26.1	—	Sarcopenic:19.0; Non-sarcopenic: 20.4	3-day dietary intake record	Sarcopenic: 72.5; Non-sarcopenic: 75.3	19
2014	Chan et al.	China	Longitudinal	Healthy	Community-dwelling	LP = 617; MP = 677; HP = 705; HP2 = 727	71.6	49.8	23.7	—	—	Semi Quantitative-Food Frequency Questionnaire (SQFFQ)	—	19
2014	Gregorio et al.	United States	Cross-sectional	Post-menopausal women	Community-dwelling	LP = 97; HP = 290	73.0	100	27.4	LP = 40.7; HP = 38.2	LP = 17.0; HP = 15.9	4-day dietary intake record	LP = 49.7; HP = 79.7	20

BMI = body mass index; HP = high protein; MP = middle protein; LP = low protein.

Table 2 provides the general characteristics of the volunteers according to their relative protein intake. All groups presented similar mean age (~73 years). The lowest sample size was observed in the middle protein intake group, followed by the very high protein intake group, low protein intake group and high protein intake group. The groups presented a similar mean lean mass and mean appendicular mass. However, it is important to observe that High protein intake and Very high protein intake groups showed a higher percentage of lean mass when compared to Low protein intake and Middle protein intake groups. In addition, a greater performance in knee extensor strength and SPPB was observed in High protein intake and Very high protein intake groups when compared to Low protein intake group. Protein, carbohydrate and fat intake increased according to relative protein intake. It should be stressed that these parameters were not reported by all the investigations.

Table 2. Characteristics of the volunteers according to relative protein intake *.

Variables	Low Protein Intake (0.67) n = 2641	Middle Protein Intake (0.88) n = 395	High Protein Intake (1.3) n = 5619	Very High Protein Intake (1.5) n = 1145
Anthropometric characteristics				
Age (years)	73.8	74.0	74.6	73.5
BMI (kg/m^2)	29.1	26.7	27	27.1
Lean Mass (kg) (% in relation to weight)	41.0 (53)	40.1 (56.1)	38.7 (58.7)	38.2 (58.1)
Appendicular Muscle Mass (kg) (% in relation to weight)	—	19.0 (25.5)	20.4 (24.7)	15.9 (24.2)
Physical functional tests				
IHG (kg)	20.4	27.5	24.3	19.1
Knee Extensor Strength (lb)	54.5	44.5	52.1	57.5
One-Leg Stand (s)	13.5	19.3	18.4	15.3
Chair Rises (s)	11.4	10.6	11.8	13.5
Tandem Walk Speed for 6 m (m/s)	0.30	0.34	0.33	—
Usual Walking Speed (m/s)	1.1	1.2	1.2	1.07
SPPB (points)	9.9	9.0	11.0	10.6
Timed 8-Foot Walk (m/s)	1	—	1.1	1.1
Dietary factors				
Protein (g/day)	58.8	67.4	85.4	87.2
Carbohydrate (g/day)	162.6	199.8	215.9	220.6
Fat (g/day)	43.6	58.6	64.4	—

BMI = body mass index; IHG = Isometric handgrip; SPPB = Short physical performance battery (i.e., combination of results in gait speed, chair stand e balance tests; The final score ranged from 0 (worst performance) to 12 (best performance). * Information was not available by all the included investigations.

Study quality results are shown in Table S1, while the point by point analysis is shown in Table S2. The overall score ranged from 17 to 20. All studies reported the items required by the STROBE criteria in relation to the abstract (items 1 and 2), clarity of the outcomes (items 7 and 15), methods of assessment (item 8), handle of quantitative variables (item 11), statistical methods and analysis (items 12, 16), discussion (items 18–21), and funding (item 22). However, 14.2% of the studies failed to clearly state specific objectives, including any prespecified hypotheses (item 3), the main aim of the investigation (item 4), describe the setting, locations and relevant dates of recruitment and data collection (item 5) [25], give the characteristics of study participants (item 14); and report other analyses done—e.g., analyses of subgroups and interactions, and sensitivity analyses (item 17). In turn, 28.5% did not properly report the eligibility criteria, and the sources and methods of selection of participants (item 6), 71.4% did not describe any efforts to address potential sources of bias (item 9), 57.1% explained how the study size was arrived at (item 10) and reported numbers of individuals at each stage of study (item 13).

3.2. High Protein Intake verses Low Protein Intake

A total of four studies provided information to investigate the association of high and low protein intake with physical function (Figure 2). It should be stressed, that Rahi et al. [32] provided their data according to gender, and the results are presented accordingly. *Upper-limb muscle strength*—Upper-limb muscle strength was measured by IHG in all studies. Three studies were added in the meta-analysis [17,20,31]. Results did not demonstrate significant differences in IHG between the groups, and a small non-significant ES was observed (ES = −0.36; 95% CI = −1.15 to 0.44, p = 0.38). Moderate heterogeneity was found across studies (χ^2 = 4.16, df = 2, p = 0.12, I^2 = 52%) (Figure 2a). *Lower-limb muscle strength*—Lower-limb muscle strength was evaluated by chair-rise and knee extensor strength. A meta-analysis of three studies—but evaluating four subgroups—observed a small non-significant difference between groups (ES = −0.09; 95% CI = −0.26 to 0.08, p = 0.30). A not important heterogeneity was found across studies (χ^2 = 3.75, df = 3, p = 0.29, I^2 = 20%) (Figure 2b).

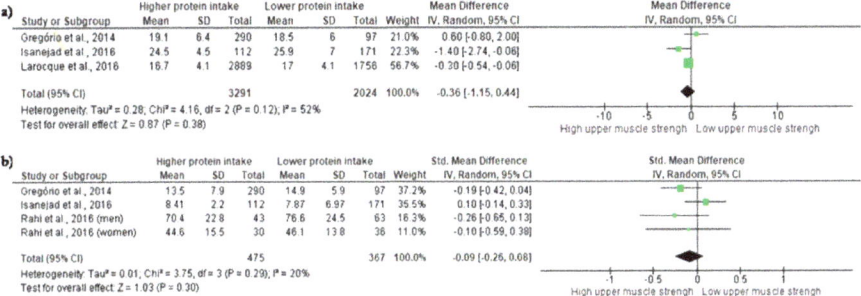

Figure 2. Mean difference in (**a**) *Upper-limb muscle strength* and Standardized mean difference in (**b**) *Lower-limb muscle strength* according to protein intake. Squares represent study-specific estimates; diamonds represent pooled estimates of random-effects meta-analyses.

3.3. Mobility

Mobility was evaluated by 10-m WS [17] and 6-m WS [34]. In the study of Chan et al. [34], three out of four groups showed a high protein intake (≥1.0 g/kg/day). In this sense, groups will be mentioned as Chan et al., 2014, 2014b, and 2014c, according to relative protein intake. In addition, the groups were evaluated alone and grouped. A small ES were observed when the analysis was performed with Chan et al. [34] (1.0 g/kg/day) and Isanejad et al. [17] (ES = 0.10; 95% CI= −0.06 to 0.27, p = 0.23, χ^2 = 20.66, df = 1, p < 0.00001, I^2 = 95%) (Figure 3a), as well as with Chan et al. (2014b) (1.4 g/kg/day) and Isanejad et al. [15] (ES = 0.11; 95% CI = −0.05 to 0.26, p = 0.18, χ^2 = 18.41, df = 1, p < 0.00001, I^2 = 95%) (Figure 3b). The combination of the groups—Chan et al. (2014 and 2014b)—changed the results, so that a small and significant ES was observed (ES = 0.07; 95% CI = 0.01 to 0.12, p = 0.02, χ^2 = 20.84, df = 2, p < 0.00001, I^2 = 90%) (Figure 3c). Significant results were also observed when Chan et al. (2014c) was evaluated alone (ES = 0.13; 95% CI = 0.01 to 0.24, p = 0.04, χ^2 = 10.29, df = 1, p = 0.01, I^2 = 90%) (Figure 3d) and with the other groups (ES = 0.06; 95% CI = 0.02 to 0.11, p = 0.003, χ^2 = 27.52, df = 3, p < 0.00001, I^2 = 89%) (Figure 3e).

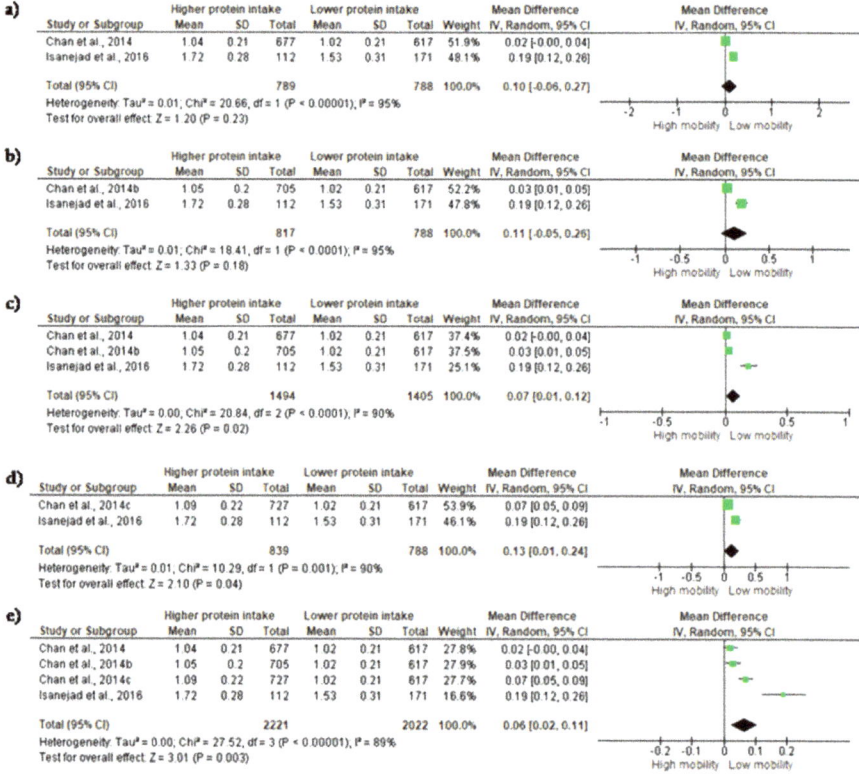

Figure 3. Mean differences in *Mobility* according to protein intake. (**a**) Chan et al., 2014, and Isanejad et al., 2016; (**b**) Chan et al., 2014b, and Isanejad et al., 2016; (**c**) Chan et al., 2014ab, and Isanejad et al., 2016; (**d**) Chan et al., 2014c, and Isanejad et al., 2016; (**e**) Chan et al., 2014abc, and Isanejad et al., 2016. Squares represent study-specific estimates; diamonds represent pooled estimates of random-effects meta-analyses.

3.4. Middle Protein Intake verses High Protein Intake

A total of four studies provided information to investigate the association of high and middle protein intake with physical function (Figure 4). *Upper-limb muscle strength*—Upper-limb muscle strength was measured by IHG in all studies. Three studies were added in the meta-analysis [17,21,33]. Results did not demonstrate significant differences in IHG between groups, and a large non-significant ES was observed (ES = 1.09; 95% CI = −3.78 to 5.96, p = 0.66). A considerable heterogeneity was found across studies (χ^2 = 25.07, df = 2, p = < 0.00001, I^2 = 92%) (Figure 4a). *Mobility*—Mobility was evaluated in three studies. Pooling of results indicated a small and non-significant ES (ES = 0.17; 95% CI= −0.12 to 0.46, p = 0.26). A considerable heterogeneity was found across studies (χ^2 = 56.46, df = 2, p = < 0.0001, I^2 = 96%) (Figure 4b). *Lower-limb muscle strength*—Lower-limb muscle strength was evaluated by chair-rise in all studies. A meta-analysis of two studies observe a moderate non-significant difference between the groups (ES = 0.49; 95% CI= −0.01 to 0.99, p = 0.05). An insignificant heterogeneity was found across studies (χ^2 = 0.72, df = 1, p = 0.40, I^2 = 0%) (Figure 4c).

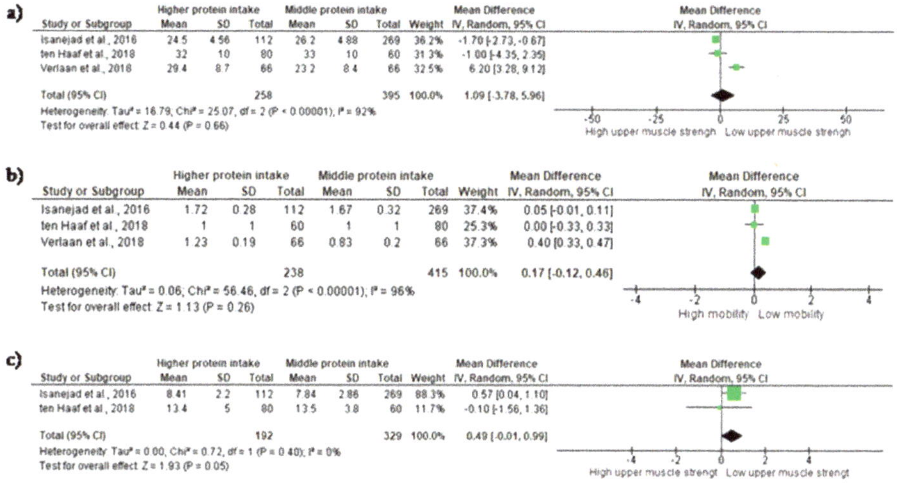

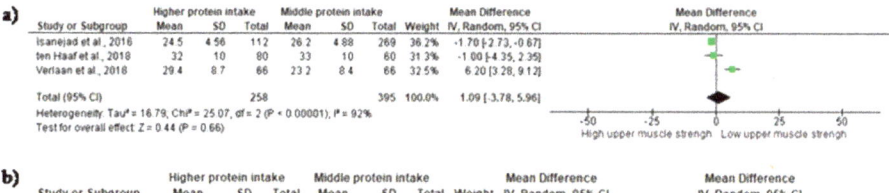

Figure 4. Mean difference in (**a**) *Upper-limb muscle strength*; (**b**) *Mobility*; and (**c**) *Lower-limb muscle strength* according to protein intake. Squares represent study-specific estimates; diamonds represent pooled estimates of random-effects meta-analyses.

3.5. Very High Protein Intake verses Low Protein Intake

A total of five investigations provided information to investigate the association of *very high protein intake* and *low protein intake* with physical function (Figure 5). Due to the lack of available evidence, we did not divide the evaluation according to the type of physical assessment, as was performed above, and studies should assess at least one lower limb physical function to be included. The evaluations included knee extensor strength [32], SPPB [20], and walking speed [34]. Pooling of results indicated a small and significant ES (ES = 0.18; 95% CI = 0.01 to 0.35, p = 0.04). A considerable heterogeneity was found across studies (χ^2 = 15.56, df = 4, p = 0.004, I^2 = 74%).

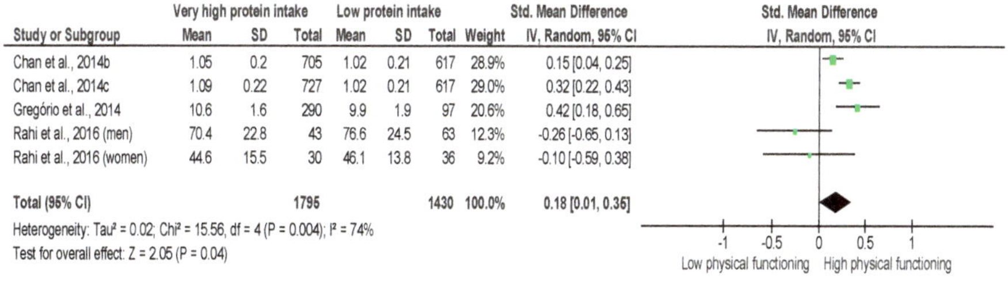

Figure 5. Standardized mean difference in *Lower-limb muscle functioning* according to protein intake. Squares represent study-specific estimates; diamonds represent pooled estimates of random-effects meta-analyses.

4. Discussion

The present study was designed to investigate the available evidence regarding the association of relative protein intake and physical function in older adults. Findings of this investigation indicate that individuals with relatively very high (≥1.2 g/kg/day) and high (≥1.0 g/kg/day) protein intakes show higher mobility and lower limb physical functioning, respectively, in comparison to those with relative low protein (<0.80 g/kg/day) intake.

The assessment of study quality demonstrated that reports were of very good quality and scored between 17 and 20. The main bias associated with the studies was the lack of adequate description about the efforts to address potential sources of bias (item 9), the design of the study size (item 10), and the report regarding the number of participants in all the phases of the study (item 13).

Although in recent years several study groups have strongly recommended that older adults consume greater levels of protein intake than the RDA, there is a lack of direct evidence testing this hypothesis [11,13]. Several observational studies have demonstrated incongruent results, so that it is possible to observe null [19,33,34] and positive [17,20,21] associations between protein intake and physical function in older adults.

To the best of our knowledge, this is the first study that directly compared the physical function of older adults with different relative protein intakes. Our findings support at least partially the need to increase protein guidelines to above the current RDA in older adults, since the very high and high protein intake groups showed better muscular health when compared to the low protein intake group. The plausibility behind these findings is based on the anabolic resistance hypothesis, according to which the muscular anabolic response to appropriate stimulation would be blunted in advanced age (to review, see Calvani et al. [14]; Landi et al. [35]). This idea is supported by the observation that the aging muscle presents diminished muscle protein synthesis in response to small amount of essential amino acids (EAAs) [36], the key nutrient for the stimulation of protein synthesis. This would eventually lead to muscle catabolism, loss on lean body mass, dynapenia, and impairment on muscle function [35]. Higher availability of EAAs, mainly leucine, seems to be necessary to reverse overcome the anabolic resistance of muscle [37]. Therefore, the greater physical performance observed in the groups with higher protein intake levels (i.e., very high and high) might be ascribed to a larger EAAs availability.

Although our findings demonstrated that very high and high protein intakes were associated with greater physical functioning in comparison to low protein intake, there were no differences between high and middle protein intake groups. These results are interesting and deserve concern because the *middle* group represented the level of protein intake recommended by the RDA.

The main motivation for considering changes from a minimum of 0.8 g/kg/day to 1.0 g/kg/day has been the findings of longitudinal studies that demonstrated preserved muscle mass [24] and lower risk of frailty [25] in older adults who had a protein intake $\geq$1.0 g/kg/day, as well as the evidence that showed a significant reduction on muscle mass of older adults who consumed the current RDA of protein for a long period [38]. However, no previous studies had directly comparing these proposed protein cutoffs, and the lack of significant differences between *high* and *middle* groups may occur, because the values of protein intake are similar, according to ten Haaf et al. [33].

Nonetheless, some researchers may argue that *very high* protein intake could be sufficient to elicit significant differences, since the studies of Vellas et al. [26] and Mustafa et al. [27] demonstrated that a very high protein intake was associated with a lower risk to poor health-related outcomes and physical disability. However, there was no available evidence to compare *very high* and *middle* protein intake groups. Taken together, these data suggest that a protein intake higher than 1.0 g/kg/day causes beneficial effects when compared to protein intake levels lower than 0.8 g/kg/day, but more studies are still necessary to precisely define the different effects of *very high* and *high* protein intakes in comparison to *middle* protein intake.

Conversely, from a practical point of view, the consumption of high protein intake by older adults has been the subject of intense scientific debate and a frequent concern of health professionals. Nowadays, has been accepted that older adults without a previous history of kidney disease show a lower risk of poor-health outcomes in response to high-protein diets [13,39]. However, although higher glomerular filtration rate seems to be a normal mechanism in response to the elevated amount of protein in the physiological system of patients with normal kidney function, an increased protein intake may collaborate to decline in the renal function of patients with a pre-existing renal disease [39]. Therefore, findings of the present study should be carefully extrapolated for other populations than healthy older adults.

On the other hand, data of the present study demonstrated that high protein intake was not associated with better performance on the IHG and chair rise when compared to low protein intake group. These findings support the inferences that a higher protein intake may be associated with better scores on some, but not all physical tests [19].

One possible explanation for these results is that a greater intake of protein might promote better functioning of systems other than the neuromuscular system. It should be stressed that the performance on the IHG and chair-rise seems to be mainly dictated by the neuromuscular system. On the other hand, walking ability needs a larger integration among the body systems in comparison with sit and stand up or tightening an object. Indeed, walking is a complex activity involving a variety of neural process (e.g., sensory, cortical cognitive, temporal) [40,41], cerebral and peripheral vascular beds [42,43], as well as lung [44], cardiac and muscular functions [45], to list a few. Consequently, walking ability represents the functioning of multiple organ systems instead of just one system [46], and marked disturbances in gait pattern may occur in response to cardiovascular, neurological and neuromuscular pathologies [40,41].

Regarding the relationship between protein intake and neural functioning, for example, evidence has demonstrated that an insufficient protein intake may impair spatial learning and memory and cause brain atrophy [47], while high protein intake decreases markers of oxidative stress (lipid peroxidation) in the brain of rats [48], and is associated with low levels of insoluble amyloid-β protein (Aβ) in older adults [49]. In addition, a systematic review showed that protein intake was positively associated with cognitive function in older adults [50]. Furthermore, increased protein intake may cause changes in the vessel wall structure and in cardiovascular control exerted by the central nervous system, consequently mediating the negative association between protein intake and blood pressure [51,52].

Physical activity levels [33], vitamin intake [31], inflammation [15], mood disorders [53], and the prevalence of chronic conditions (e.g., sarcopenia) [17] may also affect the relationship between protein intake and physical function. In the study by Isanejad et al. [17], for example, higher protein intake and physical function were significantly associated in non-sarcopenic, but not in sarcopenic older women. These inferences are in keeping with the hypothesis that individuals suffering from illness, physical stress, sarcopenia and/or frailty may require higher protein levels (1.2–1.5 g/kg) than healthy older adults [11,12,14]. In the present investigation, a considerable heterogeneity (I^2) was observed in most of the studies. Although we tried to explore heterogeneity among the studies performing the analysis with random effects, the investigations did not offer sufficient details about the samples, as indicated in the quality assessment and food intake limiting the analysis of subgroups and meta-regression (see Table 2). Therefore, our results should be taken with caution and should be confirmed with further studies.

In this context, future studies aimed at investigating the association of protein intake and physical function should collect a number of data allowing better inferences and an inclusion in future systematic reviews and meta-analysis, including total and appendicular muscle mass, the prevalence of morbidities, frailty and sarcopenia assessment, physical activity levels, and an extensive report on food consumption (e.g., amino acid content, protein source) and not just the consumption of macronutrients. Other limitations of the present study include the lack of comparison between low and middle protein intake, as well as very high and middle protein intake (due to the lack of available data), and the use of the mean protein intake to identify the groups.

In relation to the latter, we allocated the groups mentioned in the studies into low, middle, high, and very high according to the mean protein intake reported. Nevertheless, it is possible that some individuals showed higher or lower protein intake levels. One possible way to solve this problem would be that future studies designed the groups based on proposed cut-offs for older adults [11,12,14], instead of separatrix measures (e.g., quartiles), since a low quartile does not necessarily represent a low protein intake.

5. Conclusions

In conclusion, findings of the present study indicate that a very high ($\geq$1.2 g/kg/day) and high protein intake ($\geq$1.0 g/kg/day) are associated with better lower-limb physical performance when compared to low protein (<0.80 g/kg/day) intake in community-dwelling older adults. These findings add evidence regarding the potential need to increase protein guidelines to above the current recommendations. However, large randomized clinical trials are needed to confirm the addictive effects of high-protein diets ($\geq$1.0 g/kg/day) in comparison to the current recommendations on physical functioning.

Supplementary Materials: The following are available online at http://www.mdpi.com/2072-6643/10/9/1330/s1, List S1: The complete search strategy used for the PubMed. Table S1: Quality assessment analysis, Table S2: Individual quality assessment analysis of each included study.

Author Contributions: Conceptualization, H.J.C.-J., B.R., E.M. and M.U.; Methodology, H.J.C.-J., M.U., B.R. and L.M.-T; Analysis, H.J.C.-J.; Writing-Original Draft Preparation, H.J.C.-J., L.M.-T., B.R., R.B., E.M. and M.U.; Writing-Review & Editing, H.J.C.-J., L.M.-T., B.R., R.B., E.M. and M.U.; Supervision, M.U.; Project Administration, H.J.C.-J.

Funding: This research received no external funding.

Acknowledgments: The authors are grateful to the Coordenação de Aperfeiçoamento de Pessoal de Nível Superior (CAPES) for funding this research via scholarships to HJCJ (PhD visiting: 88881.190185/2018-01). BR had financial support from the Fundação de Amparo à Pesquisa do Estado de São Paulo (FAPESP) and CNPq (BPQ).

Conflicts of Interest: The authors declare no conflict of interest.

References

1. Cruz-Jentoft, A.J.; Baeyens, J.P.; Bauer, J.M.; Boirie, Y.; Cederholm, T.; Landi, F.; Martin, F.C.; Michel, J.-P.; Rolland, Y.; Schneider, S.M.; et al. Sarcopenia: European consensus on definition and diagnosis: Report of the European working group on sarcopenia in older people. *Age Ageing* **2010**, *39*, 412–423. [CrossRef] [PubMed]
2. Diz, J.B.M.; Leopoldino, A.A.O.; Moreira, B.D.S.; Henschke, N.; Dias, R.C.; Pereira, L.S.M.; Oliveira, V.C. Prevalence of sarcopenia in older Brazilians: A systematic review and meta-analysis. *Geriatr. Gerontol. Int.* **2017**, *17*, 5–16. [CrossRef] [PubMed]
3. Coelho Júnior, H.J.; Aguiar, S.D.S.; Gonçalves, I.D.O.; Sampaio, R.A.C.; Uchida, M.C.; Moraes, M.R.; Asano, R.Y. Sarcopenia is associated with high pulse pressure in older women. *J. Aging Res.* **2015**, *2015*. [CrossRef] [PubMed]
4. Kim, J.H.; Lim, S.; Choi, S.H.; Kim, K.M.; Yoon, J.W.; Kim, K.W.; Lim, J.-Y.; Park, K.S.; Jang, H.C.; Kritchevsky, S. Sarcopenia: An independent predictor of mortality in community-dwelling older Korean men. *J. Gerontol. Ser. A* **2014**, *69*, 1244–1252. [CrossRef] [PubMed]
5. Brown, J.C.; Harhay, M.O.; Harhay, M.N. Sarcopenia and mortality among a population-based sample of community-dwelling older adults. *J. Cachexia. Sarcopenia Muscle* **2016**, *7*, 290–298. [CrossRef] [PubMed]
6. Benjumea, A.-M.; Curcio, C.-L.; Duque, G.; Gómez, F. Dynapenia and sarcopenia as a risk factor for disability in a falls and fractures clinic in older persons. *Open Access Maced. J. Med. Sci.* **2018**, *6*, 344–349. [CrossRef] [PubMed]
7. Martone, A.M.; Marzetti, E.; Calvani, R.; Picca, A.; Tosato, M.; Santoro, L.; Di Giorgio, A.; Nesci, A.; Sisto, A.; Santoliquido, A.; et al. Exercise and protein intake: A synergistic approach against sarcopenia. *BioMed Res. Int.* **2017**, *2017*. [CrossRef] [PubMed]
8. Marzetti, E.; Calvani, R.; Tosato, M.; Cesari, M.; Di Bari, M.; Cherubini, A.; Collamati, A.; D'Angelo, E.; Pahor, M.; Bernabei, R.; et al. SPRINTT consortium sarcopenia: An overview. *Aging Clin. Exp. Res.* **2017**, *29*, 11–17. [CrossRef] [PubMed]
9. Nutrient Reference Values. Available online: https://www.nrv.gov.au/nutrients/protein (accessed on 26 August 2018).
10. Protein—British Nutrition Foundation. Available online: https://www.nutrition.org.uk/nutritionscience/nutrients-food-and-ingredients/protein.html?start=1 (accessed on 26 August 2018).

11. Volpi, E.; Campbell, W.W.; Dwyer, J.T.; Johnson, M.A.; Jensen, G.L.; Morley, J.E.; Wolfe, R.R. Is the optimal level of protein intake for older adults greater than the recommended dietary allowance? *J. Gerontol. Ser. A Biol. Sci. Med. Sci.* **2013**, *68*, 677–681. [CrossRef] [PubMed]
12. Landi, F.; Calvani, R.; Tosato, M.; Martone, A.M.; Ortolani, E.; Savera, G.; D'Angelo, E.; Sisto, A.; Marzetti, E. Protein intake and muscle health in old age: From biological plausibility to clinical evidence. *Nutrients* **2016**, *8*, 295. [CrossRef] [PubMed]
13. Bauer, J.; Biolo, G.; Cederholm, T.; Cesari, M.; Cruz-Jentoft, A.J.; Morley, J.E.; Phillips, S.; Sieber, C.; Stehle, P.; Teta, D.; et al. Evidence-based recommendations for optimal dietary protein intake in older people: A position paper from the prot-age study group. *J. Am. Med. Dir. Assoc.* **2013**, *14*, 542–559. [CrossRef] [PubMed]
14. Calvani, R.; Miccheli, A.; Landi, F.; Bossola, M.; Cesari, M.; Leeuwenburgh, C.; Sieber, C.C.; Bernabei, R.; Marzetti, E. Current nutritional recommendations and novel dietary strategies to manage sarcopenia. *J. Frailty Aging* **2013**, *2*, 38–53. [PubMed]
15. Bartali, B.; Frongillo, E.A.; Bandinelli, S.; Lauretani, F.; Semba, R.D.; Fried, L.P.; Ferrucci, L. Low nutrient intake is an essential component of frailty in older persons. *J. Gerontol. A. Biol. Sci. Med. Sci.* **2006**, *61*, 589–593. [CrossRef] [PubMed]
16. Lana, A.; Rodriguez-Artalejo, F.; Lopez-Garcia, E. Dairy consumption and risk of frailty in older adults: A prospective cohort study. *J. Am. Geriatr. Soc.* **2015**, *63*, 1852–1860. [CrossRef] [PubMed]
17. Isanejad, M.; Mursu, J.; Sirola, J.; Kröger, H.; Rikkonen, T.; Tuppurainen, M.; Erkkilä, A.T. Dietary protein intake is associated with better physical function and muscle strength among elderly women. *Br. J. Nutr.* **2016**, *115*, 1281–1291. [CrossRef] [PubMed]
18. Houston, D.K.; Schwartz, A.V.; Cauley, J.A.; Tylavsky, F.A.; Simonsick, E.M.; Harris, T.B.; De Rekeneire, N.; Schwartz, G.G.; Kritchevsky, S.B. Serum parathyroid hormone levels predict falls in older adults with diabetes mellitus. *J. Am. Geriatr. Soc.* **2008**, *56*, 2027–2032. [CrossRef] [PubMed]
19. Farsijani, S.; Payette, H.; Morais, J.A.; Shatenstein, B.; Gaudreau, P.; Chevalier, S. Even mealtime distribution of protein intake is associated with greater muscle strength, but not with 3-y physical function decline, in free-living older adults: The quebec longitudinal study on nutrition as a determinant of successful aging (NuAge study). *Am. J. Clin. Nutr.* **2017**, *106*, 113–124. [CrossRef] [PubMed]
20. Gregorio, L.; Brindisi, J.; Kleppinger, A.; Sullivan, R.; Mangano, K.M.; Bihuniak, J.D.; Kenny, A.M.; Kerstetter, J.E.; Insogna, K.L. Adequate dietary protein is associated with better physical performance among post-menopausal women 60–90 years. *J. Nutr. Health Aging* **2014**, *18*, 155–160. [CrossRef] [PubMed]
21. Verlaan, S.; Aspray, T.J.; Bauer, J.M.; Cederholm, T.; Hemsworth, J.; Hill, T.R.; McPhee, J.S.; Piasecki, M.; Seal, C.; Sieber, C.C.; et al. Nutritional status, body composition, and quality of life in community-dwelling sarcopenic and non-sarcopenic older adults: A case-control study. *Clin. Nutr.* **2017**, *36*, 267–274. [CrossRef] [PubMed]
22. Liberati, A.; Altman, D.G.; Tetzlaff, J.; Mulrow, C.; Gøtzsche, P.C.; Ioannidis, J.P.A.; Clarke, M.; Devereaux, P.J.; Kleijnen, J.; Moher, D. The PRISMA statement for reporting systematic reviews and meta-analyses of studies that evaluate health care interventions: Explanation and elaboration. *PLoS Med.* **2009**, *6*, e1000100. [CrossRef] [PubMed]
23. Stroup, D.F.; Berlin, J.A.; Morton, S.C.; Olkin, I.; Williamson, G.D.; Rennie, D.; Moher, D.; Becker, B.J.; Sipe, T.A.; Thacker, S.B. Meta-analysis of observational studies in epidemiology: A proposal for reporting. *JAMA* **2000**, *283*, 2008–2012. [CrossRef] [PubMed]
24. Houston, D.K.; Nicklas, B.J.; Ding, J.; Harris, T.B.; Tylavsky, F.A.; Newman, A.B.; Lee, J.S.; Sahyoun, N.R.; Visser, M.; Kritchevsky, S.B. Health ABC study dietary protein intake is associated with lean mass change in older, community-dwelling adults: The health, aging, and body composition (Health ABC) study. *Am. J. Clin. Nutr.* **2008**, *87*, 150–155. [CrossRef] [PubMed]
25. Beasley, J.M.; Lacroix, A.Z.; Neuhouser, M.L.; Huang, Y.; Tinker, L.; Woods, N.; Michael, Y.; Curb, J.D.; Prentice, R.L. Protein intake and incident frailty in the women's health initiative observational study. *J. Am. Geriatr. Soc.* **2010**, *58*, 1063–1071. [CrossRef] [PubMed]
26. Vellas, B.J.; Hunt, W.C.; Romero, L.J.; Koehler, K.M.; Baumgartner, R.N.; Garry, P.J. Changes in nutritional status and patterns of morbidity among free-living elderly persons: A 10-year longitudinal study. *Nutrition* **1997**, *13*, 515–519. [CrossRef]

27. Mustafa, J.; Ellison, R.C.; Singer, M.R.; Bradlee, M.L.; Kalesan, B.; Holick, M.F.; Moore, L.L. Dietary protein and preservation of physical functioning among middle-aged and older adults in the framingham offspring study. *Am. J. Epidemiol.* **2018**, *187*, 1411–1419. [CrossRef] [PubMed]
28. Von Elm, E.; Altman, D.G.; Egger, M.; Pocock, S.J.; Gøtzsche, P.C.; Vandenbroucke, J.P.; STROBE Initiative. The strengthening the reporting of observational studies in epidemiology (STROBE) statement: Guidelines for reporting observational studies. *Lancet* **2007**, *370*, 1453–1457. [CrossRef]
29. Green, S.; Higgins, J. *Cochrane Handbook for Systematic Reviews of Interventions*; The Cochrane Collaboratrion: London, UK, 2005.
30. Chan, R.; Leung, J.; Woo, J. Dietary patterns and risk of frailty in Chinese community-dwelling older people in Hong Kong: A prospective cohort study. *Nutrients* **2015**, *7*, 7070–7084. [CrossRef] [PubMed]
31. Larocque, S.C.; Kerstetter, J.E.; Cauley, J.A.; Insogna, K.L.; Ensrud, K.; Lui, L.-Y.; Allore, H.G. Dietary protein and vitamin D intake and risk of falls: A secondary analysis of postmenopausal women from the study of osteoporotic fractures. *J. Nutr. Gerontol. Geriatr.* **2015**, *34*, 305–318. [CrossRef] [PubMed]
32. Rahi, B.; Morais, J.A.; Gaudreau, P.; Payette, H.; Shatenstein, B. Energy and protein intakes and their association with a decline in functional capacity among diabetic older adults from the NuAge cohort. *Eur. J. Nutr.* **2016**, *55*, 1729–1739. [CrossRef] [PubMed]
33. Ten Haaf, D.; van Dongen, E.; Nuijten, M.; Eijsvogels, T.; de Groot, L.; Hopman, M. Protein intake and distribution in relation to physical functioning and quality of life in community-dwelling elderly people: acknowledging the role of physical activity. *Nutrients* **2018**, *10*, 506. [CrossRef] [PubMed]
34. Chan, R.; Leung, J.; Woo, J.; Kwok, T. Associations of dietary protein intake on subsequent decline in muscle mass and physical functions over four years in ambulant older Chinese people. *J. Nutr. Health Aging* **2014**, *18*, 171–177. [CrossRef] [PubMed]
35. Landi, F.; Calvani, R.; Cesari, M.; Tosato, M.; Martone, A.M.; Ortolani, E.; Savera, G.; Salini, S.; Sisto, A.; Picca, A.; et al. Sarcopenia: An overview on current definitions, diagnosis and treatment. *Curr. Protein Pept. Sci.* **2018**, *19*, 633–638. [CrossRef] [PubMed]
36. Katsanos, C.S.; Kobayashi, H.; Sheffield-Moore, M.; Aarsland, A.; Wolfe, R.R. Aging is associated with diminished accretion of muscle proteins after the ingestion of a small bolus of essential amino acids. *Am. J. Clin. Nutr.* **2005**, *82*, 1065–1073. [CrossRef] [PubMed]
37. Katsanos, C.S.; Kobayashi, H.; Sheffield-Moore, M.; Aarsland, A.; Wolfe, R.R. A high proportion of leucine is required for optimal stimulation of the rate of muscle protein synthesis by essential amino acids in the elderly. *Am. J. Physiol. Metab.* **2006**, *291*, E381–E387. [CrossRef] [PubMed]
38. Campbell, W.W.; Trappe, T.A.; Wolfe, R.R.; Evans, W.J. The recommended dietary allowance for protein may not be adequate for older people to maintain skeletal muscle. *J. Gerontol. A. Biol. Sci. Med. Sci.* **2001**, *56*, M373–M380. [CrossRef] [PubMed]
39. Martin, W.F.; Armstrong, L.E.; Rodriguez, N.R. Dietary protein intake and renal function. *Nutr. Metab.* **2005**, *2*, 25. [CrossRef] [PubMed]
40. Hamacher, D.; Herold, F.; Wiegel, P.; Hamacher, D.; Schega, L. Brain activity during walking: A systematic review. *Neurosci. Biobehav. Rev.* **2015**, *57*, 310–327. [CrossRef] [PubMed]
41. Paraskevoudi, N.; Balcı, F.; Vatakis, A. "Walking" through the sensory, cognitive, and temporal degradations of healthy aging. *Ann. N. Y. Acad. Sci.* **2018**. [CrossRef] [PubMed]
42. El Khoudary, S.R.; Chen, H.-Y.; Barinas-Mitchell, E.; McClure, C.; Selzer, F.; Karvonen-Gutierrez, C.; Jackson, E.A.; Ylitalo, K.R.; Sternfeld, B. Simple physical performance measures and vascular health in late midlife women: The study of women's health across the nation. *Int. J. Cardiol.* **2015**, *182*, 115–120. [CrossRef] [PubMed]
43. Su, N.; Zhai, F.-F.; Zhou, L.-X.; Ni, J.; Yao, M.; Li, M.-L.; Jin, Z.-Y.; Gong, G.-L.; Zhang, S.-Y.; Cui, L.-Y.; et al. Cerebral small vessel disease burden is associated with motor performance of lower and upper extremities in community-dwelling populations. *Front. Aging Neurosci.* **2017**, *9*, 313. [CrossRef] [PubMed]
44. Nolan, C.M.; Maddocks, M.; Maher, T.M.; Canavan, J.L.; Jones, S.E.; Barker, R.E.; Patel, S.; Jacob, J.; Cullinan, P.; Man, W.D.-C. Phenotypic characteristics associated with slow gait speed in idiopathic pulmonary fibrosis. *Respirology* **2018**, *23*, 498–506. [CrossRef] [PubMed]
45. Vandervoort, A.A. Aging of the human neuromuscular system. *Muscle Nerve* **2002**, *25*, 17–25. [CrossRef] [PubMed]

46. Rosso, A.L.; Sanders, J.L.; Arnold, A.M.; Boudreau, R.M.; Hirsch, C.H.; Carlson, M.C.; Rosano, C.; Kritchevsky, S.B.; Newman, A.B. Multisystem physiologic impairments and changes in gait speed of older adults. *J. Gerontol. Ser. A Biol. Sci. Med. Sci.* **2015**, *70*, 319–324. [CrossRef] [PubMed]
47. Reyes-Castro, L.A.; Padilla-Gómez, E.; Parga-Martínez, N.J.; Castro-Rodríguez, D.C.; Quirarte, G.L.; Díaz-Cintra, S.; Nathanielsz, P.W.; Zambrano, E. Hippocampal mechanisms in impaired spatial learning and memory in male offspring of rats fed a low-protein isocaloric diet in pregnancy and/or lactation. *Hippocampus* **2018**, *28*, 18–30. [CrossRef] [PubMed]
48. Madani, Z.; Malaisse, W.J.; Ait-Yahia, D. A comparison between the impact of two types of dietary protein on brain glucose concentrations and oxidative stress in high fructose-induced metabolic syndrome rats. *Biomed. Rep.* **2015**, *3*, 731–735. [CrossRef] [PubMed]
49. Fernando, W.M.A.D.; Rainey-Smith, S.R.; Gardener, S.L.; Villemagne, V.L.; Burnham, S.C.; Macaulay, S.L.; Brown, B.M.; Gupta, V.B.; Sohrabi, H.R.; Weinborn, M.; et al. Associations of dietary protein and fiber intake with brain and blood amyloid-β. *J. Alzheimer's Dis.* **2018**, *61*, 1589–1598. [CrossRef] [PubMed]
50. Koh, F.; Charlton, K.; Walton, K.; McMahon, A.-T. Role of dietary protein and thiamine intakes on cognitive function in healthy older people: A systematic review. *Nutrients* **2015**, *7*, 2415–2439. [CrossRef] [PubMed]
51. Liu, R.; Dang, S.; Yan, H.; Wang, D.; Zhao, Y.; Li, Q.; Liu, X. Association between dietary protein intake and the risk of hypertension: A cross-sectional study from rural western China. *Hypertens. Res.* **2013**, *36*, 972. [CrossRef] [PubMed]
52. Tielemans, S.M.A.J.; Altorf-van der Kuil, W.; Engberink, M.F.; Brink, E.J.; van Baak, M.A.; Bakker, S.J.L.; Geleijnse, J.M. Intake of total protein, plant protein and animal protein in relation to blood pressure: A meta-analysis of observational and intervention studies. *J. Hum. Hypertens.* **2013**, *27*, 564–571. [CrossRef] [PubMed]
53. Guligowska, A.; Pigłowska, M.; Fife, E.; Kostka, J.; Sołtysik, B.K.; Kroc, Ł.; Kostka, T. Inappropriate nutrients intake is associated with lower functional status and inferior quality of life in older adults with depression. *Clin. Interv. Aging* **2016**, *11*, 1505–1517. [CrossRef] [PubMed]

© 2018 by the authors. Licensee MDPI, Basel, Switzerland. This article is an open access article distributed under the terms and conditions of the Creative Commons Attribution (CC BY) license (http://creativecommons.org/licenses/by/4.0/).

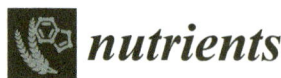 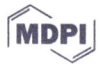

Review

Low Protein Intake Is Associated with Frailty in Older Adults: A Systematic Review and Meta-Analysis of Observational Studies

Hélio José Coelho-Júnior [1,2,*], Bruno Rodrigues [1], Marco Uchida [1] and Emanuele Marzetti [2]

[1] Applied Kinesiology Laboratory–LCA, School of Physical Education, University of Campinas, Av. Érico Veríssimo, 701, Cidade Universitária "Zeferino Vaz", Barão Geraldo, Campinas-SP 13083-851, Brazil; prof.brodrigues@gmail.com (B.R.); uchida@g.unicamp.br (M.U.)
[2] Department of Geriatrics, Neurosciences and Orthopedics, Teaching Hospital "Agostino Gemelli", Catholic University of the Sacred Heart, 00168 Rome, Italy; emarzetti@live.com
* Correspondence: coelhojunior@hotmail.com.br; Tel.: +55-1194-9398-302

Received: 23 July 2018; Accepted: 14 September 2018; Published: 19 September 2018

Abstract: (1) Background: Several factors have been suggested to be associated with the physiopathology of frailty in older adults, and nutrition (especially protein intake) has been attributed fundamental importance in this context. The objective of this study was to conduct a systematic review and meta-analysis to investigate the relationship between protein intake and frailty status in older adults. (2) Methods: A search of scientific studies was conducted in the main databases (Medline, Scopus, Cochrane library), and in the reference lists of selected articles. The search terms included synonyms and Medical Subject Headings and involved the use of Boolean operators which allowed the combination of words and search terms. Observational studies—cross-sectional and longitudinal—that met the eligibility criteria were included in the review. Article selection and data extraction were performed by two independent reviewers. Meta-analyses with random effects were performed. Publication bias was measured using the Strengthening the Reporting of Observational Studies in Epidemiology instrument. (3) Results: In the final sample, 10 articles, seven cross-sectional and three longitudinal, were included in the present study. Overall, studies investigated a total of 50,284 older adults from three different continents between 2006 and 2018. Four cross-sectional studies were included in the meta-analyses. The results demonstrated that a high protein intake was negatively associated with frailty status in older adults (odds ratio: 0.67, confidence interval = 0.56 to 0.82, $p = 0.0001$). (4) Conclusions: Our findings suggest that a high consumption of dietary protein is inversely associated with frailty in older adults.

Keywords: frailty; protein intake; older adults

1. Introduction

The aging process is a continuous phenomenon characterized by alterations in major physiological systems, accompanied by the development of chronic diseases and geriatric syndromes, such as frailty. Frailty may be conceptualized as a multidimensional geriatric clinical state that involves multiple signs and symptoms leading to extreme vulnerability to stressors and resulting in increased risk of negative health-related outcomes (e.g., functional decline, disability, falls, hospitalization, institutionalization, death) [1,2].

Nutrition is acknowledged as a major factor in the context of frailty. In fact, malnutrition is considered one of the pillars for the development of this condition [3], since it can influence all diagnostic criteria for frailty (i.e., unintentional weight loss, low muscle strength, exhaustion, reduced physical activity levels, and slow walking speed) [4]. Three previous systematic reviews have been conducted on the association between nutrition and frailty. Authors observed that several factors might be responsible for this close relationship between frail and nutrition, including oral health, nutritional status, dietary patterns, diet quality, the antioxidant capacity of the diet, micronutrients and macronutrients intake [3,5]. Nevertheless, protein intake might be the main factor behind this relationship, through its actions on muscle mass and strength.

Indeed, human skeletal muscle protein turnover comprises the process of muscle protein synthesis and muscle protein breakdown [6–8]. On one hand, muscle hypertrophy occurs when the rates of protein synthesis exceed protein breakdown, which may be elicited by hyper amino acidemia induced by dietary protein intake; on the other hand, an inadequate protein intake leads to lower protein synthesis rate, resulting in net protein breakdown and muscle catabolism [6–8]. During aging, numerous process collaborate to a reduced protein intake, such as lack of hunger, impaired oral health, and loss of acuity in taste, smell and sight, to quote a few [9]; consequently, collaborating to muscle catabolism [9]. In addition, evidence has demonstrated that the anabolic response to hyper aminoacidemia may be blunted in older adults [10,11], which indicate that this population should consume larger amounts of protein in comparison to young adults in an attempt to maintain muscle protein synthesis. Nevertheless, over time, the lack of adequate protein intake leads to a state called as sarcopenia [9,12,13], which is characterized by marked muscle atrophy, dynapenia, and reduced physical function, all variables encompassed on frailty definition [14]. If there is no immediate intervention to reduce sarcopenia and frailty progression, as well as improve protein intake, the patients will develop a severe physical disability and consequently exhaustion and sedentary behavior [1,15].

It should be stressed that other pathways besides sarcopenia may be also responsible for the association between protein intake and frailty, since evidence has demonstrated that protein intake is associated with dementia, global cognitive scores, visuospatial skill, nonverbal memory, and logical memory in older adults [16–18]; all aspects linked with frailty [1].

However, investigations on the association between protein intake and frailty have shown positive, negative and even null results. In addition, to the best of our knowledge, there is a lack of systematic reviews and meta-analysis dedicated to investigating the relationship between protein intake and frailty in older adults.

Therefore, the present study was conducted to perform a systematic review to identify and compare studies reporting the relationship between frailty status and protein intake in older adults. Additionally, data were combined to calculate the pooled overall relationship between frailty status and protein intake.

2. Materials and Methods

We conducted a systematic review and meta-analysis of observational studies to investigate and quantify the association between protein intake and frailty in older adults. The study was fully performed by investigators and no librarian was part of the team. This study complies with the criteria of the Primary Reporting Items for Systematic Reviews and Meta-analyses (PRISMA) Statement [19] and the Meta-analysis of Observational Studies in Epidemiology (MOOSE) guidelines [20].

2.1. Eligibility Criteria

The inclusion criteria of the present study consisted of: (a) observational studies, including cross-sectional, case-control and longitudinal studies, which investigated as primary or secondary outcome the association of protein intake and frailty in older adults; (b) study sample 60 years or older; (c) frailty defined by a validated scale; (d) reported information on the proportion of frailty among those with high and low levels of protein intake; (e) published studies (English language). To be included in the meta-analysis, in addition to the aforementioned inclusion criteria, the investigations had to provide: (f) at least two groups divided according to protein intake (e.g., high and low), (g) the prevalence of frailty in each group, (h) and the total sample size in each group. We excluded randomized-clinical trials (RCTs), quasi-experimental, cross-over studies and any kind of investigation which examined the effects of a nutritional intervention associated or not with other interventions (e.g., physical exercise) on frailty. Studies that classified the volunteers as frail according to reduced physical/or cognitive function were also excluded.

2.2. Search Strategy and Selection Criteria

Studies published on or before July 2018 were retrieved from the following three electronic databases by one investigator: (1) PubMed, (2) the Cochrane Library, and (3) SCOPUS. Reference lists for reviews and retrieved articles for additional studies were checked and citation searches on key articles were performed on Google Scholar and ResearchGate for additional reports. Initially, a search strategy was designed using keywords, MeSH terms, and free text words such as protein intake, frailty, older adults. Additionally, keywords and subject headings were exhaustively combined using Boolean operators. The complete search strategy used for the PubMed can be shown in List S1. Only eligible full texts in English language were considered for review. Authors were contacted if necessary.

2.3. Data Extraction and Quality Assessment

Titles and abstracts of retrieved articles were screened for eligibility by two researchers. If an abstract did not provide enough information for evaluation, the full-text was retrieved. Disagreements were solved by a third reviewer. Reviewers were not blinded to authors, institutions, or manuscript journals. Data extraction was independently performed by two reviews using a standardized coding form. Disagreements were solved by a third reviewer. Coded variables included methodological quality and the characteristics of the studies. The quality of reporting for each study was performed by two researchers using the Strengthening the Reporting of Observational Studies in Epidemiology (STROBE) instrument [21]. The agreement rate between reviewers was κ = 0.98 for quality assessment.

2.4. Statistical Analysis

The meta-analysis was conducted using Revman V.5. Effect sizes (ESs) were measured using odds ratio (OR) and 95% confidence intervals (CIs). The OR indicates the risk for frailty according to protein intake, high in relation to low. A significant OR is required to have a 95% confidence interval (CI 95%) that did not include the value of 1 and a p value for the test of significance of the total overall effect (Z) lower than 0.05. An inverse variance random-effect model was used to calculate the pooled ES since the studies demonstrated different characteristics regarding the main aspects associated with frailty (e.g., modified frailty criteria), protein intake (e.g., different cut-offs for high and low protein intake definition), and covariates (e.g., energy intake). Funnel plots and Egger's regression analysis were used to evaluate the publication bias. Heterogeneity across studies was tested using the Q-statistics and I^2 index was used to assess inconsistency [22]. Additionally, I^2 index was classified as might not be important (0–40%), may represent moderate heterogeneity (30–60%), may represent substantial heterogeneity (50–90%), and considerable heterogeneity (75–100%) [22]. Forest plots were used to illustrate summary statistics and the variation (heterogeneity) across studies.

3. Results

3.1. Literature Search

Of the 2555 registers recovered from electronic databases and hand search, 2523 records were excluded based on duplicate data, title or abstract. Thirty-two studies were fully reviewed and assessed for eligibility. Finally, 10 studies met the inclusion criteria (Figure 1).

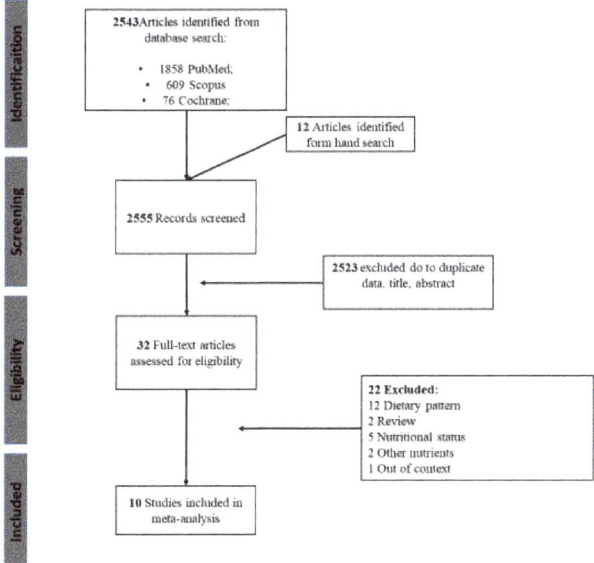

Figure 1. Flow chart of the present study.

3.2. Characteristics of the Included Studies

Table 1 provides a general description of the included studies. Overall, a total of 18,120 community-dwelling older adults from five different countries (France, Germany, Italy, Japan, and the United States of America) were investigated between 2006 and 2018 in the cross-sectional studies. Frailty assessment was performed with two tools. The frailty phenotype proposed by Fried et al. (2001) was used in six of the seven studies [23–28], while one study used the Kihon checklist (KCL) [29]. However, it is important to mention that the frailty phenotype [14] was modified in 5 of the 6 studies. Indeed, weight loss criterion was modified in the studies of Rahi et al. [28] and Shikany et al. [27], while Bartali et al. [23] removed this variable. In turn, in the investigations performed by Kobayashi et al. [24,25], slowness and weakness were indirectly measured based on a questionnaire. Slowness assessment was also modified in the study of Rahi et al. [28]. Dietary intake was primarily assessed by population-specific food-frequency questionnaires (FFQ) (57.1%) [23,26,27], followed by self-administered diet history questionnaires (28.6%) [24,25], and the 24 h dietary recall (14.3%) [28]. High and low protein intake was differently defined in the investigations. Measures of centrality (e.g., tertiles, quartiles, quintiles) were used in 6 of the 7 studies [23–27], while Rahi et al. [28] performed the analysis based on a pre-established cut-off (i.e., protein intake levels ≥ 1 g/kg of body weight). Regarding longitudinal studies, 32,164 community-dwelling older adults were investigated between 2010 and 2016. The studies were conducted in North America (United States of America) and Europe (Spain). The mean duration of follow-up was 3.7 years (3.0–4.6 years). The frailty phenotype was used in all studies for frailty assessment. However, as was observed in cross-sectional studies, the frailty phenotype was modified in 2 of the 3 longitudinal studies. Shikany et al. [27] considered the loss of appendicular lean mass as a measurement of weight loss. In turn, Beasley et al. [30] used a modified version of frailty phenotype as they measured muscle weakness and slowness using the Rand-36 Physical function scale. FFQ (66.6%) and computerized face-to-face diet history (33.3%) were used for a dietary intake assessment. In longitudinal studies, all investigations used measures of centrality (i.e., quartile and quintile) to determine the levels of protein intake.

Table 1. General description of the included studies.

Year	Authors	Country	Study Design	Setting	n	Mean Age (age range; min–max)	Sex Ratio of Participants (female/male) by frail vs. non-frail	Frailty Assessment Method	Dietary Intake Assessment Method	Protein Intake (g/day)	Protein Intake Level Definition	Outcomes	Covariates Included in Models	Quality Analysis Score
Cross-sectional														
2006	Bartali et al. [23]	Italy	Cross-sectional	Community-dwelling	802	74.1	1.2	CHS frailty index (a)	Food-frequency questionnaire	-	Dichotomous	Low protein intake is associated with frailty	Results were adjusted for age, sex, education, economic status, household composition, smoking status, number of diseases, cognitive function, body mass index, and "happiness."	22
2013	Kobayashi et al. [24]	Japan	Cross-sectional	Community-dwelling	2108	74.7	-	CHS frailty index (b)	Self-administered diet history questionnaire	74.0	Quintile (≤62.9 g/day, 63–69.8 g/day, 69.8–76.1 g/day, 76.1–84.3 g/day, ≥84.3 g/day)	Protein intake was inversely associated with frailty	Results were energy-adjusted and for age, BMI, residential block, size of residential area, living alone, current smoking, alcohol drinking, dietary supplement use, history of chronic disease, depression symptoms, and energy intake.	20
2013	Bollwein et al. [26]	Germany	Cross-sectional	Community-dwelling	194	83.0 (75–96)	6.5 vs. 1.3	CHS frailty index	Food-frequency questionnaire	76.6	Quartiles (≤0.90, 0.91–1.07, 1.08, ≥1.27)	Protein intake was not associated with frailty	Results were adjusted for age and sex, instrumental activities of the daily living score, number of medications, and chewing difficulties	19
2014	Shikany et al. [27]	United States of America	Cross-sectional	Community-dwelling	5925	75.0	-	CHS frailty index (c)	Food-frequency questionnaire	-	Quintile (≤6.0–13.7%, 13.8–15.2%, 15.3–16.5%, 16.6%–18.3%, 18.4–29.3%)	Protein intake was not associated with frailty	Results were adjusted for age, race, center, education, marital status, smoking, health status, medical conditions, body mass index, and energy intake	20
2016	Rahi et al. [28]	France	Cross-sectional	Community-dwelling	1345	75.6	4.0 vs. 1.46	CHS frailty index (d)	24 h dietary recall	70.4	Dichotomous <1g/kg body weight/day and ≥1g/kg body weight	Protein intake was associated with frailty	The model 1 was adjusted for age, sex, and educational level, and the model 2 was additionally adjusted for BMI, diabetes, cardiovascular history, depression, cognitive performance, number of drugs, and total energy intake.	20
2017	Kobayashi et al. [25]	Japan	Cross-sectional	Community-dwelling	2108	74.0	-	CHS frailty index (b)	Self-administered diet history questionnaire	73.1	Tertile (≤67.6 g/day, 67.6–78.3 g/day, ≥78.3 g/day)	Protein intake was inversely associated with frailty	Dietary total antioxidant capacity	20
2018	Nanri et al. [29]	Japan	Cross-sectional	Community-dwelling	5638	73.2	0.88 vs. 1.05 *	KCL	Food-frequency questionnaire	-	Men = quartiles (≤48.8 g/day, 48.8–56.1 g/day, 56.1–65.4 g/day, >65.4 g/day); Women = quartiles (<43.8 g/day, 43.8–51.1 g/day, 51.1–59.5 g/day, >59.5 g/day)	Protein intake was inversely associated with frailty	For men, the model 1 was adjusted for age, body mass index, total energy intake, alcohol status, smoking status and history of disease and the model 2 was adjusted for family structure, educational attainment, population density, and self-related health.	20

Table 1. Cont.

Year	Authors	Country	Study Design	Setting	n	Mean Age (age range; min–max)	Sex Ratio of Participants (female/male) by frail vs. non-frail	Frailty Assessment Method	Dietary Intake Assessment Method	Protein Intake (g/day)	Protein Intake Level Definition	Outcomes	Covariates Included in Models	Quality Analysis Score
Longitudinal														
2010	Beasley et al. [8]	United States of America	Longitudinal (3.0 years follow-up)	Community-dwelling	24,417	65–79	-	CHS frailty index (e)	Food-frequency questionnaire	72.8	Quintiles of protein intake (% kilocalories)	Protein intake was significantly associated with the odds of becoming frail	Results were adjusted for age, ethnicity, BMI, income, education, having a current health care provider, smoking, alcohol, general health status, history of comorbid conditions, history of hormone therapy use, number of falls, whether participant lives alone, disabled defined by at least 1 activity of daily living affected, depressive symptoms, log-transformed calibrated energy intake	20
2014	Shikany et al. [27]	United States of America	Longitudinal (4.6 years follow-up)	Community-dwelling	5925	75.0	-	CHS frailty index (c)	Food-frequency questionnaire	-	Quintile (≤ 6.0–13.7%, 13.8–15.2%, 15.3–16.5%, 16.6–18.3%, 18.4–29.3%)	Protein intake was not associated with the odds of becoming frail	Results were adjusted for age, race, center, education, marital status, smoking, health status, medical conditions, body mass index, and energy intake	20
2016	Sandoval-Insausti et al. [33]	Spain	Longitudinal (3.5 years follow-up)	Community-dwelling	1822	68.7	0.9 vs. 2.4	CHS frailty index	Computerized face-to-face diet history	76.6	Quartiles of protein intake	Protein intake was associated with the odds of becoming frail	Results were adjusted for age, energy intake, ethanol, lipids, animal or vegetal protein, level of education, marital status, tobacco consumption, BMI, abdominal obesity, and dietary fiber, diseases.	20

CHS = Cardiovascular Health Study; KCL = Kihon checklist; bw/d = body weight/day; BMI= Body mass index; (a) Bartali et al. used a modified version of the CHS frailty index, since weight loss was removed; (b) Kobayashi et al. used the CHS frailty index version modified by Woods et al as they did not have direct measures of gait speed and strength; (c) Shikany et al., used a modified version of the CHS frailty index as they measured weight loss criterion based on loss of appendicular lean mass; (d) Rahi et al., used a modified version of the CHS frailty index as a loss of 3 kg and a reduced BMI (<21 kg/m^2) were both accepted as measures of weight loss criterion, slowness was determined based on the Rosow-Breslau test, and weakness was identified using the chair standing method (e) Beasley et al., used a modified version of the CHS frailty index as they measured muscle weakness and slow walking speed using the Rand-36 Physical function scale; * frail vs non-frail.

3.3. Quality Assessment

The overall score of the quality assessment of cross-sectional and longitudinal studies is shown in Table 1 and the analysis of each variable is detailed in Tables S1 and S2, respectively. The point by point analysis is shown in Table S3. The overall score of cross-sectional studies ranged from 19 to 22. All studies reported the items required by the STROBE criteria in relation to the abstract (items 1 and 2), objectives and hypothesis (items 3 and 4), described the settings, locations, relevant dates, eligibility criteria and the source and methods of selection of participants (items 5 and 6), clarity of the outcomes (items 7), methods of assessment (item 8), handle of the quantitative variables (item 11), give the characteristics of study participants (item 14), reported the number of outcome events (item 15), statistical methods and analysis (items 12, 16, 17), and discussion (items 18–21). However, 57.1% of the studies failed to clearly report the efforts performed to address potential sources of bias (item 9) [24,26–28], 42.9% did not properly explain how the study size arrived at (item 10) [26–28], and 14.3% did not show the number of individuals at each stage of study (item 13) [26].

Similar results were seen in longitudinal studies, in which all investigations received a STROBE score of 20. None of the studies adequately presented a description of how the study was arrived at (item 10), while 66.6% failed to describe any efforts to address potential sources of bias (item 9) [27,31], and 33.3% did not show the number of individuals at each stage of study (item 13) [30].

3.4. Association between Protein Intake and Frailty

3.4.1. Protein Intake and Frailty Prevalence (i.e., Cross-Sectional Studies)

A total of four studies provided information regarding different intakes of protein in at least two groups, the prevalence of frailty in each group, and the total sample size in each group; therefore, they were added in the meta-analysis (Figure 2). Two aspects should be mentioned before the presentation of data. First of all, Nanri et al. [29] provided the data according to gender, and the results are presented accordingly. In turn, the investigations performed by Kobayashi et al. [24,25] used the same database (i.e., Three-generation Study of Women on Diets and Health), so that the studies were not analyzed in combination. The overall meta-analysis results showed a 0.67 OR (Figure 2a) and a 0.66 OR (Figure 2b) for frailty (95% CI = 0.56 to 0.82, p = 0.0001; 95% CI = 0.54 to 0.80, p = 0.0001) in older adults with high protein intake compared with low protein intake according to the inclusion of Kobayashi et al. [24] or Kobayashi et al. [25], respectively. When the study of Kobayashi et al. [25] was not in the analysis, it was possible to observe an I^2 lower than 40% accompanied by a p = 0.18, indicating that this heterogeneity might not be important [22]. However, when the study of Kobayashi et al. [24] was removed, the I^2 increased to 49% and p value was of 0.12, which can indicate a moderate heterogeneity [22].

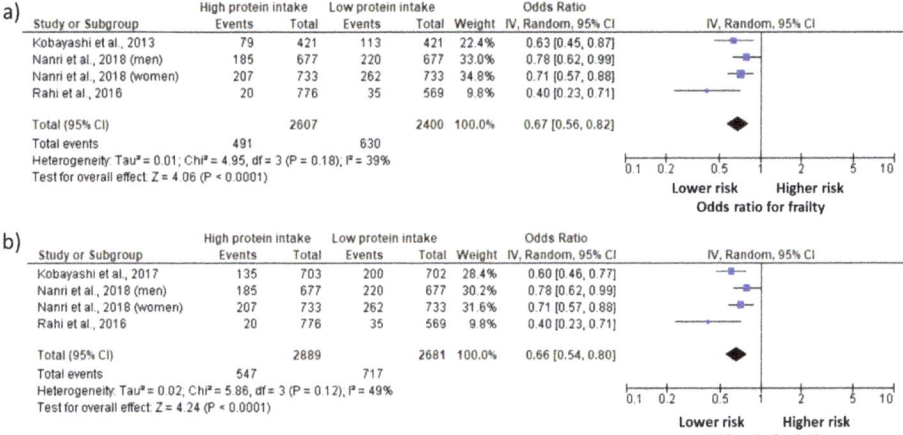

Figure 2. Odds ratio (OR) of the prevalence of frailty in older adults with high and low protein intake. Squares represent study-specific estimates; diamonds represent pooled estimates of random-effects meta-analyses. (**a**) The analysis was performed included Kobayashi et al. 2013; (**b**) The analysis was performed included Kobayashi et al. 2017.

Figure 3 shows the funnel plots (a) and (b) based on the primary outcome according to the inclusion of Kobayashi et al. [24] or Kobayashi et al. [25], respectively. The figures are asymmetrical indicating that potential publication bias might influence the results of this review. Egger's linear regression test indicated possible publication bias for the association when the study of Kobayashi et al. [24] was included ($p = 0.02$), but not Kobayashi et al. [25] ($p = 0.09$).

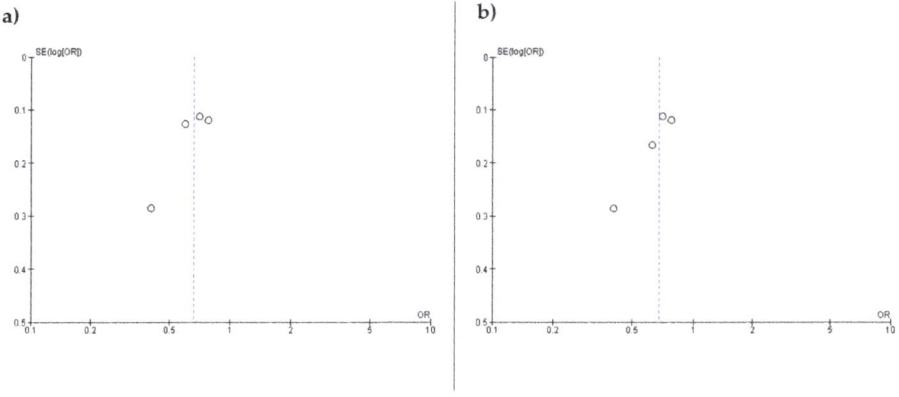

Figure 3. Funnel plots including (**a**) Kobayashi et al. 2013 and (**b**) Kobayashi et al. 2017 OR.

3.4.2. Protein Intake and Frailty Risk (i.e., Longitudinal Studies)

We found three studies that evaluated the longitudinal relationship between protein intake and frailty risk. The findings demonstrate that two of the three studies observed that higher protein intake was negatively associated with frailty risk.

4. Discussion

Frailty is a multifactorial condition associated with poor prognosis. Low protein intake has been proposed among the factors possibly involved in the pathogenesis of frailty. We, therefore, performed a systematic review and meta-analysis to investigate the relationship between protein intake and frailty in older adults. The main findings of the present study indicate that low protein intake is associated with frailty prevalence in older adults.

Study quality assessment demonstrated that reports were of very good quality, such that cross-sectional studies scored between 19 and 22 and all longitudinal studies scored 20. Interestingly, cross-sectional and longitudinal studies did not provide the same items, including efforts to address potential sources of bias (item 9), the design of the study size (item 10), and the report regarding the number of participants in all the phases of the study (item 13).

Some recent systematic and descriptive reviews have investigated the relationship between nutrition and frailty [3,4,32,33]. However, none of these studies was specifically designed to investigate the role of protein intake in this phenomenon and the findings were not quantitatively assessed. Thus, to the best of our knowledge, this is the first systematic review and meta-analysis designed to investigate the relationship between protein intake and frailty in older adults.

The results of the present study may be at least partially explained by the theoretical overlap between sarcopenia and physical frailty [34,35]. Indeed, physical frailty, as measured by the Fried's criteria [14,36], encompasses features as slowness, weakness, exhaustion, and sedentary behavior, which are strongly associated with the sarcopenia condition [34,35]. Slowness (i.e., slow walking speed) and weakness (i.e., low upper-limb muscle strength), for example, are proposed as diagnostic criteria for sarcopenia by the European Working Group on Sarcopenia in Older Persons (EWGSOP) [15], while exhaustion and sedentary behavior are common consequences of sarcopenia progression [37]. Indeed, Landi et al. [35] suggested that sarcopenia may be envisioned as a central mechanism for the development of physical frailty. In another word, physical frailty may be the final pathway of sarcopenia progression [35]. This idea is further supported by the higher prevalence of sarcopenia in pre-frail and frail older adults when compared to non-frail peers [38,39].

Sufficient protein consumption may cause a shifting on net balance in favor of muscle protein synthesis [7,40]. Protein supplementation *per se* has been shown to prevent the progression of physical decline in frail older adults [30,41]. In addition, protein intake has a key role in the physiological adaptations elicited by the resistance training on the neuromuscular apparatus since a greater muscle protein synthesis is expected when both non-pharmacological therapies are offered in combination [6,7]. Taken together, these findings suggest that sufficient protein intake may reverse or at least prevent functional decline in frail older adults.

However, this kind of inference deserves caution since not all evidence has demonstrated the positive effects of protein supplementation on the sarcopenia aspects associated with frailty, such as muscle mass, muscle strength and physical function [42,43]. Finally, it should be noted that the changes observed after protein supplementation may be different from those observed in response to dietary protein intake.

It is worth mentioning, that our main findings are based on cross-sectional studies and causal extrapolations should be performed carefully. Unfortunately, there were no available data from longitudinal studies to perform a meta-analysis. Overall, findings are still controversial. Shikany et al. [27] observed that protein intake was inversely associated with the risk of transitioning from robust to pre-frail status in a range of 4.6 years, while there were no significant associations between protein and frailty status. However, Sandoval-Insausti et al. [31] reported that total protein and animal protein intake were inversely associated with frailty and its components (i.e., slowness) over a mean follow-up of 3.5 years. Similarly, Beasley et al. [30] concluded that higher protein intake was associated with reduced risk of frailty in community-dwelling older women.

Interestingly, the main variables investigated in the present study were differently defined across the investigations. Regarding frailty, although this variable was assessed using the frailty phenotype in most investigations, adaptations of some of the criteria were observed in 5 of the 6 cross-sectional studies, as well as in 2 of the 3 longitudinal studies. In fact, weight loss criterion was modified in the trial of Rahi et al. [28], in which researchers included volunteers with self-reported unintentional loss > 3 kg or as a body mass index < 21 kg/m^2, while Shikany et al. [27] included subjects who lost appendicular muscle mass. In turn, Bartali et al. [23] removed the weight loss criterion of their investigation. Slowness and weakness were also modified. In this case, Kobayashi et al. [24,25], Beasley et al. [30], and Rahi et al. [28] (only slowness) used self-reported questionnaires instead of direct evaluations. It is also possible to observe that different cutoffs to define high a low protein intake (i.e., tertiles, quartiles, quintiles and pre-established values) were used in the investigations.

These modifications have direct implications in the findings of the present study. Although scales and questionnaires may offer more information in a shorter period when compared to performance-based measurements, evidence has demonstrated the limited capacity of these tools to reflect different measures of physical status [44,45]. This probably occurs because the results of patient-reported questionnaires may be biased due to mood, motivation, fatigue, health status, fluctuations in memory, and the specific knowledge and familiarity with the questionnaires and scales [44,45]. In this sense, different results than those observed in the present study could occur if the investigations were performance based on direct measures, as proposed by Fried et al. [14]. Furthermore, the use of different cut-offs to define protein intake levels leads to disagreements and restrict the proposal of public health recommendations to older adults due to the range of approaches used by the studies.

Taken together, these differences may also explain the heterogeneity of results observed among the longitudinal studies. Nevertheless, different settings, eligibility criteria, gender, sarcopenia status, dietary assessment methods, and follow-up periods of the various studies may also explain this variability. In this sense, more well-controlled cross-sectional and longitudinal studies are still necessary to improve the actual knowledge about frailty and protein intake in older adults, as well as to confirm our findings.

We should state the absence of subgroup analyses as the major limitation of the present study. Indeed, the use of crude OR limits interpretation of our meta-analysis, since the influence of important covariates (e.g., age, type of protein [animal, vegetal], sarcopenia) were not taken into consideration in the results, and we recommend that readers interpret our results carefully. The main aspect that prevented us to perform the analysis was the lack of available data in the included studies. Regarding dietary assessment, it is worth mentioning that total protein intake, which was used in all studies for comparisons, is probably not the best parameter to represent adequate protein consumption, since investigations in the context of physical function and sarcopenia have used relative protein intake (g/kg/day) [46–48]. In addition, recent evidence has demonstrated that a spread distribution of protein intake during the main meals is better associated with gait speed than relative protein intake [49]. Providing support to the importance of the distribution of protein intake, Loenneke et al. [50] observed that a frequent consumption of meals containing at least 30 g of protein was associated with greater lean mass and lower-limb muscle strength in middle-aged and older adults. The role of animal and plant-based protein sources on variables associated with frailty has also been the object of discussion among researchers [51,52]. Therefore, although future investigations are still necessary to confirm our findings, the present study may serve as a guide for future studies in this field; so that investigation should include more information regarding the factors that may interfere in the relationship between protein intake and frailty, taking into account the variables that have been investigated by other studies.

In addition, funnel plots and Egger's linear regression test indicated that biases from publications and other factors may have had a significant influence on the results of our meta-analysis mainly when the study of Kobayashi et al. [24] was included. Possible explanations for this publication bias included the small number of studies investigated, multiple publication bias, and heterogeneity [22].

Finally, another aspect of the present study that deserves concerns is the use of STROBE instrument as a tool to quality assessment. As discussed by da Costa et al. [53], STROBE was primarily developed to improve the reporting of observational studies. Thus, some may argue that another tool should have been used in the present study. However, it should be stressed that there is no gold standard tool to assess the risk of bias in non-randomized studies, as well as some of the STROBE questions may represent an evaluation of risk of bias; consequently, making it a tool commonly used in systematic reviews and meta-analysis [53].

In conclusion, our findings support the need for increased protein intake in older adults in an attempt to avoid frailty development.

Supplementary Materials: The following are available online at http://www.mdpi.com/2072-6643/10/9/1334/s1, List S1. The complete search strategy used for the PubMed, Table S1. Quality assessment of cross-sectional studies, Table S2. Quality assessment of longitudinal studies, Table S3 Point by point analysis.

Author Contributions: H.J.C.-J., B.R., E.M., and M.U.; Methodology, H.J.C.-J, B.R, E.M. and M.U.; Analysis, H.J.C.-J.; Writing-Original Draft Preparation, H.J.C.-J, B.R, E.M. and M.U; Writing-Review & Editing, H.J.C.-J. and E.M. Supervision, E.M. Project Administration, H.J.C.-J.

Funding: This research received no external funding.

Acknowledgments: The authors are grateful to the Coordenação de Aperfeiçoamento de Pessoal de Nível Superior (CAPES) for funding this research via scholarships to HJCJ (PhD visiting: 88881.190185/2018-01). BR had financial support from the Fundação de Amparo à Pesquisa do Estado de São Paulo (FAPESP) and CNPq (BPQ).

Conflicts of Interest: The authors declare no conflict of interest.

References

1. Morley, J.E.; Vellas, B.; Abellan van Kan, G.; Anker, S.D.; Bauer, J.M.; Bernabei, R.; Cesari, M.; Chumlea, W.C.; Doehner, W.; Evans, J.; et al. Frailty Consensus: A Call to Action. *J. Am. Med. Dir. Assoc.* **2013**, *14*, 392–397. [CrossRef] [PubMed]
2. Cesari, M.; Calvani, R.; Marzetti, E. Frailty in Older Persons. *Clin. Geriatr. Med.* **2017**, *33*, 293–303. [CrossRef] [PubMed]
3. Artaza-Artabe, I.; Sáez-López, P.; Sánchez-Hernández, N.; Fernández-Gutierrez, N.; Malafarina, V. The relationship between nutrition and frailty: Effects of protein intake, nutritional supplementation, vitamin D and exercise on muscle metabolism in the elderly. A systematic review. *Maturitas* **2016**, *93*, 89–99. [CrossRef] [PubMed]
4. Yannakoulia, M.; Ntanasi, E.; Anastasiou, C.A.; Scarmeas, N. Frailty and nutrition: From epidemiological and clinical evidence to potential mechanisms. *Metabolism* **2017**, *68*, 64–76. [CrossRef] [PubMed]
5. Kaiser, M.; Bandinelli, S.; Lunenfeld, B. Frailty and the role of nutrition in older people. A review of the current literature. *Acta. Biomed.* **2010**, *81* (Suppl. 1), 37–45. [PubMed]
6. Phillips, S.M. The science of muscle hypertrophy: Making dietary protein count. *Proc. Nutr. Soc.* **2011**, *70*, 100–103. [CrossRef] [PubMed]
7. Stokes, T.; Hector, A.J.; Morton, R.W.; McGlory, C.; Phillips, S.M. Recent Perspectives Regarding the Role of Dietary Protein for the Promotion of Muscle Hypertrophy with Resistance Exercise Training. *Nutrients* **2018**, *10*, 180. [CrossRef] [PubMed]
8. Tipton, K.D.; Phillips, S.M. Dietary Protein for Muscle Hypertrophy. In *Nestle Nutrition Institute Workshop Series*; Karger Publishers: Basel, Switzerland, 2013; Volume 76, pp. 73–84.
9. Robinson, S.M.; Reginster, J.Y.; Rizzoli, R.; Shaw, S.C.; Kanis, J.A.; Bautmans, I.; Bischoff-Ferrari, H.; Bruyere, O.; Cesari, M.; Dawson-Hughes, B.; et al. Does nutrition play a role in the prevention and management of sarcopenia? *Clin. Nutr.* **2018**, *37*, 1121–1132. [CrossRef] [PubMed]
10. Katsanos, C.S.; Kobayashi, H.; Sheffield-Moore, M.; Aarsland, A.; Wolfe, R.R. Aging is associated with diminished accretion of muscle proteins after the ingestion of a small bolus of essential amino acids. *Am. J. Clin. Nutr.* **2005**, *82*, 1065–1073. [CrossRef] [PubMed]
11. Katsanos, C.S.; Kobayashi, H.; Sheffield-Moore, M.; Aarsland, A.; Wolfe, R.R. A high proportion of leucine is required for optimal stimulation of the rate of muscle protein synthesis by essential amino acids in the elderly. *Am. J. Physiol. Metab.* **2006**, *291*, E381–E387. [CrossRef] [PubMed]
12. Yanai, H. Nutrition for Sarcopenia. *J. Clin. Med. Res.* **2015**, *7*, 926–931. [CrossRef] [PubMed]

13. Phillips, S.M. Current Concepts and Unresolved Questions in Dietary Protein Requirements and Supplements in Adults. *Front. Nutr.* **2017**, *4*, 13. [CrossRef] [PubMed]
14. Fried, L.P.; Tangen, C.M.; Walston, J.; Newman, A.B.; Hirsch, C.; Gottdiener, J.; Seeman, T.; Tracy, R.; Kop, W.J.; Burke, G.; et al. Cardiovascular Health Study Collaborative Research Group Frailty in older adults: Evidence for a phenotype. *J. Gerontol. A Biol. Sci. Med. Sci.* **2001**, *56*, M146–M156. [CrossRef] [PubMed]
15. Cruz-Jentoft, A.J.; Baeyens, J.P.; Bauer, J.M.; Boirie, Y.; Cederholm, T.; Landi, F.; Martin, F.C.; Michel, J.-P.; Rolland, Y.; Schneider, S.M.; et al. Sarcopenia: European consensus on definition and diagnosis: Report of the European Working Group on Sarcopenia in Older People. *Age Ageing* **2010**, *39*, 412–423. [CrossRef] [PubMed]
16. La Rue, A.; Koehler, K.M.; Wayne, S.J.; Chiulli, S.J.; Haaland, K.Y.; Garry, P.J. Nutritional status and cognitive functioning in a normally aging sample: A 6-year reassessment. *Am. J. Clin. Nutr.* **1997**, *65*, 20–29. [CrossRef] [PubMed]
17. Roberts, R.O.; Roberts, L.A.; Geda, Y.E.; Cha, R.H.; Pankratz, V.S.; O'Connor, H.M.; Knopman, D.S.; Petersen, R.C. Relative Intake of Macronutrients Impacts Risk of Mild Cognitive Impairment or Dementia. *J. Alzheimer's Dis.* **2012**, *32*, 329–339. [CrossRef] [PubMed]
18. Koh, F.; Charlton, K.; Walton, K.; McMahon, A.-T. Role of dietary protein and thiamine intakes on cognitive function in healthy older people: A systematic review. *Nutrients* **2015**, *7*, 2415–2439. [CrossRef] [PubMed]
19. Liberati, A.; Altman, D.G.; Tetzlaff, J.; Mulrow, C.; Gøtzsche, P.C.; Ioannidis, J.P.A.; Clarke, M.; Devereaux, P.J.; Kleijnen, J.; Moher, D. The PRISMA Statement for Reporting Systematic Reviews and Meta-Analyses of Studies That Evaluate Health Care Interventions: Explanation and Elaboration. *PLoS Med.* **2009**, *6*, e1000100. [CrossRef] [PubMed]
20. Stroup, D.F.; Berlin, J.A.; Morton, S.C.; Olkin, I.; Williamson, G.D.; Rennie, D.; Moher, D.; Becker, B.J.; Sipe, T.A.; Thacker, S.B. Meta-analysis of observational studies in epidemiology: A proposal for reporting. Meta-analysis Of Observational Studies in Epidemiology (MOOSE) group. *JAMA* **2000**, *283*, 2008–2012. [CrossRef] [PubMed]
21. Von Elm, E.; Altman, D.G.; Egger, M.; Pocock, S.J.; Gøtzsche, P.C.; Vandenbroucke, J.P.; Strobe, I. The Strengthening the Reporting of Observational Studies in Epidemiology (STROBE) statement: Guidelines for reporting observational studies. *Lancet* **2007**, *370*, 1453–1457. [CrossRef]
22. Green, S.; Higgins, J. Cochrane handbook for systematic reviews of interventions. 2005.
23. Bartali, B.; Frongillo, E.A.; Bandinelli, S.; Lauretani, F.; Semba, R.D.; Fried, L.P.; Ferrucci, L. Low nutrient intake is an essential component of frailty in older persons. *J. Gerontol. A Biol. Sci. Med. Sci.* **2006**, *61*, 589–593. [CrossRef] [PubMed]
24. Kobayashi, S.; Asakura, K.; Suga, H.; Sasaki, S. High protein intake is associated with low prevalence of frailty among old Japanese women: A multicenter cross-sectional study. *Nutr. J.* **2013**, *12*, 164. [CrossRef] [PubMed]
25. Kobayashi, S.; Suga, H.; Sasaki, S. Diet with a combination of high protein and high total antioxidant capacity is strongly associated with low prevalence of frailty among old Japanese women: A multicenter cross-sectional study. *Nutr. J.* **2017**, *16*, 29. [CrossRef] [PubMed]
26. Bollwein, J.; Diekmann, R.; Kaiser, M.J.; Bauer, J.M.; Uter, W.; Sieber, C.C.; Volkert, D. Distribution but not amount of protein intake is associated with frailty: A cross-sectional investigation in the region of Nurnberg. *Nutr. J.* **2013**, *12*, 109. [CrossRef] [PubMed]
27. Shikany, J.M.; Barrett-Connor, E.; Ensrud, K.E.; Cawthon, P.M.; Lewis, C.E.; Dam, T.-T.L.; Shannon, J.; Redden, D.T. Macronutrients, diet quality, and frailty in older men. *J. Gerontol. A Biol. Sci. Med. Sci.* **2014**, *69*, 695–701. [CrossRef] [PubMed]
28. Rahi, B.; Colombet, Z.; Gonzalez-Colaco Harmand, M.; Dartigues, J.-F.; Boirie, Y.; Letenneur, L.; Feart, C. Higher Protein but Not Energy Intake Is Associated with a Lower Prevalence of Frailty Among Community-Dwelling Older Adults in the French Three-City Cohort. *J. Am. Med. Dir. Assoc.* **2016**, *17*, 672.e7–672.e11. [CrossRef] [PubMed]
29. Nanri, H.; Yamada, Y.; Yoshida, T.; Okabe, Y.; Nozawa, Y.; Itoi, A.; Yoshimura, E.; Watanabe, Y.; Yamaguchi, M.; Yokoyama, K.; et al. Sex Difference in the Association Between Protein Intake and Frailty: Assessed Using the Kihon Checklist Indexes Among Older Adults. *J. Am. Med. Dir. Assoc.* **2018**, *19*, 801–805. [CrossRef] [PubMed]

30. Beasley, J.M.; Lacroix, A.Z.; Neuhouser, M.L.; Huang, Y.; Tinker, L.; Woods, N.; Michael, Y.; Curb, J.D.; Prentice, R.L. Protein intake and incident frailty in the women's health initiative observational study. *J. Am. Geriatr. Soc.* **2010**, *58*, 1063–1071. [CrossRef] [PubMed]
31. Sandoval-Insausti, H.; Perez-Tasigchana, R.F.; Lopez-Garcia, E.; Garcia-Esquinas, E.; Rodriguez-Artalejo, F.; Guallar-Castillon, P. Macronutrients Intake and Incident Frailty in Older Adults: A Prospective Cohort Study. *J. Gerontol. A Biol. Sci. Med. Sci.* **2016**, *71*, 1329–1334. [CrossRef] [PubMed]
32. Bonnefoy, M.; Berrut, G.; Lesourd, B.; Ferry, M.; Gilbert, T.; Guerin, O.; Hanon, C.; Jeandel, C.; Paillaud, E.; Raynaud-Simon, A.; et al. Frailty and nutrition: Searching for evidence. *J. Nutr. Health Aging* **2015**, *19*, 250–257. [CrossRef] [PubMed]
33. Lorenzo-Lopez, L.; Maseda, A.; de Labra, C.; Regueiro-Folgueira, L.; Rodriguez-Villamil, J.L.; Millan-Calenti, J.C. Nutritional determinants of frailty in older adults: A systematic review. *BMC Geriatr.* **2017**, *17*, 108. [CrossRef] [PubMed]
34. Cederholm, T. Overlaps between Frailty and Sarcopenia Definitions. In *Nestle Nutrition Institute Workshop Series*; Karger Publishers: Basel, Switzerland, 2015; Volume 83, pp. 65–70.
35. Landi, F.; Calvani, R.; Cesari, M.; Tosato, M.; Martone, A.M.; Bernabei, R.; Onder, G.; Marzetti, E. Sarcopenia as the Biological Substrate of Physical Frailty. *Clin. Geriatr. Med.* **2015**, *31*, 367–374. [CrossRef] [PubMed]
36. Marzetti, E.; Calvani, R.; Cesari, M.; Tosato, M.; Cherubini, A.; Di Bari, M.; Pahor, M.; Savera, G.; Collamati, A.; D'Angelo, E.; et al. Operationalization of the physical frailty & sarcopenia syndrome: Rationale and clinical implementation. *Transl. Med. UniSa.* **2015**, *13*, 29. [PubMed]
37. Ziaaldini, M.M.; Marzetti, E.; Picca, A.; Murlasits, Z. Biochemical Pathways of Sarcopenia and Their Modulation by Physical Exercise: A Narrative Review. *Front. Med.* **2017**, *4*, 167. [CrossRef] [PubMed]
38. Frisoli, A.; Chaves, P.H.; Ingham, S.J.M.; Fried, L.P. Severe osteopenia and osteoporosis, sarcopenia, and frailty status in community-dwelling older women: Results from the Women's Health and Aging Study (WHAS) II. *Bone* **2011**, *48*, 952–957. [CrossRef] [PubMed]
39. Mijnarends, D.M.; Schols, J.M.G.A.; Meijers, J.M.M.; Tan, F.E.S.; Verlaan, S.; Luiking, Y.C.; Morley, J.E.; Halfens, R.J.G. Instruments to assess sarcopenia and physical frailty in older people living in a community (care) setting: Similarities and discrepancies. *J. Am. Med. Dir. Assoc.* **2015**, *16*, 301–308. [CrossRef] [PubMed]
40. McGlory, C.; Devries, M.C.; Phillips, S.M. Skeletal muscle and resistance exercise training; the role of protein synthesis in recovery and remodeling. *J. Appl. Physiol.* **2016**, *122*, 541–548. [CrossRef] [PubMed]
41. Kim, C.-O.; Lee, K.-R. Preventive effect of protein-energy supplementation on the functional decline of frail older adults with low socioeconomic status: A community-based randomized controlled study. *J. Gerontol. A Biol. Sci. Med. Sci.* **2013**, *68*, 309–316. [CrossRef] [PubMed]
42. Tieland, M.; van de Rest, O.; Dirks, M.L.; van der Zwaluw, N.; Mensink, M.; van Loon, L.J.C.; de Groot, L.C. Protein Supplementation Improves Physical Performance in Frail Elderly People: A Randomized, Double-Blind, Placebo-Controlled Trial. *J. Am. Med. Dir. Assoc.* **2012**, *13*, 720–726. [CrossRef] [PubMed]
43. Dominguez, L.J.; Barbagallo, M. Perspective: Protein supplementation in frail older persons: Often necessary but not always sufficient. *J. Am. Med. Dir. Assoc.* **2013**, *14*, 72–73. [CrossRef] [PubMed]
44. Hoeymans, N.; Feskens, E.J.; van den Bos, G.A.; Kromhout, D. Measuring functional status: Cross-sectional and longitudinal associations between performance and self-report (Zutphen Elderly Study 1990–1993). *J. Clin. Epidemiol.* **1996**, *49*, 1103–1110. [CrossRef]
45. Cress, M.E.; Buchner, D.M.; Questad, K.A.; Esselman, P.C.; deLateur, B.J.; Schwartz, R.S. Exercise: Effects on physical functional performance in independent older adults. *J. Gerontol. A Biol. Sci. Med. Sci.* **1999**, *54*, M242–M248. [CrossRef] [PubMed]
46. Gregorio, L.; Brindisi, J.; Kleppinger, A.; Sullivan, R.; Mangano, K.M.; Bihuniak, J.D.; Kenny, A.M.; Kerstetter, J.E.; Insogna, K.L. Adequate dietary protein is associated with better physical performance among post-menopausal women 60–90 years. *J. Nutr. Health Aging* **2014**, *18*, 155–160. [CrossRef] [PubMed]
47. Verlaan, S.; Aspray, T.J.; Bauer, J.M.; Cederholm, T.; Hemsworth, J.; Hill, T.R.; McPhee, J.S.; Piasecki, M.; Seal, C.; Sieber, C.C.; et al. Nutritional status, body composition, and quality of life in community-dwelling sarcopenic and non-sarcopenic older adults: A case-control study. *Clin. Nutr.* **2017**, *36*, 267–274. [CrossRef] [PubMed]
48. Isanejad, M.; Mursu, J.; Sirola, J.; Kröger, H.; Rikkonen, T.; Tuppurainen, M.; Erkkilä, A.T. Dietary protein intake is associated with better physical function and muscle strength among elderly women. *Br. J. Nutr.* **2016**, *115*, 1281–1291. [CrossRef] [PubMed]

49. Ten Haaf, D.; van Dongen, E.; Nuijten, M.; Eijsvogels, T.; de Groot, L.; Hopman, M. Protein Intake and Distribution in Relation to Physical Functioning and Quality of Life in Community-Dwelling Elderly People: Acknowledging the Role of Physical Activity. *Nutrients* **2018**, *10*, 506. [CrossRef] [PubMed]
50. Loenneke, J.P.; Loprinzi, P.D.; Murphy, C.H.; Phillips, S.M. Per meal dose and frequency of protein consumption is associated with lean mass and muscle performance. *Clin. Nutr.* **2016**, *35*, 1506–1511. [CrossRef] [PubMed]
51. Imai, E.; Tsubota-Utsugi, M.; Kikuya, M.; Satoh, M.; Inoue, R.; Hosaka, M.; Metoki, H.; Fukushima, N.; Kurimoto, A.; Hirose, T.; et al. Animal Protein Intake Is Associated with Higher-Level Functional Capacity in Elderly Adults: The Ohasama Study. *J. Am. Geriatr. Soc.* **2014**, *62*, 426–434. [CrossRef] [PubMed]
52. Tieland, M.; Borgonjen-Van den Berg, K.; Van Loon, L.; de Groot, L. Dietary Protein Intake in Dutch Elderly People: A Focus on Protein Sources. *Nutrients* **2015**, *7*, 9697–9706. [CrossRef] [PubMed]
53. Da Costa, B.R.; Cevallos, M.; Altman, D.G.; Rutjes, A.W.S.; Egger, M. Uses and misuses of the STROBE statement: Bibliographic study. *BMJ Open* **2011**, *1*, e000048. [CrossRef] [PubMed]

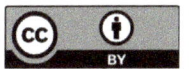

© 2018 by the authors. Licensee MDPI, Basel, Switzerland. This article is an open access article distributed under the terms and conditions of the Creative Commons Attribution (CC BY) license (http://creativecommons.org/licenses/by/4.0/).

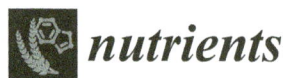

Article

A Distinct Pattern of Circulating Amino Acids Characterizes Older Persons with Physical Frailty and Sarcopenia: Results from the BIOSPHERE Study

Riccardo Calvani [1,2], Anna Picca [1,2,*], Federico Marini, Alessandra Biancolillo [3], Jacopo Gervasoni [1,2], Silvia Persichilli [1,2], Aniello Primiano [2], Hélio José Coelho-Junior [2,4], Maurizio Bossola [1,2], Andrea Urbani [1,2], Francesco Landi [1,2], Roberto Bernabei [1,2] and Emanuele Marzetti [1]

[1] Fondazione Policlinico Universitario Agostino Gemelli, IRCCS, Rome 00168, Italy; riccardo.calvani@gmail.com (R.C.); jacopo.gervasoni@policlinicogemelli.it (J.G.); silvia.persichilli@policlinicogemelli.it (S.P.); mauriziobossola@gmail.com (M.B.); andrea.urbani@unicatt.it (A.U.); francesco.landi@unicatt.it (F.L.); roberto.bernabei@unicatt.it (R.B.); emanuele.marzetti@policlinicogemelli.it (E.M.)
[2] Università Cattolica del Sacro Cuore, Rome 00168, Italy; anielloprim@gmail.com (A.P.); coelhojunior@hotmail.com.br (H.J.C.-J.)
[3] Department of Chemistry, Sapienza University of Rome, Rome 00168, Italy; federico.marini@uniroma1.it (F.M.); alessandra.biancolillo@uniroma1.it (A.B.)
[4] Applied Kinesiology Laboratory–LCA, School of Physical Education, University of Campinas, Campinas-SP 13.083-851, Brazil
* Correspondence: anna.picca1@gmail.com; Tel.: +39-06-3015-5559

Received: 17 September 2018; Accepted: 1 November 2018; Published: 6 November 2018

Abstract: Physical frailty and sarcopenia (PF&S) are hallmarks of aging that share a common pathogenic background. Perturbations in protein/amino acid metabolism may play a role in the development of PF&S. In this initial report, 68 community-dwellers aged 70 years and older, 38 with PF&S and 30 non-sarcopenic, non-frail controls (nonPF&S), were enrolled as part as the "BIOmarkers associated with Sarcopenia and Physical frailty in EldeRly pErsons" (BIOSPHERE) study. A panel of 37 serum amino acids and derivatives was assayed by UPLC-MS. Partial Least Squares–Discriminant Analysis (PLS-DA) was used to characterize the amino acid profile of PF&S. The optimal complexity of the PLS-DA model was found to be three latent variables. The proportion of correct classification was $76.6 \pm 3.9\%$ ($75.1 \pm 4.6\%$ for enrollees with PF&S; $78.5 \pm 6.0\%$ for nonPF&S). Older adults with PF&S were characterized by higher levels of asparagine, aspartic acid, citrulline, ethanolamine, glutamic acid, sarcosine, and taurine. The profile of nonPF&S participants was defined by higher concentrations of α-aminobutyric acid and methionine. Distinct profiles of circulating amino acids and derivatives characterize older people with PF&S. The dissection of these patterns may provide novel insights into the role played by protein/amino acid perturbations in the disabling cascade and possible new targets for interventions.

Keywords: aging; muscle; protein; metabolism; metabolomics; profiling; biomarkers; multi-marker; physical performance; multivariate

1. Introduction

Over the last decades, sarcopenia, the progressive and generalized decline in skeletal muscle mass and function with age, has become a "blockbuster" condition in geriatrics, given its increasing prevalence in a globally aging world and its clinical relevance [1–4]. Indeed, this condition conveys a broad spectrum of negative health-related outcomes, including disability, loss of independence, institutionalization, and mortality [5,6]. Frailty has been defined as a geriatric "multidimensional syndrome characterized by decreased reserve and diminished resistance to stressors," and is often envisioned as a pre-disability condition [7]. Sarcopenia overlaps with the clinical picture of frailty, especially in its physical domain, and may represent both the biological substratum of physical frailty (PF) and the pathophysiologic basis upon which the negative health outcomes of PF develop [8,9]. The two conditions have therefore been merged into a new entity (i.e., PF and sarcopenia; PF&S) [10] that was operationalized in the context of the "Sarcopenia and Physical fRailty IN older people: multi-componenT Treatment strategies" (SPRINTT) project [11,12].

Although the pathophysiology of PF&S is complex and multifactorial, the central role attributed to muscle wasting suggests that biomarkers related to sarcopenia may be used to support the diagnosis and track the evolution of PF&S, unveil its underlying mechanisms, and identify meaningful targets for interventions [13,14].

Dietary protein intake and circulating amino acids play a pivotal role in muscle plasticity and trophism [15], but also modulate several biological processes (including inflammation, insulin sensitivity, and redox homeostasis) that may be involved in age-related muscle atrophy and dysfunction [16,17]. Hence, perturbations in protein-amino acid metabolism may represent a major mechanism in sarcopenia [18,19].

Amino acid profiling, especially when coupled with multivariate statistical analysis, may serve as a powerful analytical approach to explore the possible role of protein-amino acid networks in PF&S [20]. Recently, distinct amino acid signatures were associated with muscle mass in older adults with functional limitations [21] and low muscle quality [22] in the Baltimore Longitudinal Study of Aging. Moreover, reduced non-fasting plasma concentrations of the branched-chain amino acids (BCAAs) leucine and isoleucine were detected in Norwegian older community-dwellers with sarcopenia [23], while higher proline concentrations were independently associated with sarcopenia in older Japanese people [24]. Finally, low plasma levels of essential amino acids (EAAs) characterized the amino acid profile of severely frail Japanese older people compared with non-frail peers [25].

The "BIOmarkers associated with Sarcopenia and Physical frailty in EldeRly pErsons" (BIOSPHERE) study was designed to determine and validate a panel of PF&S biomarkers encompassing systemic inflammation, oxidative stress, muscle remodeling, neuromuscular junction dysfunction, and amino acid metabolism through multivariate statistical modeling [26]. In the present work, we report the initial results obtained through the simultaneous analysis of an array of circulating amino acids and derivatives coupled with Partial Least Squares–Discriminant Analysis (PLS-DA). This innovative approach allowed identifying distinct patterns of circulating amino acids and derivatives that characterize older adults with and without PF&S. This may represent a first relevant step towards the integration of specific biochemical measurements into the assessment of PF&S in research and clinical settings.

2. Materials and Methods

2.1. Study Design and Population

BIOSPHERE was conceived as a cross-sectional, case-control study [26]. The study protocol was approved by the Ethics Committee of the Università Cattolica del Sacro Cuore (Rome, Italy; protocol number: 8498/15) and is thoroughly described elsewhere [26]. Briefly, after obtaining written informed consent, 200 older persons, 100 cases (individuals with PF&S) and 100 non-physically frail, non-sarcopenic (nonPF&S) controls aged 70+ were enrolled. Selection criteria are reported in Table S1. Candidates were diagnosed with PF&S when presenting the following parameters: (a) low physical performance, defined as a summary score on the Short Physical Performance Battery (SPPB) [27] between 3 and 9; (b) low appendicular muscle mass (aLM) according to the criteria recommended by the Foundation for the National Institutes of Health (FNIH) sarcopenia project [28]; and (c) absence of major mobility disability, operationalized as an inability to walk 400 m in 15 min at a usual pace [29].

This initial analysis involved 68 participants (38 cases and 30 controls) in whom circulating amino acids and derivatives were measured.

2.2. Measurement of Appendicular Lean Mass by Dual X-Ray Absorptiometry (DXA)

Whole-body DXA scans were obtained on a Hologic Discovery A densitometer (Hologic, Inc., Bedford, MA, USA). Scan acquisition and analysis were performed according to manufacturer's directions. Candidates were considered to be eligible if presenting with an aLM to body mass index (BMI) ratio (aLM$_{BMI}$) <0.789 or <0.512 in men and women, respectively. When the aLM$_{BMI}$ criterion was not met, candidates were tested with the alternative criterion (i.e., crude aLM < 19.75 kg in men and <15.02 kg in women) [28].

2.3. Blood Sample Collection

Blood samples were collected in the morning by venipuncture of the median cubital vein after overnight fasting, using commercial collection tubes (BD Vacutainer®; Becton, Dickinson and Co., Franklin Lakes, NJ, USA). For serum separation, samples were left at room temperature for 20 min and subsequently centrifuged at 1000× g for 10 min at 4 °C. Aliquots of serum were subsequently stored at −80 °C until analysis.

2.4. Amino Acids Profiling

Thirty-seven amino acids and derivatives (1-methylhistidine, 3-methylhistidine, 4-hydroxyproline, α-aminobutyric acid, β-alanine, β-aminobutyric acid, γ-aminobutyric acid, alanine, aminoadipic acid, anserine, arginine, asparagine, aspartic acid, carnosine, citrulline, cystathionine, cystine, ethanolamine, glutamic acid, glycine, histidine, isoleucine, leucine, lysine, methionine, ornithine, phenylalanine, phosphoethanolamine, phosphoserine, proline, sarcosine, serine, taurine, threonine, tryptophan, tyrosine, valine) were measured in serum through a ultraperformance liquid chromatography/mass spectrometry (UPLC/MS) validated methodology. Briefly, 50 μL of sample were mixed with 100 μL 10% (w/v) sulfosalicylic acid containing an internal standard mix (50 μM) (Cambridge Isotope Laboratories, Inc., Tewksbury, MA, USA) and centrifuged at 1000× g for 15 min. Ten microliters of the supernatant were transferred into a vial containing 70 μL of borate buffer to which 20 μL of AccQ Tag reagents (Waters Corporation, Milford, MA, USA) were subsequently added. Samples were then vortexed for 10 s and heated at 55 °C for 10 min. The chromatographic separation was performed by ACQUITY H-Class (Waters Corporation) using a CORTECS UPLC C18 column 1.6 μm 2.1 × 150 mm (Waters Corporation) eluted at a flow rate of 500 μL/min with a linear gradient (9 min) from 99 to 1 water 0.1% formic acid in acetonitrile 0.1% formic acid. The mass spectrometer was an ACQUITY QDa single quadrupole equipped with electrospray source operating in positive mode (Waters Corporation). The analytical process was monitored using amino acid controls (level 1 and level 2) manufactured by the MCA laboratory of the Queen Beatrix Hospital (Winterswijk, The Netherlands).

2.5. Statistical Analysis

All analyses were performed using in-house routines running under MATLAB R2015b environment (The MathWorks, Natick, MA, USA).

2.5.1. Descriptive Statistics

Differences in demographic, anthropometric, clinical, and functional characteristics between cases and controls were assessed via t-test statistics and χ^2 or Fisher exact tests, for continuous and categorical variables, respectively. All tests were two-sided, with statistical significance set at $p < 0.05$.

2.5.2. Partial Least Squares–Discriminant Analysis

The strategy for the identification and validation of potential biomarkers for PF&S relied on the building of discriminant models to differentiate cases from controls. The approach chosen for the present study was based on PLS-DA [30], because of its versatility and ability to deal with highly correlated predictors. Briefly, PLS-DA is a classification method based on the PLS regression algorithm [31]. PLS-DA builds the linear relation between a set of responses Y and a matrix of predictors X by projecting the latter onto a low-dimensional space of latent (abstract) variables (LVs) that are characterized by having the highest covariance with the responses to be predicted. The statistical reliability of the PLS-DA model was subsequently verified by a double cross-validation (DCV) procedure and by means of randomization tests [32]. Three figures of merit were considered in the present study: (i) the number of misclassifications (NMC); (ii) the area under the receiver operating characteristic (ROC) curve (AUROC); and (iii) the value of the discriminant Q2 (DQ2) [33].

For the identification of potential biomarkers, two approaches aimed at highlighting the experimental variables contributing the most to the classification model were followed, and they involved inspecting variable importance in projection (VIP) indices [31] and rank product (RP) [34], respectively. A more detailed description of the PLS-DA statistics is provided as supplementary material.

3. Results

3.1. Descriptive Characteristics of the Study Population

The study population included 38 older adults with PF&S and 30 nonPF&S controls. The main demographic, anthropometric, clinical, and functional characteristics of the study population according to the presence of PF&S are presented in Table 1. No differences between groups were observed with regard to age, gender distribution, number of co-morbid conditions, and number of prescription medications. The distribution of specific disease conditions and the prevalence of use of individual drug classes are shown in Table S2. As expected, physical performance, as assessed by the SPPB, was lower in PF&S participants (SPPB score: 7.4 ± 1.5) relative to controls (11.3 ± 0.9) ($p < 0.0001$). Similarly, aLM, either absolute or adjusted for BMI, was smaller in the PF&S group compared with nonPF&S enrollees.

Table 1. Main characteristics of BIOmarkers associated with Sarcopenia and Physical frailty in EldeRly pErsons (BIOSPHERE) participants according to the presence of physical frailty and sarcopenia (PF&S).

	PF&S ($n = 38$)	nonPF&S ($n = 30$)	p
Age, years (mean $\pm$ SD)	76.4 ± 4.9	74.6 ± 4.3	0.1067
Gender (female), n (%)	25 (65.8)	16 (53.3)	0.4280
BMI, kg/m^2 (mean $\pm$ SD)	29.1 ± 4.4	26.7 ± 2.4	0.0112
SPPB (mean $\pm$ SD)	7.4 ± 1.5	11.3 ± 0.9	<0.0001
aLM, kg (mean $\pm$ SD)	16.2 ± 3.2	19.4 ± 3.9	0.0004
aLM$_{BMI}$ (mean $\pm$ SD)	0.554 ± 0.120	0.795 ± 0.264	<0.0001
Number of disease conditions * (mean $\pm$ SD)	2.3 ± 1.5	1.8 ± 1.4	0.1448
Number of medications (mean $\pm$ SD)	3.2 ± 1.8	2.8 ± 1.9	0.4115

* Includes hypertension, coronary artery disease, prior stroke, peripheral vascular disease, diabetes, chronic obstructive pulmonary disease, and osteoarthritis. BMI: body mass index; SPPB: Short Physical Performance Battery; aLM: appendicular lean mass; PF&S: physical frailty and sarcopenia; nonPF&S: non physically frail, non sarcopenic; SD: standard deviation.

3.2. Participant Classification According to PLS-DA

In order to verify the existence of a specific pattern of amino acids in participants with PF&S, a PLS-DA classification model was constructed and validated. The optimal PLS-DA model was built using three LVs that accounted for more than 44% of the variance originally present in the X block.

As indicated by the DCV procedure, the model allowed to correctly predict the presence of PF&S in 95.7 ± 2.1% of participants in the calibration phase (94.7 ± 3.8% for PF&S and 96.7 ± 4.6% for controls), 84.1 ± 2.7% in the internal validation stage (82.6 ± 3.6% for PF&S and 86.0 ± 4.8% for controls), and 76.6 ± 3.9% in external validation (75.1 ± 4.6% for PF&S; 78.5 ± 6.0% for nonPF&S). Figure 1, which depicts the projection of participants onto the space spanned by the first two LVs of the PLS-DA model, shows a clear separation between participants with and without PF&S.

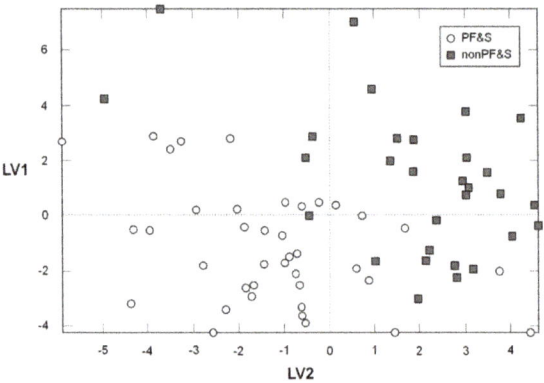

Figure 1. Scores plot showing the separation of participants according to the serum concentrations of amino acids and derivatives in the space spanned by the two latent variables (LV1 and LV2), as determined by Partial Least Squares–Discriminant Analysis (PLS-DA).

The classification ability of the PLS-DA model was further validated by comparing the results of the DCV with the distributions of NMC, AUROC and DQ2 under the null hypothesis (Figure 2). For each of the three figures of merits considered, the values obtained on the real dataset fell outside of the corresponding null hypothesis distribution, which corresponds to a $p < 0.05$.

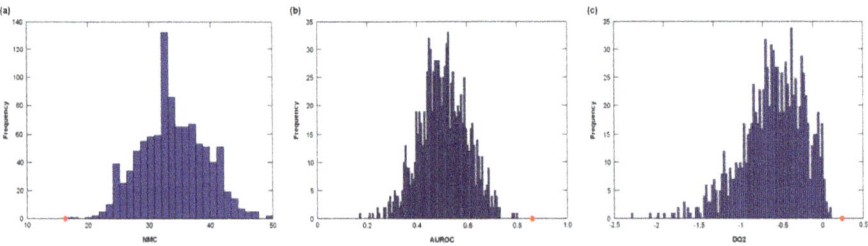

Figure 2. Distribution of (a) number of misclassifications (NMC), (b) area under the receiver operating characteristic (ROC) curve (AUROC), and (c) discriminant Q2 (DQ2) values under their respective null hypothesis as estimated by permutation tests (blue histograms) and the corresponding values obtained by the PLS-DA model on unpermuted data (red circles). Values obtained on the real dataset (red circles) fall outside of the corresponding null hypothesis distribution (blue histograms), corresponding to a $p < 0.05$.

In order to identify the metabolites that were mostly involved in discriminating between cases and controls, the values of the VIP indices were inspected. The variables corresponding to a VIP greater than one are reported in Table 2. Nine amino acids were found to contribute significantly to the discrimination model. Participants with PF&S were characterized by higher levels of asparagine, aspartic acid, citrulline, ethanolamine, glutamic acid, sarcosine, and taurine. Conversely, the profile of non-PF&S individuals was defined by higher levels of α-aminobutyric acid (AABA) and methionine. Serum concentrations of non-discriminant amino acids are reported in Table S3.

Table 2. Serum concentrations of discriminant analytes, variable importance in projection (VIP) values, and rank product (RP) values in BIOSPHERE participants with and without physical frailty and sarcopenia (PF&S). Serum concentrations are shown as mean ± standard deviation.

	PF&S (n = 38)	nonPF&S (n = 30)	VIP	RP
α-aminobutyric acid (μmol/L)	20.0 ± 4.9	22.3 ± 5.7	2.2	8.0
Asparagine (μmol/L)	91.0 ± 12.6	77.8 ± 13.4	3.4	2.0
Aspartic Acid (μmol/L)	24.6 ± 5.4	17.0 ± 4.0	5.8	2.6
Citrulline (μmol/L)	44.8 ± 12.1	36.8 ± 11.5	2.1	2.8
Ethanolamine (μmol/L)	10.3 ± 1.7	9.0 ± 2.2	1.7	9.9
Glutamic acid (μmol/L)	71.7 ± 16.6	54.3 ± 21.2	2.3	8.5
Methionine (μmol/L)	22.6 ± 2.8	23.4 ± 5.7	1.3	6.3
Sarcosine (μmol/L)	1.9 ± 0.6	1.5 ± 0.5	1.4	8.0
Taurine (μmol/L)	220.1 ± 36.5	189.5 ± 47.2	1.8	6.7

4. Discussion

In the present study, we report the first results from the BIOSPHERE study. The most relevant finding was that older individuals with PF&S showed a distinct profile of circulating amino acids characterized by higher serum levels of asparagine, aspartic acid, citrulline, ethanolamine, glutamic acid, sarcosine, and taurine. Conversely, the profile of nonPF&S participants was defined by higher levels of AABA and methionine.

The existence of an amino acid signature in the setting of PF&S suggests that specific metabolic alterations might be involved in the pathogenesis of this condition. Indeed, PF&S was associated with lower circulating levels of the EAA methionine. EAAs are defined as those amino acids that must be provided with the diet to meet optimal requirements [35]. The reduction of serum concentrations of a number of EAAs (including methionine) with age was reported in both genders and was purportedly associated with decreases in total energy and protein intake [36]. In addition, low plasma levels of EAA were found in severely frail older people [25]. These findings may be linked to malnutrition (both quantitative and qualitative), a common causative factor of frailty and sarcopenia [37,38]. The concomitant low serum concentration of the non-essential non-proteinogenic amino acid AABA seems to corroborate the previous finding since AABA may derive from the catabolism of methionine [39]. Furthermore, plasma levels of AABA were found to be associated with both the quality and amount of dietary protein [40,41]. Although these findings seem to point towards a poor-quality protein diet or (selective) malabsorption, further studies are needed to clarify the relationship between diet and circulating EAA levels in the context of PF&S.

Methionine is also involved in one-carbon metabolism, a crucial pathway that modulates multiple physiologic processes, including nucleotide biosynthesis, amino acid homeostasis, epigenetic maintenance, and redox balance [42]. Not surprisingly, alterations in one-carbon metabolism were observed in aging and age-related diseases, such as cancer, cardiovascular disease, and neurodegeneration [42,43]. Sarcosine, the N-methyl-derivative of glycine, is another relevant intermediate of one-carbon metabolism [42]. Sarcosine is formed from dietary choline and the metabolism of methionine [44,45], and can be found in muscles and other body tissues. A recent metabolomics study showed that circulating sarcosine levels were reduced with aging both in rodents and humans, while dietary restriction prevented this decline in both species [46]. Counterintuitively, sarcosine levels were higher in persons with PF&S relative to controls. However, circulating sarcosine may increase in case of folate deficiency, because folate mediates the conversion of sarcosine to glycine [45]. Thus, this finding might be linked to insufficient folate ingestion and/or perturbation in folate/one-carbon metabolism.

Sarcosine also activates autophagy in mouse fibroblasts in a dose-dependent manner [46], and alterations in myocyte quality control mechanisms (including autophagy) may contribute to sarcopenia [47–49]. In particular, defective autophagic clearance of damaged cellular constituents, alterations in mitochondrial proteostasis and dynamics, and impaired mitochondriogenesis are thought to be critically involved in age-related muscle degeneration [50]. In this context, the presence of ethanolamine among the most discriminant metabolites for PF&S classification is of particular interest. Ethanolamine is a naturally occurring amino alcohol that plays a pivotal role in the synthesis of phosphatidylethanolamine, a central intermediate of lipid metabolism and a major component of biological membranes [51]. Phosphatidylethanolamine is also directly involved in the regulation of autophagy [52], and it is postulated that ethanolamine treatment or the consumption of ethanolamine-rich foods may increase cellular phosphatidylethanolamine levels, induce autophagy, and provide beneficial anti-aging effects across species [52]. While serum ethanolamine levels were different between PF&S and controls, this did not result in a corresponding difference in serum phosphatidylethanolamine concentrations, suggesting alterations in CDP-ethanolamine pathway, the major route of phosphatidylethanolamine production [53]. Interestingly, the disruption of CDP-ethanolamine pathway in muscle was associated with alterations in mitochondrial biogenesis and muscle atrophy in mice [54].

Taurine is a ubiquitous non-proteinogenic sulfur-containing amino acid that represents the most abundant free amino acid in the heart, retina, skeletal muscle, brain, and leukocytes, accounting for approximately 0.1% of total body weight [55]. In skeletal muscle, which contains 70% of total body taurine, this amino acid is involved in the regulation of ion channel function, membrane stability, mitochondrial quality control, and calcium homeostasis [56–59]. In muscle, taurine also serves osmoregulatory, anti-oxidant, and anti-inflammatory functions [56–59]. Given these multiple actions, taurine has recently been proposed as a candidate therapeutic agent against sarcopenia [60]. While it is reported that serum taurine concentrations decline with age in men [36], increased levels of serum taurine have been retrieved in the metabolic profiles of old wild-type mice from different genetic backgrounds [61]. Circulating levels of taurine are regulated by the balance among different factors, including dietary intake, intestinal absorption, bile acid conjugation, urinary excretion, and endogenous synthesis from methionine and cysteine [55]. Taurine may be released from cells following osmotic perturbations, oxidative stress, and (chronic) inflammatory stimulation [58]. Further studies are needed to unveil the mechanisms responsible for the high circulating taurine levels observed in older adults with PF&S.

Citrulline is a non-essential non-protein amino acid with a key role in nitrogen homeostasis [62]. Citrulline is an end product of glutamine metabolism and an endogenous precursor of arginine [63]. For its capacity of promoting endothelial nitric oxide availability and vasodilation, "sparing" arginine and glutamine from hepatic catabolism and the supposed ability to activate mTORC1 signaling [64], citrulline was proposed as a pharmaconutrient to counteract sarcopenia [65]. Several reports have shown that serum citrulline increases with age [36,66,67]. In addition, in a metabolomics study assessing the individual variability in human blood metabolites [68], citrulline was among the circulating molecules that exhibit a remarkable age-related increase. The authors attributed this finding to impairment in urea cycle efficiency due to the progressive decline of liver and renal function with age [68]. However, no differences in kidney or liver function were observed between participants belonging to the two BIOSPHERE study groups. Further investigation on interorgan nitrogen homeostasis pathways are needed to explain the higher circulating values of citrulline found in older adults with PF&S.

Asparagine, aspartic acid, and glutamic acid are among the six amino acids that are metabolized in resting muscles [69]. These amino acids provide the amino groups and the ammonia required for the synthesis of glutamine and alanine, which are released following protein meals and in the post-absorptive state [69]. The carbon skeletons of these metabolites may be used solely for de novo synthesis of TCA-cycle intermediates and glutamine [70]. The higher levels of asparagine, aspartic acid, and glutamic acid observed in persons with PF&Ss may be suggestive of perturbations in muscle energy metabolism associated with muscle wasting. Interestingly, a pattern of metabolic changes accompany muscle remodeling after disuse, including energy substrate accumulation (e.g., asparagine) in atrophied muscles [71,72].

As opposed to EAAs, no significant differences were observed between groups in the serum levels of BCAAs. It should however be considered that the absorption of dietary proteins is influenced by several factors, which may impact their bioavailability and circulating concentrations. In particular, whether PF&S is associated with changes in the expression of amino acid transporters and gastrointestinal physicochemical properties is presently unknown. Furthermore, the lower splanchnic extraction of BCAAs might offset subtle differences in their systemic concentrations between groups [73]. Notwithstanding, our finding on BCAAs is not consistent with previous investigations that reported changes in BCAA concentrations in relation to sarcopenia, low muscle mass, and functional limitation [21–23]. These discrepancies may be due to differences in operational definitions adopted and experimental designs among studies. In addition, heterogeneity in eating habits among participants of the different studies may contribute to the contrasting results.

The present study has some limitations that should be acknowledged. First, the study population was relatively small, and a great number of experimental variables were included in the analyses. However, the innovative analytical approach implemented in the study, based on PLS-DA plus DCV, is an ideal strategy to cope with this issue. The study sample was exclusively comprised of Caucasian individuals, which impedes generalizing the findings to other ethnic groups. Other factors that might affect circulating amino acid levels include lifestyle and eating habits [74,75]. For instance, regular participation in physical activity has been associated with reduced circulating levels of BCAAs as well as alanine and proline across a wide age spectrum [76]. Furthermore, exercise training has shown to increase the plasma levels of glycine and citrulline in overweight adults [77]. Although only people not engaged in regular exercise were enrolled in the present study, the amount of physical activity of participants was not quantified. Hence, the possible influence of physical activity on amino acid profiles in the context of PF&S could not be established. The same applies to the possible influence of different nutritional patterns and amino acid intakes. However, as recently highlighted, differences in circulating amino acids are less marked than those between amino acid intakes [74]. The cross-sectional design of the study does not allow inference to be drawn on the time course of changes of the variables considered and on cause-effect relationships. Finally, although a fairly large number of amino acids and derivatives was assayed, it cannot be excluded that more powerful biomarkers of PF&S might be obtained through the analysis of a larger range of biomediators.

5. Conclusions

In the present study, a PLS-DA-based approach allowed distinct patterns of circulating amino acids and derivatives to be identified in older persons with and without PF&S. The pathways unveiled by this initial investigation may be used to generate new mechanistic hypotheses on the pathophysiology of PF&S. Furthermore, the longitudinal implementation of the proposed analytical strategy could facilitate the tracking of PF&S condition over time and the monitoring of response to treatments. This may represent a first relevant step towards the integration of specific biochemical measurements into the assessment of PF&S, both in clinical and research settings.

Supplementary Materials: The following are available online at http://www.mdpi.com/2072-6643/10/11/1691/s1, Partial Least Squares–Discriminant Analysis; Table S1: Eligibility criteria in BIOSPHERE; Table S2: Distribution of co-morbid conditions and prevalence of use of individual drug classes in BIOSPHERE participants with and without physical frailty & sarcopenia (PF&S); Table S3: Serum concentrations of non-discriminant analytes in BIOSPHERE participants with and without of physical frailty & sarcopenia (PF&S).

Author Contributions: Conceptualization, A.P. (Anna Picca), E.M., and R.C.; methodology, A.P. (Aniello Primiano), J.G., and S.P.; software, A.B. and F.M.; validation, A.P. (Anna Picca), F.L., E.M., H.J.C.-J., and R.C.; formal analysis, A.B. and F.M.; investigation, A.P. (Anna Picca), E.M., and R.C.; resources, A.U., F.M., and R.B.; data curation, A.P. (Anna Picca), M.B., and R.C.; writing—original draft preparation, E.M. and R.C.;

writing—review and editing, A.P. (Anna Picca), F.M., H.J.C.-J., J.G., and M.B.; visualization: A.P. (Aniello Primiano), J.G., and S.P.; supervision, A.U., F.L., and R.B.; funding acquisition, R.B.

Funding: This research was funded by a grant from Fondazione Roma (NCDs Call for Proposals 2013). The work was also partly supported by a grant from the Innovative Medicines Initiative—Joint Undertaking (IMI-JU 115621), the nonprofit research foundation "Centro Studi Achille e Linda Lorenzon", and by intramural research grants from the Università Cattolica del Sacro Cuore (D3.2 2013 and D3.2 2015).

Acknowledgments: The authors thank Vincenzo Brandi, Marianna Broccatelli, Carilia Celesti, Emanuela D'Angelo, Mariaelena D'Elia, Anna Maria Martone, Giulia Savera, and Elisabetta Serafini for their invaluable help with participant screening and assessment. The authors also thank Luca Mariotti for administrative management of the BIOSPHERE project.

Conflicts of Interest: E.M., F.L., R.B. and R.C. are partners of the SPRINTT consortium, which is partly funded by the European Federation of Pharmaceutical Industries and Associations (EFPIA). The other authors declare no conflict of interest.

References

1. Dodds, R.M.; Roberts, H.C.; Cooper, C.; Sayer, A.A. The epidemiology of sarcopenia. *J. Clin. Densitom.* **2015**, *18*, 461–466. [CrossRef] [PubMed]
2. Cao, L.; Morley, J.E. Sarcopenia is recognized as an independent condition by an International Classification of Disease, Tenth Revision, Clinical Modification (ICD-10-CM) code. *J. Am. Med. Dir. Assoc.* **2016**, *17*, 675–677. [CrossRef] [PubMed]
3. Rosenberg, I.H. Sarcopenia: Origins and clinical relevance. *Clin. Geriatr. Med.* **2011**, *27*, 337–339. [CrossRef] [PubMed]
4. Landi, F.; Calvani, R.; Cesari, M.; Tosato, M.; Martone, A.M.; Ortolani, E.; Savera, G.; Salini, S.; Sisto, A.; Picca, A.; et al. Sarcopenia: An overview on current definitions, diagnosis and treatment. *Curr. Protein Pept. Sci.* **2018**, *19*, 633–638. [CrossRef] [PubMed]
5. Hirani, V.; Blyth, F.; Naganathan, V.; Le Couteur, D.G.; Seibel, M.J.; Waite, L.M.; Handelsman, D.J.; Cumming, R.G. Sarcopenia is associated with incident disability, institutionalization, and mortality in community-dwelling older men: The Concord Health and Ageing in Men project. *J. Am. Med. Dir. Assoc.* **2015**, *16*, 607–613. [CrossRef] [PubMed]
6. Marzetti, E.; Calvani, R.; Tosato, M.; Cesari, M.; Di Bari, M.; Cherubini, A.; Collamati, A.; D'Angelo, E.; Pahor, M.; Bernabei, R.; et al. Sarcopenia: An overview. *Aging Clin. Exp. Res.* **2017**, *29*, 11–17. [CrossRef] [PubMed]
7. Cesari, M.; Calvani, R.; Marzetti, E. Frailty in older persons. *Clin. Geriatr. Med.* **2017**, *33*, 293–303. [CrossRef] [PubMed]
8. Landi, F.; Calvani, R.; Cesari, M.; Tosato, M.; Martone, A.M.; Bernabei, R.; Onder, G.; Marzetti, E. Sarcopenia as the biological substrate of physical frailty. *Clin. Geriatr. Med.* **2015**, *31*, 367–374. [CrossRef] [PubMed]
9. Cesari, M.; Landi, F.; Vellas, B.; Bernabei, R.; Marzetti, E. Sarcopenia and physical frailty: Two sides of the same coin. *Front. Aging Neurosci.* **2014**, *6*, 192. [CrossRef] [PubMed]
10. Cesari, M.; Landi, F.; Calvani, R.; Cherubini, A.; Di Bari, M.; Kortebein, P.; Del Signore, S.; Le Lain, R.; Vellas, B.; Pahor, M.; et al. Rationale for a preliminary operational definition of physical frailty and sarcopenia in the SPRINTT trial. *Aging Clin. Exp. Res.* **2017**, *29*, 81–88. [CrossRef] [PubMed]
11. Marzetti, E.; Calvani, R.; Landi, F.; Hoogendijk, E.O.; Fougère, B.; Vellas, B.; Pahor, M.; Bernabei, R.; Cesari, M.; SPRINTT Consortium. Innovative Medicines Initiative: The SPRINTT project. *J. Frailty Aging* **2015**, *4*, 207–208. [CrossRef] [PubMed]
12. Cesari, M.; Marzetti, E.; Calvani, R.; Vellas, B.; Bernabei, R.; Bordes, P.; Roubenoff, R.; Landi, F.; Cherubini, A.; SPRINTT Consortium. The need of operational paradigms for frailty in older persons: The SPRINTT project. *Aging Clin. Exp. Res.* **2017**, *29*, 3–10. [CrossRef] [PubMed]
13. Calvani, R.; Marini, F.; Cesari, M.; Tosato, M.; Anker, S.D.; von Haehling, S.; Miller, R.R.; Bernabei, R.; Landi, F.; Marzetti, E.; et al. Biomarkers for physical frailty and sarcopenia: State of the science and future developments. *J. Cachexia Sarcopenia Muscle* **2015**, *6*, 278–286. [CrossRef] [PubMed]

14. Calvani, R.; Marini, F.; Cesari, M.; Tosato, M.; Picca, A.; Anker, S.D.; von Haehling, S.; Miller, R.R.; Bernabei, R.; Landi, F.; et al. Biomarkers for physical frailty and sarcopenia. *Aging Clin. Exp. Res.* **2017**, *29*, 29–34. [CrossRef] [PubMed]
15. Brook, M.S.; Wilkinson, D.J.; Phillips, B.E.; Perez-Schindler, J.; Philp, A.; Smith, K.; Atherton, P.J. Skeletal muscle homeostasis and plasticity in youth and ageing: Impact of nutrition and exercise. *Acta Physiol. (Oxf.)* **2016**, *216*, 15–41. [CrossRef] [PubMed]
16. Zhenyukh, O.; Civantos, E.; Ruiz-Ortega, M.; Sánchez, M.S.; Vázquez, C.; Peiró, C.; Egido, J.; Mas, S. High concentration of branched-chain amino acids promotes oxidative stress, inflammation and migration of human peripheral blood mononuclear cells via mTORC1 activation. *Free Radic. Biol. Med.* **2017**, *104*, 165–177. [CrossRef] [PubMed]
17. Yoon, M.-S. The Emerging Role of Branched-Chain Amino Acids in Insulin Resistance and Metabolism. *Nutrients* **2016**, *8*, 405. [CrossRef] [PubMed]
18. Landi, F.; Calvani, R.; Tosato, M.; Martone, A.M.; Ortolani, E.; Savera, G.; D'Angelo, E.; Sisto, A.; Marzetti, E. Protein intake and muscle health in old age: From biological plausibility to clinical evidence. *Nutrients* **2016**, *8*, 295. [CrossRef] [PubMed]
19. Pasini, E.; Corsetti, G.; Aquilani, R.; Romano, C.; Picca, A.; Calvani, R.; Dioguardi, F.S. Protein-amino acid metabolism disarrangements: The hidden enemy of chronic age-related conditions. *Nutrients* **2018**, *10*, 391. [CrossRef] [PubMed]
20. He, Q.; Yin, Y.; Zhao, F.; Kong, X.; Wu, G.; Ren, P. Metabonomics and its role in amino acid nutrition research. *Front. Biosci. (Landmark Ed.)* **2011**, *16*, 2451–2460. [CrossRef] [PubMed]
21. Lustgarten, M.S.; Price, L.L.; Chale, A.; Phillips, E.M.; Fielding, R.A. Branched chain amino acids are associated with muscle mass in functionally limited older adults. *J. Gerontol. A Biol. Sci. Med. Sci.* **2014**, *69*, 717–724. [CrossRef] [PubMed]
22. Moaddel, R.; Fabbri, E.; Khadeer, M.A.; Carlson, O.D.; Gonzalez-Freire, M.; Zhang, P.; Semba, R.D.; Ferrucci, L. Plasma biomarkers of poor muscle quality in older men and women from the Baltimore Longitudinal Study of Aging. *J. Gerontol. A Biol. Sci. Med. Sci.* **2016**, *71*, 1266–1272. [CrossRef] [PubMed]
23. Ottestad, I.; Ulven, S.M.; Øyri, L.K.L.; Sandvei, K.S.; Gjevestad, G.O.; Bye, A.; Sheikh, N.A.; Biong, A.S.; Andersen, L.F.; Holven, K.B. Reduced plasma concentration of branched-chain amino acids in sarcopenic older subjects: A cross-sectional study. *Br. J. Nutr.* **2018**, *120*, 445–453. [CrossRef] [PubMed]
24. Toyoshima, K.; Nakamura, M.; Adachi, Y.; Imaizumi, A.; Hakamada, T.; Abe, Y.; Kaneko, E.; Takahashi, S.; Shimokado, K. Increased plasma proline concentrations are associated with sarcopenia in the elderly. *PLoS ONE* **2017**, *12*, e0185206. [CrossRef] [PubMed]
25. Adachi, Y.; Ono, N.; Imaizumi, A.; Muramatsu, T.; Andou, T.; Shimodaira, Y.; Nagao, K.; Kageyama, Y.; Mori, M.; Noguchi, Y.; et al. Plasma amino acid profile in severely frail elderly patients in Japan. *Int. J. Gerontol.* **2018**. [CrossRef]
26. Calvani, R.; Picca, A.; Marini, F.; Biancolillo, A.; Cesari, M.; Pesce, V.; Lezza, A.M.S.; Bossola, M.; Leeuwenburgh, C.; Bernabei, R.; et al. The "BIOmarkers associated with Sarcopenia and PHysical frailty in EldeRly pErsons" (BIOSPHERE) study: Rationale, design and methods. *Eur. J. Intern. Med.* **2018**, *56*, 19–25. [CrossRef] [PubMed]
27. Guralnik, J.M.; Simonsick, E.M.; Ferrucci, L.; Glynn, R.J.; Berkman, L.F.; Blazer, D.G.; Scherr, P.A.; Wallace, R.B. A short physical performance battery assessing lower extremity function: Association with self-reported disability and prediction of mortality and nursing home admission. *J. Gerontol.* **1994**, *49*, M85–M94. [CrossRef] [PubMed]
28. Studenski, S.A.; Peters, K.W.; Alley, D.E.; Cawthon, P.M.; McLean, R.R.; Harris, T.B.; Ferrucci, L.; Guralnik, J.M.; Fragala, M.S.; Kenny, A.M.; et al. The FNIH sarcopenia project: Rationale, study description, conference recommendations, and final estimates. *J. Gerontol. A Biol. Sci. Med. Sci.* **2014**, *69*, 547–558. [CrossRef] [PubMed]
29. Newman, A.B.; Simonsick, E.M.; Naydeck, B.L.; Boudreau, R.M.; Kritchevsky, S.B.; Nevitt, M.C.; Pahor, M.; Satterfield, S.; Brach, J.S.; Studenski, S.A.; et al. Association of long-distance corridor walk performance with mortality, cardiovascular disease, mobility limitation, and disability. *JAMA* **2006**, *295*, 2018–2026. [CrossRef] [PubMed]
30. Barker, M.; Rayens, W. Partial least squares for discrimination. *J. Chemom.* **2003**, *17*, 166–173. [CrossRef]

31. Wold, S.; Martens, H.; Wold, H. The multivariate calibration problem in chemistry solved by the PLS method. In *Matrix Pencils*; Lecture Notes in Mathematics; Springer: Berlin, Germany, 1983; Volume 973, pp. 286–293. ISBN 978-3-540-11983-8.
32. Westerhuis, J.A.; Hoefsloot, H.C.J.; Smit, S.; Vis, D.J.; Smilde, A.K.; van Velzen, E.J.J.; van Duijnhoven, J.P.M.; van Dorsten, F.A. Assessment of PLSDA cross validation. *Metabolomics* **2008**, *4*, 81–89. [CrossRef]
33. Szymańska, E.; Saccenti, E.; Smilde, A.K.; Westerhuis, J.A. Double-check: Validation of diagnostic statistics for PLS-DA models in metabolomics studies. *Metabolomics* **2012**, *8*, 3–16. [CrossRef] [PubMed]
34. Smit, S.; van Breemen, M.J.; Hoefsloot, H.C.J.; Smilde, A.K.; Aerts, J.M.F.G.; de Koster, C.G. Assessing the statistical validity of proteomics based biomarkers. *Anal. Chim. Acta* **2007**, *592*, 210–217. [CrossRef] [PubMed]
35. Wu, G. Amino acids: Metabolism, functions, and nutrition. *Amino Acids* **2009**, *37*, 1–17. [CrossRef] [PubMed]
36. Kouchiwa, T.; Wada, K.; Uchiyama, M.; Kasezawa, N.; Niisato, M.; Murakami, H.; Fukuyama, K.; Yokogoshi, H. Age-related changes in serum amino acids concentrations in healthy individuals. *Clin. Chem. Lab. Med.* **2012**, *50*, 861–870. [CrossRef] [PubMed]
37. Cruz-Jentoft, A.J.; Kiesswetter, E.; Drey, M.; Sieber, C.C. Nutrition, frailty, and sarcopenia. *Aging Clin. Exp. Res.* **2017**, *29*, 43–48. [CrossRef] [PubMed]
38. Calvani, R.; Miccheli, A.; Landi, F.; Bossola, M.; Cesari, M.; Leeuwenburgh, C.; Sieber, C.C.; Bernabei, R.; Marzetti, E. Current nutritional recommendations and novel dietary strategies to manage sarcopenia. *J. Frailty Aging* **2013**, *2*, 38–53. [CrossRef] [PubMed]
39. Matsuo, Y.; Greenberg, D.M. Metabolic formation of homoserine and alpha-aminobutyric acid from methionine. *J. Biol. Chem.* **1955**, *215*, 547–554. [PubMed]
40. Haschke-Becher, E.; Kainz, A.; Bachmann, C. Reference values of amino acids and of common clinical chemistry in plasma of healthy infants aged 1 and 4 months. *J. Inherit. Metab. Dis.* **2016**, *39*, 25–37. [CrossRef] [PubMed]
41. Kar, S.K.; Jansman, A.J.M.; Schokker, D.; Kruijt, L.; Harms, A.C.; Wells, J.M.; Smits, M.A. Amine metabolism is influenced by dietary protein source. *Front. Nutr.* **2017**, *4*, 41. [CrossRef] [PubMed]
42. Ducker, G.S.; Rabinowitz, J.D. One-carbon metabolism in health and disease. *Cell Metab.* **2017**, *25*, 27–42. [CrossRef] [PubMed]
43. Suh, E.; Choi, S.-W.; Friso, S. One-carbon metabolism: An unsung hero for healthy aging. *Mol. Basis Nutr. Aging* **2016**, 513–522. [CrossRef]
44. Mudd, S.H.; Ebert, M.H.; Scriver, C.R. Labile methyl group balances in the human: The role of sarcosine. *Metabolism* **1980**, *29*, 707–720. [CrossRef]
45. Allen, R.H.; Stabler, S.P.; Lindenbaum, J. Serum betaine, N,N-dimethylglycine and N-methylglycine levels in patients with cobalamin and folate deficiency and related inborn errors of metabolism. *Metabolism* **1993**, *42*, 1448–1460. [CrossRef]
46. Walters, R.O.; Fontana, L.; Kurland, I.; Diaz, A.; Arias-Perez, E.; Cuervo, A.; Promislow, D.; Huffman, D. Sarcosine is uniquely modulated by aging and dietary restriction in rodents and humans. *Innov. Aging* **2017**, *1*, 1208–1209. [CrossRef]
47. Marzetti, E.; Calvani, R.; Lorenzi, M.; Tanganelli, F.; Picca, A.; Bossola, M.; Menghi, A.; Bernabei, R.; Landi, F. Association between myocyte quality control signaling and sarcopenia in old hip-fractured patients: Results from the Sarcopenia in HIp FracTure (SHIFT) exploratory study. *Exp. Gerontol.* **2016**, *80*, 1–5. [CrossRef] [PubMed]
48. Calvani, R.; Joseph, A.-M.; Adhihetty, P.J.; Miccheli, A.; Bossola, M.; Leeuwenburgh, C.; Bernabei, R.; Marzetti, E. Mitochondrial pathways in sarcopenia of aging and disuse muscle atrophy. *Biol. Chem.* **2013**, *394*, 393–414. [CrossRef] [PubMed]
49. Picca, A.; Calvani, R.; Lorenzi, M.; Menghi, A.; Galli, M.; Vitiello, R.; Randisi, F.; Bernabei, R.; Landi, F.; Marzetti, E. Mitochondrial dynamics signaling is shifted toward fusion in muscles of very old hip-fractured patients: Results from the Sarcopenia in HIp FracTure (SHIFT) exploratory study. *Exp. Gerontol.* **2017**, *96*, 63–67. [CrossRef] [PubMed]
50. Picca, A.; Calvani, R.; Bossola, M.; Allocca, E.; Menghi, A.; Pesce, V.; Lezza, A.M.S.; Bernabei, R.; Landi, F.; Marzetti, E. Update on mitochondria and muscle aging: All wrong roads lead to sarcopenia. *Biol. Chem.* **2018**, *399*, 421–436. [CrossRef] [PubMed]

51. Vance, J.E. Phosphatidylserine and phosphatidylethanolamine in mammalian cells: Two metabolically related aminophospholipids. *J. Lipid Res.* **2008**, *49*, 1377–1387. [CrossRef] [PubMed]
52. Rockenfeller, P.; Koska, M.; Pietrocola, F.; Minois, N.; Knittelfelder, O.; Sica, V.; Franz, J.; Carmona-Gutierrez, D.; Kroemer, G.; Madeo, F. Phosphatidylethanolamine positively regulates autophagy and longevity. *Cell Death Differ.* **2015**, *22*, 499–508. [CrossRef] [PubMed]
53. van der Veen, J.N.; Kennelly, J.P.; Wan, S.; Vance, J.E.; Vance, D.E.; Jacobs, R.L. The critical role of phosphatidylcholine and phosphatidylethanolamine metabolism in health and disease. *Biochim. Biophys. Acta* **2017**, *1859*, 1558–1572. [CrossRef] [PubMed]
54. Selathurai, A.; Kowalski, G.M.; Burch, M.L.; Sepulveda, P.; Risis, S.; Lee-Young, R.S.; Lamon, S.; Meikle, P.J.; Genders, A.J.; McGee, S.L.; et al. The CDP-ethanolamine pathway regulates skeletal muscle diacylglycerol content and mitochondrial biogenesis without altering insulin sensitivity. *Cell Metab.* **2015**, *21*, 718–730. [CrossRef] [PubMed]
55. Huxtable, R.J. Physiological actions of taurine. *Physiol. Rev.* **1992**, *72*, 101–163. [CrossRef] [PubMed]
56. Conte Camerino, D.; Tricarico, D.; Pierno, S.; Desaphy, J.-F.; Liantonio, A.; Pusch, M.; Burdi, R.; Camerino, C.; Fraysse, B.; De Luca, A. Taurine and skeletal muscle disorders. *Neurochem. Res.* **2004**, *29*, 135–142. [CrossRef] [PubMed]
57. De Luca, A.; Pierno, S.; Camerino, D.C. Taurine: The appeal of a safe amino acid for skeletal muscle disorders. *J. Transl. Med.* **2015**, *13*, 243. [CrossRef] [PubMed]
58. Lambert, I.H.; Kristensen, D.M.; Holm, J.B.; Mortensen, O.H. Physiological role of taurine–from organism to organelle. *Acta Physiol. (Oxf.)* **2015**, *213*, 191–212. [CrossRef] [PubMed]
59. Ito, T.; Yoshikawa, N.; Inui, T.; Miyazaki, N.; Schaffer, S.W.; Azuma, J. Tissue depletion of taurine accelerates skeletal muscle senescence and leads to early death in mice. *PLoS ONE* **2014**, *9*, e107409. [CrossRef] [PubMed]
60. Scicchitano, B.M.; Sica, G. The beneficial effects of taurine to counteract sarcopenia. *Curr. Protein Pept. Sci.* **2018**, *19*, 673–680. [CrossRef] [PubMed]
61. Tomás-Loba, A.; Bernardes de Jesus, B.; Mato, J.M.; Blasco, M.A. A metabolic signature predicts biological age in mice. *Aging Cell* **2013**, *12*, 93–101. [CrossRef] [PubMed]
62. Breuillard, C.; Cynober, L.; Moinard, C. Citrulline and nitrogen homeostasis: An overview. *Amino Acids* **2015**, *47*, 685–691. [CrossRef] [PubMed]
63. Papadia, C.; Osowska, S.; Cynober, L.; Forbes, A. Citrulline in health and disease. Review on human studies. *Clin. Nutr.* **2017**. [CrossRef] [PubMed]
64. Le Plénier, S.; Walrand, S.; Noirt, R.; Cynober, L.; Moinard, C. Effects of leucine and citrulline versus non-essential amino acids on muscle protein synthesis in fasted rat: A common activation pathway? *Amino Acids* **2012**, *43*, 1171–1178. [CrossRef] [PubMed]
65. Martone, A.M.; Lattanzio, F.; Abbatecola, A.M.; Carpia, D.L.; Tosato, M.; Marzetti, E.; Calvani, R.; Onder, G.; Landi, F. Treating sarcopenia in older and oldest old. *Curr. Pharm. Des.* **2015**, *21*, 1715–1722. [CrossRef] [PubMed]
66. Sarwar, G.; Botting, H.G.; Collins, M. A comparison of fasting serum amino acid profiles of young and elderly subjects. *J. Am. Coll. Nutr.* **1991**, *10*, 668–674. [CrossRef] [PubMed]
67. Pitkänen, H.T.; Oja, S.S.; Kemppainen, K.; Seppä, J.M.; Mero, A.A. Serum amino acid concentrations in aging men and women. *Amino Acids* **2003**, *24*, 413–421. [CrossRef] [PubMed]
68. Chaleckis, R.; Murakami, I.; Takada, J.; Kondoh, H.; Yanagida, M. Individual variability in human blood metabolites identifies age-related differences. *Proc. Natl. Acad. Sci. USA* **2016**, *113*, 4252–4259. [CrossRef] [PubMed]
69. Wagenmakers, A.J. Muscle amino acid metabolism at rest and during exercise: Role in human physiology and metabolism. *Exerc. Sport Sci. Rev.* **1998**, *26*, 287–314. [CrossRef] [PubMed]
70. Wagenmakers, A.J. Protein and amino acid metabolism in human muscle. *Adv. Exp. Med. Biol.* **1998**, *441*, 307–319. [CrossRef] [PubMed]
71. Stein, T.P.; Wade, C.E. Metabolic consequences of muscle disuse atrophy. *J. Nutr.* **2005**, *135*, 1824S–1828S. [CrossRef] [PubMed]
72. Ilaiwy, A.; Quintana, M.T.; Bain, J.R.; Muehlbauer, M.J.; Brown, D.I.; Stansfield, W.E.; Willis, M.S. Cessation of biomechanical stretch model of C2C12 cells models myocyte atrophy and anaplerotic changes in metabolism using non-targeted metabolomics analysis. *Int. J. Biochem. Cell Biol.* **2016**, *79*, 80–92. [CrossRef] [PubMed]

73. Soultoukis, G.A.; Partridge, L. Dietary protein, metabolism, and aging. *Annu. Rev. Biochem.* **2016**, *85*, 5–34. [CrossRef] [PubMed]
74. Schmidt, J.A.; Rinaldi, S.; Scalbert, A.; Ferrari, P.; Achaintre, D.; Gunter, M.J.; Appleby, P.N.; Key, T.J.; Travis, R.C. Plasma concentrations and intakes of amino acids in male meat-eaters, fish-eaters, vegetarians and vegans: A cross-sectional analysis in the EPIC-Oxford cohort. *Eur. J. Clin. Nutr.* **2016**, *70*, 306–312. [CrossRef] [PubMed]
75. Fukai, K.; Harada, S.; Iida, M.; Kurihara, A.; Takeuchi, A.; Kuwabara, K.; Sugiyama, D.; Okamura, T.; Akiyama, M.; Nishiwaki, Y.; et al. Metabolic profiling of total physical activity and sedentary behavior in community-dwelling men. *PLoS ONE* **2016**, *11*, e0164877. [CrossRef] [PubMed]
76. Kujala, U.M.; Mäkinen, V.-P.; Heinonen, I.; Soininen, P.; Kangas, A.J.; Leskinen, T.H.; Rahkila, P.; Würtz, P.; Kovanen, V.; Cheng, S.; et al. Long-term leisure-time physical activity and serum metabolome. *Circulation* **2013**, *127*, 340–348. [CrossRef] [PubMed]
77. Glynn, E.L.; Piner, L.W.; Huffman, K.M.; Slentz, C.A.; Elliot-Penry, L.; AbouAssi, H.; White, P.J.; Bain, J.R.; Muehlbauer, M.J.; Ilkayeva, O.R.; et al. Impact of combined resistance and aerobic exercise training on branched-chain amino acid turnover, glycine metabolism and insulin sensitivity in overweight humans. *Diabetologia* **2015**, *58*, 2324–2335. [CrossRef] [PubMed]

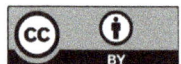

© 2018 by the authors. Licensee MDPI, Basel, Switzerland. This article is an open access article distributed under the terms and conditions of the Creative Commons Attribution (CC BY) license (http://creativecommons.org/licenses/by/4.0/).

MDPI
St. Alban-Anlage 66
4052 Basel
Switzerland
Tel. +41 61 683 77 34
Fax +41 61 302 89 18
www.mdpi.com

Nutrients Editorial Office
E-mail: nutrients@mdpi.com
www.mdpi.com/journal/nutrients

www.ingramcontent.com/pod-product-compliance
Lightning Source LLC
LaVergne TN
LVHW071954080526
838202LV00064B/6744